OSTEOPOROSIS

The Alternatives

A Guide to Myth and Reality, Hype and Facts

"You Shall Know the Truth, and the Truth Shall Make You Free"

Eva Lee Snead, M.D.

For permissions, or serializations, condensations, adaptations, or for our catalog of other publications, write the Publisher at the address below.

Library of Congress Cataloging-in-Publication Data

Snead, Eva Lee, 1942-
Osteoporosis: the alternatives: a guide to myth and reality, hype and facts: you shall know the truth, and the truth shall make you free / Eva Lee Snead.

p. cm.
Includes bibliographical references and index

ISBN 1-893157-00-8

1. Osteoporosis—Popular works. I. Title
RC931.O73 S665 1999
616.7'16--dc21   99-047037

Published by
BRIDGER HOUSE PUBLISHERS, INC
P.O. Box 2208, Carson City, NV 89702, 1-800-729-4131

Cover design by The Right Type
Printed in the United States of America
10 9 8 7 6 5 4 3 2 1

PREFACE

Acknowledgments

I wish to thank my friends, my patients, and the hundreds of researchers before me, who gave generously of their time and knowlege to make this book possible. A special thanks to Adrian and Mike for scrificing many a stack of pancakes because I took time away from them to write.

A NOTE TO ANIMAL LOVERS

(The animals' Viet Nam Memorial Wall)

Because of my respect for animal activists, and my high regard for their cause, I want to state my position on the animal abuse perpetrated under the guise of scientific necessity, in order to avoid the ill feelings and confusion which ensued the publication of some of my previous work.

I have previously written and published "Some Call it "AIDS",...I Call it Murder" in which I feel to have clearly expounded on how unscientific, cowardly and dangerous it is to experiment on animals. Some individuals of the anti-vivisection movement did not believe I went far enough, and gave me a very bad rap; knowing that many readers are animal lovers, I want to mention and explain why this book talks about animal experiements, and cites them.

I do not endorse animal experimentation, I find it to be abhorrent and abusive. I feel that recognizing animals' involuntary contributions to science is my best tribute to our little and big friends from the animal kingdom, a kind of zoological "memorial wall" like the one we dedicate to those fallen in Viet Nam.

I hope that we can establish a healthier, more animal respecting world.

FOREWORD

Eva Lee Snead, M.D. has been a strong promoter of health and healing, an educator and guide in the field of alternative health, for many years. She has had extensive medical training, with emphasis on endocrinology, the science of glands and hormones, in which she served an externship. She has been in the practice of Medicine, Nutrition and Chelation therapy for the beter part of 34 years. During these years she dealt with numerous degenerative illnesses, iuncluding that of osteoporosis.

This is not only the age of Aquarius, but also the era of "The Graying of America". Population growth has slowed down and the elderly are living longer, but not necessarily healthier lives. They are often living dead suffering from an assortment of degenerative conditions such as Alzheimer's the various forms of arthritis, cardiovascular conditions, etc.. One of the most crippling and tragic conditions they are afflicted with is the weakening of their bone structure, the disease known as osteoporosis.

During the last decade, she has become increasingly concerned with the total lack of understanding of nutrition by the traditional health practitioners, and the haphazard dealings with endocrinology by the alternative practitioners. These flaws, she thought, held the population hostage of ignorance, prejudice and fear, making them more and more vulnerable to the destruction of their skeletons and connective tissues.

This book is an attempt to offer solutions to this serious problem.

Michael A. Moczygemba
Aum Publications, Health and Nutrition Books

INTRODUCTION

To paraphrase Gibran's "The Prophet", I must say that this book was born out of its need for itself, spurred on by the pain and misery of the millions who suffer unnecessarily of weakened, brittle bones. I have been interested in this malady since the early years of my practice, and had the satisfaction of improving the lot of those who came to me with bone and joint problems, without unnecessary side effects and secondary problems.

With the graying of America, degenerative illnesses were highlighted, and many products were advertised on the shaky basis of unsubstantiated research, inducing many women to opt for ineffective, random treatments, more seriously flawed than the establishment's synthetic hormone approaches. were touted as calcium supplements. Many believed to become instant authorities in the science of Endocrinology (hormones and glands), and strictly technical knowledge was replaced by hype and wishful thinking. I thought it was time to share reliable knowledge with the public.

"Osteoporosis: The Alternatives" is a digest of information regarding the following areas:
1. what constitutes osteoporosis
2. what you need to know about bone growth
3. what *establishment medicine* has to offer, as far as testing,
4. what *establishment medicine* has to offer as far as medications: the pluses and minuses of this, and, last, but not least,
5. the many alternative ways in which to prevent, arrest or reverse osteoporosis. Some of these alternatives are "self help" measures, others do require the assistance of a holistic health professional.

The information has been gathered from many sources, preferably original studies and articles, from reputable universities and centers for the learning of healing. Much information has been validated by my own clinical experience since 1968.

Establishment medicine and alternative healing sciences are the main approaches used in addressing disease problems and prevention. I have tried to extrapolate the best and most reliable information from both these sources: my selectioons were made on the basis of consistency, reproducibility, proper methods, etc. I did my best to avoid mere opinion, guesses and prejudice. I hope that the readers will find the material informative and helpful.

Without any further squandering of time, I invite all to partake and enjoy, and better still, be whole!

Eva Lee Snead, M.D.

TABLE OF CONTENTS

CHAPTER I

OSTEOPOROSIS: GENERALITIES

WHAT IS OSTEOPOROSIS?

It is a condition which affects the skeleton, the bones of the body, a decrease in **bone mass** and **bone density** due to improper replacement of bone proteins and calcium, usually occurring after menopause, or due to the side effects of some medication, eating disorders and hormonal problems, causing bones to be weak and more susceptible to fracture. It is a major underlying cause of bone fractures in post-menopausal women and older persons in general. A fall, blow, or lifting action that would not bruise or strain the average person can easily cause one or more bones to break in a person with severe *osteoporosis*. This is why osteoporosis is sometimes called brittle bone disease. The bones most frequently affected are the *vertebrae* (backbones), *wrist and hip*. By the time it becomes obvious to an individual that osteoporosis has developed, up to 30 % of the sufferer's bone mass may have been lost.

> **OSTEOPOROSIS IS A DECREASE BOTH IN BONE MASS AND BONE DENSITY**

HOW DOES IT MANIFEST?

It usually is a *silent disease* that progresses for decades, sometimes without any outward signs, until a sufferer has a fracture. However, people may often gradually lose height due to collapsed vertebrae without realizing they have osteoporosis. "In addition to causing hip fractures, osteoporosis is also responsible for loss of bone in the jaw, gum recession (both of which are early signs of this condition), dowager's hump, back pain due to compression and fractures of the vertebra, and fractures of the wrist [also called *Colles fracture*]."[L000] [emphasis added] In fact, back pain is probably the most common symptom.

DIAGNOSTIC CRITERIA

According to the WHO (World Health Organization), osteoporosis is a condition where the bone is at least 2.5 *SD* (*standard deviations*)— a certain measurement criterion—below the mean normal value for healthy young adults. Based on this definition, approximately 30% of women older than 50 have osteoporosis. *Osteopenia* (bone deficiency) is a less serious or intermediate abnormality in bone density, defined as a *BMD* [*bone mineral density*] of greater than 1 and less than 2.5 SD below the healthy young adult mean value."[B051]

A PRACTICAL WAY TO CLASSIFY OSTEOPOROSIS

One practical way to classify the "osteoporosis" is by their *bio-mechanical* problems instead of by their severity or their accompanying medical conditions.

- *true* osteoporosis, bone fragility would increase to such an extent that normal physical activity would cause spontaneous fractures and/or a bone pain syndrome, mainly affecting the spine...falls could also cause extremity bone fractures.

- *physiologic osteopenia*, reduced bone strength and mass would fit correspondingly reduced physical activities and muscle strength so well that fractures would not happen without falls or other injuries. Those fractures would affect extremity bones more than the vertebrae.

- *combination states*, features of the other two would combine in various ways.

- *transient osteopenias* are conditions of temporary thinning of bone, as occurs during prolonged periods of inactivity (space exploration?), lactation, etc.

HOW COMMON IS IT?

Since osteoporosis develops as a function of aging, the ever growing older population generates a constant increase in the numbers of victims. According to current information, an estimated 75 million people suffer from osteoporosis in Europe, Japan, and the United States, as many as 200 million worldwide. If present trends continue, the prevalence of osteoporosis is expected to double by 2020.

Broken bones, a consequence of osteoporosis, are also on the increase. Over 1,600,000 hip fractures occur world-wide every year due to osteoporosis. Predictions have it that a third of all European women will suffer an osteoporosis-related fracture in later life. Among those who live to age 90, 32% of women and 17% of men will suffer a hip fracture, most due to osteoporosis. The staggering cost of osteoporosis in the United States has been estimated at $3.8 billion annually.

WHO IS AT RISK, AND HOW DOES IT DEVELOP?

Bone mass is built up during childhood and young adulthood, through the ages of between 25-35, with proteins forming the *matrix* (the soft, pliable, proteinaceous bed for bone structure), and calcium giving it density and strength. After the age of 35, bones begin to lose some of their calcium, and eventually the production of protein is impaired. Therefore, people of older age develop osteoporosis.

> **PEOPLE OF OLDER AGE, ESPECIALLY POST-MENOPAUSAL WOMEN, DEVELOP OSTEOPOROSIS**

Post-menopausal women represent the largest group at risk. Before menopause, the ovaries produce abundant *hormones* which stimulate the production of the *protein matrix* of the bone mass. At menopause, the ovaries slow or stop producing hormones, and the estrogen levels drop. Estrogen has a protective effect on bones. Also, women who already have low levels of estrogen before their menopause, due to over-dieting, extreme levels of exercise, or who lose their supply of estrogen early as a result of surgery to remove their ovaries, are often at risk of bone loss earlier in life.

OSTEOPOROSIS IN MEN: FACTORS OF INCREASED RISK

Certain groups of males also have a high incidence of osteoporosis. A case-control study involving 20 hospitals in Philadelphia, Pennsylvania, and 14 hospitals in Kaiser Permanente Medical Care Program of northern California evaluated factors that determine an increased risk of first hip fracture in males. Men in the lowest one fifth (*quintile*) of body mass had a greatly increased risk of hip fracture compared with men in the heaviest quintile.[G120] The factors for an increased risk included:

■ lower body mass

■ lower limb dysfunction

■ smoking cigarettes or a pipe, even in people with a voluminous body mass

■ use of *cimetidine* (*Tagamet*®), an acid blocker

■ use of *psychotropic* drugs (tranquilizers, antidepressants)

Physical activity may be a particularly promising preventive measure for men.

I could add other risk factors, such as the use of progressive hair coloring based on **lead acetate pigments**, and the use of **sunscreens** robbing the body of health giving, wonderful sunshine.

OTHER CHANGES ASSOCIATED WITH LOW HORMONES AND/OR OSTEOPOROSIS

The loss of hormonal support affects not only the bones and teeth but other structural elements of the body such as the joints, muscles, body shape, skin, and hair. Although bone loss may occur silently for many years, women notice changes in these other structural elements within a few years of entering menopause.

For instance, the incidence of *osteoarthritis* increases at the time of menopause; women who have never experienced joint pain suddenly become symptomatic. In addition, women with pre-existing arthritis find that their symptoms get worse. Many women reaching menopause complain of increased stiffness in their hands and shoulders as well as low back pain.

The lack of sex hormones also affects *muscle tone*. Muscles throughout the body tend to sag and lose tone after menopause. Women tend to be very conscious of pelvic muscle tone loss, as well as sagging of the facial and arm muscles. The loss of pelvic muscle tone can affect sexual pleasure and the ability to hold urine. Facial drooping can appear fairly rapidly within a year or two of menopause. This change can be a cause of distress in many women who don't like this visible sign of aging. Other tissues, such as the breasts, lose their tone and droop more. The lack of estrogen is probably also responsible for the increase in low back and pelvic pain that women experience around this time.

Another visible sign of aging for many women after menopause is a *change in body shape* as the distribution of weight on the body changes. The waist and upper back get thicker, while the hips and breasts tend to lose some of their fat. The result is that the female shape changes from an hourglass figure to a pear shape. Many women find that not only does their figure shape change, but they gain weight more easily (10 to 15 pounds in the year or two following menopause isn't unusual). This can occur no matter how diligently they diet or how much they exercise. The lack of female hormonal support plus the slowing of the metabolism are probably responsible for these changes. Women after menopause don't burn calories as efficiently as during their younger years. Careful attention to diet and regular exercise can certainly help, but may not entirely correct, these physical changes.

Aging is not funny. I will always be reminded of a short, personal anecdote from the "Reader's Digest", many years ago: a lady who was trying to overcome the effect of the ravages of time with humor, stated that she always counted her blessings, and, at that moment, was thinking how wonderful it was that wrinkles did not hurt! Yet, they do hurt most people, even if this pain is not physical. The skin and hair undergo many changes after menopause, due to loss of estrogen. There is a gradual tendency towards progressive thinning and dryness of the skin. Skin pigmentation becomes uneven, which affects coloration. Some women may lose their even skin tone and notice patches of lighter and darker skin. As *collagen* (gelatinous support tissue) production slows down, the skin loses its elasticity. The muscle and fat tissues that help give skin its underlying support begin to shrink. There is also a reduction in sweat gland activity with decreased tolerance to temperature changes. As a result, many visible signs of skin aging become apparent, such as pronounced wrinkling and creasing. Many women find these changes cosmetically unappealing and employ a variety of dermatologic aids in an attempt to make their skin look younger and healthier.

Women who smoke, have poor nutritional habits, or have had excessive exposure to sunlight are more likely to show signs of skin aging at a younger age. Conversely, women who tend to carry a little extra weight or have reached menopause at a later age will have better looking skin. This is because they have had higher circulating levels of estrogen in their bodies for more years than a thin woman who enters menopause at an early age.

Lack of estrogen also affects the hair. With menopause, hair on the head and in the pubic area becomes drier, coarser, and sparser. Leg, arm and underarm hair grows slower, and thins out. Women may also notice the growth of darker or coarser hair in areas where they've never had hair before, such as the chin, upper lip, chest, or abdomen. This unusual growth of hair is due to the stimulation of the hair *follicles* (the bulb shaped hair root under the skin) by low amounts of male hormones (*androgens*). High estrogen levels block the action of these male hormones on hair follicle receptors. However, after menopause, these low amounts of androgen may not decrease to the same extent that estrogen does in certain women. These unopposed androgens can then affect the pattern of hair growth and hair loss, taking on a more male like pattern.

OTHER BONE DAMAGING DISEASES

There are many different types, not to be confused with osteoporosis; it is good for the public to understand this, so they can avoid inappropriate diagnoses. Information is available from the ARTHRITIS FOUNDATION (800-542-0295).

OSTEOPOROSIS AND OSTEOARTHRITIS (OSTEOARTHROSIS)

Although the words are similar, and many lay as well as professional people are not quite clear about the distinctions between arthritis, osteoarthritis, osteoporosis, etc., it is worth mentioning that there are pronounced *anthropometric* (body structure) distinctions between sufferers of Osteoporosis and *osteoarthritis*.

In a study (in 1983) of 27 women with osteoporosis (of the post-menopausal type), and 25 women with general arthritis, researchers found that the osteoporotic women were shorter, leaner, had less fat, muscle girth, and strength. The women with osteoarthritis (of comparable age and skeletal size) were fatter [sic] and had more muscle mass and strength.[D040]

SOMATIC CHARACTERISTICS OF WOMEN WHO HAVE EITHER

OSTEOPOROSIS	OR	OSTEOARTHRITIS
thinner		fatter
less muscle		more muscle
shorter		taller
weaker		stronger

PAGET'S DISEASE OF THE BONE

In *Paget's disease,* bone formation is accelerated, changing both the strength and shape of the bone. It most often affects the pelvis, lumbar spine (lower back), sacrum (tail bone), skull, and the femur or the tibia (long bones in the legs), usually centering in one or more of these areas. Once established, however, it rarely spreads to other areas.

Similarly to osteoporosis, the disease affects mostly Caucasians of north-western European ancestry. In the United States, Paget's disease is also seen occasionally in African-Americans. Contrary to the distribution of osteoporosis, Paget's disease is slightly more common in men than in women, usually beginning between the ages of 50 and 70. Sometimes it runs in families.

The cause is unknown. One of the most accepted theories points to an early viral infection which lies inactive for many years. [M061]

RHEUMATOID ARTHRITIS

In a Danish study of patients with rheumatoid arthritis, the concentration of minerals in the bone tissue, or *bone mineral density* (*BMD*) in the lumbar spine did not differ from age-matched healthy controls, but the bone density of the forearm and hand were significantly lower in the rheumatoid arthritis patients. This happened early in the disease. Patients who had better function-ality and grip strength also had better bone mass. Impaired physical activity, related to disease activity, seems to impinge on bone mass. In this study, it was not the use of the cortisone preparations that decreased the bone mass, as had been expected, and the authors concluded that the anti-inflammatory effect of steroids actually lead to clinical improvement, which counteracted the expect-ed negative effect of these drugs on bone in rheumatoid arthritis. [H040]

WHAT ARE FACTORS OF
INCREASED OR DECREASED RISK?

Risk factors for an increased chance to develop osteoporosis can be arranged into three categories:

■ Genetic
  Caucasian or Asian race
  Diabetes
  Family history of disease

Lactose intolerance
Small body build
Premature graying

■ Hormone-related
Age (greatly increased risk over the age of 70)
Bilateral ovarian removal (*oophorectomy*)
Early onset of menopause (before age of 45)
Female sex (women are four times more likely than men to develop osteoporosis)
Hyperparathyroidism (a condition in which the small *parathyroid* glands, located on both sides of the thyroid gland, overproduce a bone-modifying hormone)
Hyperprolactinemia (a condition in which the *pituitary* gland, located in the skull directly above the nose, and under the brain, overproduces the milk releasing hormone *prolactin*)
Immobilization and prolonged bed rest
Late onset of menstrual periods
Nulliparity (not having had any babies)

■ Lifestyle/health-related
Acid blockers (*cimetidine, Tagamet®, etc.*)
Anorexia nervosa (prolonged, abnormal fasting or minimal eating)
Certain types of diseases, e.g. chronic liver disease
Chronic infections
Certain types of medicines, e.g. long-term use of *corticosteroids* (drugs such as *prednisone* and *cortisone*)
Cigarette smoking
Cosmetics
Cushing's syndrome (a condition where the adrenal glands overproduce *cortisone*)
Diabetes
Dialysis (kidney machines)
Excessive alcohol consumption
Excessive exercise (enough to stop the periods of young women)
Failure/surgical removal of ovaries, resulting in lower level of estrogen production

Fluid pill use (***Lasix®***, ***furosemide***)
Inadequate calcium intake
Inappropriate diet
Lack of exercise
Mercury (silver) amalgam dental fillings (may interfere by inhibiting the change of the inactive thyroid hormone T4 to the active form, T3)
Pancreatic insufficiency
Pernicious anemia (an anemia associated to low stomach acid and lack of vitamin **B12**
Radiation, X-Rays
Thyroid diseases, including ***hypothyroidism***, ***hyperthyroidism***, and ***Thyrotoxicosis*** (a condition in which the ***thyroid*** gland overproduces hormone)
Transplant surgery
Type 1 diabetes

A CLOSER LOOK AT SOME FACTORS OF INCREASED RISK

Some factors for an increase in the risk for osteoporosis, pertain to women, others, to both sexes.

THE OSTEOPOROSIS GENE (THE "VDR" GENE)

It has been known for many years that there are ethnic differences in bone mass and fracture rates. We also know that a family history of osteoporosis carries an increased risk, as does being female, blond, and tall, all of which are genetic traits:

FACTORS OF INCREASED RISK FOR OSTEOPOROSIS

family history	female
tall	blond
body build	VDR type

Until recently, the understanding of the role of genetics in the development of osteoporosis was purely based upon population observations. That has changed with Australian scientists' discovery of a single gene that appears to play a crucial role in determining a persons risk of developing osteoporosis.[U090]

According to the Australian study, confirmed by others, there are two variants of a gene that allows cells to absorb calcium. The first version of the gene (*"b"*) is linked with stronger skeletons, while the other (*"B"*) is linked with weaker ones. **VDR** stands for *vitamin D receptor*. This gene is responsible for building vitamin D receptor sites on cells. Vitamin D responsive cells are widespread, and are involved in many physiologic processes including calcium absorption, bone mineralization, and calcium excretion. It may be somewhat controlled by vitamin D intake. Research suggests that the risk of developing osteoporosis depends greatly on which version of the vitamin D receptor gene an individual inherits.

When a test for the VDR gene will be commercially available, doctors may someday be able to identify people who are at higher risk for developing osteoporosis very early, and implement therapies at a younger age. Individuals receive one VDR gene from each parent, resulting in one of three possible combinations: **BB, bb,** or **Bb**. In studies of twins the BB combination was associated with the lowest bone densities, the bb combination with the highest, and the Bb combination with values of bone density somewhere in between. The B gene's effect is expressed (manifested) somewhat differently in different ethnic groups, suggesting that other genetic factors such as race and sex may also play a role.

One's total genetic makeup (race, sex, body build, complexion, and VDR type) probably determines one's maximal potential for bone density. Diet and exercise are critically important in determining how close we actually come to achieving that potential.

HORMONE DEFICIENCIES AND DISORDERS

Sex hormone deficiency is a problem. Low calcium intake worsens the consequences of sex hormone deficiency. One study suggested that calcium supplementation can decrease the minimum estrogen dosage required to maintain bone mass in post-menopausal women. However, oral calcium alone does not prevent the post-menopausal bone loss resulting from estrogen deficiency. In addition to estrogen, other hormones enhance net calcium absorption:

- *human growth hormone (HGH)*
- *insulin-like growth factor-I*
- *parathyroid hormone*

HYPERPROLACTINEMIA

"Hyperprolactinemia is associated with decreased bone mineral density."[T061] Women who are not ovulating as a consequence of suffering from an elevated milk producing hormone (*prolactin*) level have premature loss of bone mass.[K120] The treatment of this fairly common problem with the medication *bromocriptine* or *Parlodel*, corrects this hormonal imbalance and improves bone quality.[T061]

EARLY MENOPAUSE DUE TO HYSTERECTOMY

If we are convinced that the severity of typical menopausal complaints (hot flushes and vaginal dryness) are related to hormone imbalances, which can lead to osteoporosis, it must follow that these must be worse in hysterectomized women (one or both ovaries present), than in normal women (uterus and both ovaries present) who have reached menopause. Does this hypothesis bear out when statistics are performed? "Hysterectomized women, especially those aged 39 to 41 years, report significantly more *vasomotor* [flushing] complaints, vaginal dryness, and atypical complaints than do normal *climacteric* [menopausal] women of the same age. The higher prevalence of typical climacteric complaints in hysterectomized women largely explains their higher level of atypical complaints...the literature indicates that hysterectomized women with ovarian conservation are *overrepresented* with regard to osteoporosis, cardiovascular disease, osteoarthritis, depression, and sexual problems."[O050] [emphasis added]

PREMATURE GRAYING MAY BE A SIGN OF BONE DISEASE

If only your operator knows for sure, your bones may be at risk! An NIH Healthline report from October/November 1994 by Judy Folkenberg tells of a recently discovered factor which indicates a person's increased risk for the development of osteoporosis.

> ### A GRAY AREA...CAN PREMATURE GRAYING BE A SIGN OF BONE DISEASE? [N030]

For the purpose of this study, *osteopenia*— bone thinning—was measured by spinal scans. The scientists found that persons with premature graying (hair turned more than 50 % gray before the age of 40) were over 4 times more likely to have varying degrees of osteopenia when compared to the control group—those individuals without premature gray hair. The younger the hair had turned gray, the greater the chance of a history of osteoporosis in the family. Individuals with premature graying in their teens and twenties had a stronger family history of the disorder than those who had premature graying in their thirties.

The scientists weren't sure why premature graying and increased risk for osteoporosis were linked, but thought that perhaps the gene that controls premature graying was next to the gene that regulates bone density (genes in close proximity sometimes act together); or perhaps one gene influenced the other. However, if we take a peek at the connection between graying, and the levels of the vitamin PABA (see under that heading), we may gain some insight into the subject.

THE INFLUENCE OF SKIN PIGMENTATION
Even among similar groups, the risk is lower with women who have darker skin. For example, in Israel the darker skin Sephardic Jews have a lower rate of fractures than do Jewish women of European origin.

THE INFLUENCE OF FAMILY HISTORY
If your close female relatives suffered from osteoporosis, you have a higher risk of developing this problem. Many women who have seen their mothers or grandmothers develop a dowager's hump or become disabled after suffering a hip fracture, upsetting the entire family who must deal with the long term disability, will go through the same pattern, in turn.

THE INFLUENCE OF AGE

THE OLDER THE MENOPAUSE, THE SWEETER THE HORMONES

Bone density is affected by the age at which women begin their menopause and how much hormonal support they maintain during their post-menopausal years. Women who have had a surgical menopause before age 40, by hysterectomy with removal of their ovaries, or just ovary removal (*oophorectomy*) are at high risk of osteoporosis because of the abrupt withdrawal of estrogen at a young age. Similarly, women who go through an early natural menopause are at high risk. A woman going through early menopause at age 35 or 40 has as much as 10 to 15 years less estrogen protection for her bones than a woman going through menopause at age 50. Thus, the older you are when going through menopause, the more years of hormonal protection are provided for your bones.[O050] In my own experience, the same results can be expected from the tubal ligations done for contraceptive purposes. Women who underwent these surgeries have a 25% or better chance of developing *disfunctional menstrual bleeding* (clotting, irregular periods, etc.) which are linked to hormonal deficiencies. Although the mechanism is not clear, there have been suggestions that the ovarian circulation is impaired by the surgical procedure.

DIABETES AND OSTEOPOROSIS

It is a well known fact that *insulin dependent diabetes mellitus* (*IDDM*) cases can be complicated with decrease in bone mass, or osteopenia. This has been tested by the diagnostic methods previously mentioned, single photon absorptiometry, and dual energy X-ray absorptiometry (DXA), a method that is excellent for very precise measurements of bone mineralization. Osteoarthritis and *osteophytes* (outgrowth of bones) of unknown origin in the lumbar vertebrae are also often observed in elderly *non-insulin dependent diabetes mellitus* (*NIDDM*) patients. The BMD in the head and spine especially decreased in women after menopause.[K010]

A study performed in Korea confirmed some of these findings. Before menopause, the density of minerals concentrated in bone was higher in diabetics than in non-diabetics. Then, bone loss related to menopause started before the onset of menopause in diabetics, and the minerals of postmenopausal women showed a definite decrease with aging; there was abrupt bone loss after 55 years of age.[K130]

Diabetics have quirky patterns of decrease of bone mineral density. Although diabetics have decreased skin and muscle blood flow, according to a German study in 1955, "bone blood flow is increased in the distal limb of diabetic patients, which is believed to increase osteoclastic activity."[K130] Bone mineral density testing revealed that in the diabetic group studied there was a 10% reduction of bone mineral density in the femoral neck, and a 12% reduction in the distal limb, compared with the control group. No significant difference was found in the lumbar spine. The German doctors noticed the incidence of peripheral bone mass decrease or osteopenia in Insulin Dependent Diabetic patients, even if it was not osteoporosis. A link also exists between *diabetic neuropathy* (a form of nerve damage), and decreased bone mineral density for the femoral neck, but not for the distal limb or axial skeleton. They stated that "Whether there [was] a common causal link or a casual connection between diabetic neuropathy and bone mineral density ha[d] still to be determined."[M270] [emphasis added]

MICROVASCULAR COMPLICATIONS

Diabetics frequently suffer from *Microvascular complications*, (damage to tiny blood vessels), which are a critical factor in the progression of diabetic osteopenia. What is behind these blood vessel problems? It must be remembered that vascular complications not only are due to diabetes itself, but probably to the severe danger caused by the fish protein contained in preparations of NPH, lente and semi-lente insulin. This fish protein suppresses the formation of small blood vessels, a fact totally unknown to the bulk of the medical profession and the public. Other risk factors for osteoporosis (nutritional status and smoking) must be taken into account.

Does a normal insulin supply promote stronger bones? Since osteoporosis is a known complication of diabetes, this suggests a role for insulin in bone maintenance. In studies on rat bone tumor cells, which have not yet been confirmed in humans, bone cells appear to bind insulin and bone-specific enzymes such as alkaline phosphatase are inhibited by insulin, all of which may have important bone protective consequences.[L070]

INSULIN AND HORMONAL INTERACTIONS IN DIABETES

Does *insulin* help strengthen bones? It may, but it is very important to realize that only *regular* insulin which does not contain the fish proteins that actually *decrease* circulation, may be of benefit. Insulin may be a natural fighter of bone resorption by affecting osteoblasts and osteoclasts, through an interaction between insulin and PTH. In addition, insulin is known to promote collagen production by osteoblasts. These findings imply that efficient insulin activity may exert an anabolic [protein building] effect on bone, and rationalize the many clinical studies demonstrating reduced bone density in Type I diabetes.[M090]

LACTOSE MALDIGESTION

Lactose (milk sugar) maldigestion causes non-specific abdominal symptoms such as bloating, *borborygmus* (gurgling), colic, flatulence, and diarrhea. The degree of discomfort depends not only on the amount of lactose consumed, but also on an individual sensitivity to lactose. The symptoms of *irritable bowel syndrome* (*IBS*) and lactose maldigestion are similar.

Consequently, most reports indicate an increased frequency of lactose maldigestion in patients suffering from IBS. *Recurrent abdominal pain (RAP)* in children corresponds to IBS in adults. Lactose maldigestion is a frequent cause of RAP in regions with a high prevalence of lactose maldigestion in early childhood. Diffuse small-intestinal damage in *celiac disease* or *kwashiorkor* leads to a proportional decrease of all disaccharidase (double sugars such as lactose) activities, the most pronounced being a decrease of the lactose digesting enzyme *lactase*. The consumption of milk may then cause abdominal discomfort and increased diarrhea.[G130]

Several studies have indicated an increased frequency of lactose maldigestion in patients with osteoporosis. A connection between lactose maldigestion and decreased absorption of calcium has not been proven, however. Researchers have, tentatively, concluded that the increased tendency toward osteoporosis is more likely caused by a lower calcium intake because of milk intolerance, than by the maldigestion itself. Milk and dairy products with reduced lactose content are better tolerated by patients with lactose maldigestion.

In a Great Britain study from the mid-nineteen-eighties, the daily intake of calcium derived from milk was significantly lower in osteoporotic patients. The malabsorption of lactose can be easily diagnosed, because blood sugar normally rises when lactose is given, but when absorption of lactose is poor, the sugar rises much more slowly. When tested, the fasting blood glucose concentration was higher in the osteoporotic patients than in the controls, although body weight was significantly lower.

Absorption of lactose is significantly impaired in women with "idiopathic" (cause undetermined) osteoporosis; this, combined with low consumption of milk, and disorders of glucose metabolism without overt symptoms, may be a major factor in the development of osteoporosis in women.[F030]

DEFICIENCY OF STOMACH ACID

Whereas we used to be totally convinced that people with insufficient stomach acid do not absorb calcium well, today the answer is not so clear. However, the design of the few available studies is so ambiguous and bizarre, that one must wonder whether this is by design or by accident, and whether there are special interest groups that refuse to aim for a clear answer. Those who would benefit from the sale of anti-acids (SUCH AS

TUMS) as calcium replacement, would certainly, at least in my humble opinion, not want it made clear that a low acid situation impairs calcium absorption..[B180]

"Since calcium solubility is a prerequisite to calcium absorption, and since solubility of calcium is highly...dependent [on the presence of stomach acid], it has been generally assumed that gastric acid secretion and gastric acidity play an important role in the intestinal absorption of calcium from ingested food or calcium salts such as *CaCO3* [*calcium carbonate*]." [emphasis added] However, studies performed in 1973 showed that the acid content of the stomach was not a significant contributor to calcium absorption. In older patients, who may have achlorhydria...other, better absorbed forms of calcium should be used."[T070] Since I do not have to worry about the impact of my words on the calcium carbonate industry, I will, wholeheartedly, say that I believe that better absorbable forms should always be the option.

CHRONIC PANCREATIC INSUFFICIENCY AND OSTEOPOROSIS

Low bone mineral density (BMD) has been demonstrated in some patients with chronic intestinal disorders accompanied by diarrhea and malabsorption. However, very few studies have evaluated BMD in patients with *pancreatic insufficiency* (a condition with inadequate production of digestive enzymes in the pancreas gland) due to *cystic fibrosis* (a disease of the lungs), or patients with pancreatic insufficiency as a consequence of *chronic pancreatitis* (a long standing inflammatory and scarring condition of the pancreas gland). In an Argentine study reported in 1997, ten patients of fourteen demonstrated osteopenia in the lumbar spine and in the femoral neck. Three patients displayed osteoporosis in the lumbar spine and two in the femoral neck. Serum calcium, serum parathyroid hormone, and alkaline phosphatase were in the normal range in all patients. Serum vitamin D (*25-(OH)D3*) was below normal range in 7 of 12 patients. Scores of patients with pancreatitis of alcoholic origin were similar to those of nonalcoholic patients. Most patients with pancreatic insufficiency as a consequence of chronic pancreatitis exhibit osteopenia, and some show evidence of osteoporosis.[M250]

EXERCISE AND OSTEOPOROSIS

Do rock hard bodies promote rock hard bones? Although we have always heard that exercise is an excellent tool for the development of strong bones, in a European evaluation of certain athletes there were some surprising results. In a study of 40 international top ranked, high performance sport champs of different disciplines (28 weight-lifters, 6 sports-boxers and 6 bicycle- racers), bone density measurements of the lumbar spine and the left hip were performed by dual-photon-absorptiometry (DEXA; QDR 2000, Siemens) and evaluated by an interactive software-programme (Hologic Inc.). The results were compared to the measurements of 21 age-matched male control individuals. It came as no surprise that in the high performance weight lifters there was an increase of bone density of 23%, compared to the control individuals . The sports-boxers had an increase up to 17% (lumbar spine), 9% (hip) and 7% over all. But it was an absolutely unexpected finding, that in the third athletes group (Tour de France-bikers) BMD was decreased 10% in the lumbar spine, 14% in the hip, and 17% over all.[S010] The final conclusions were that while

■ training programs stressing axial loads of the skeletal system may lead to an increase of BMD in the spine and the hip of young individuals

■ the BMD of endurance athletes may decrease

Is "Olé! OK? Not where it pertains to future osteoporosis. In a contemporary study in Spanish ballet dancers, an evaluation of their mineral nutrition and bone mass, revealed that, although both male and female dancers had a slimmer figure and lighter diet, "The...trunk bone mass observed in the female dancers [was lower and] is a risk factor for eventual osteoporosis.[C141]

OBESITY
Although obesity is considered a factor of increased risk for many diseases such as osteoarthritis and uterine cancer, being overweight is associated with protection against osteoporosis in post-menopausal women. This is because the fat cells produce a type of estrogen called estrone, through conversion of an adrenal hormone called *androstenedione*. This type of estrogen provides some support for the bones once the ovarian source of estrogen has dwindled.[R040]

PERNICIOUS ANEMIA
Pernicious anemia is a disease that occurs as a consequence of a vitamin B12 deficiency. The symptoms include *achlorhydria* (the total absence of naturally occurring stomach acid). It has been a long held belief among medical people that gastric (stomach) acid is necessary for the absorption of dietary calcium, therefore researchers expected that "the total absence

of gastric acid secretion that occurs in pernicious anaemia could result in bone loss....[In a study at Mayo clinic, comparing normal women to pernicious anemia women]...the bone mineral density of the lumbar spine was decreased by 16% in women with pernicious anaemia."[E000] However, the absorption of calcium was similar to healthy individuals. The lumbar spine bone mineral quantities went hand in hand, not with acid, but with the serum concentration of a group of proteins (*group 1 pepsinogen*), produced by the *gastric fundus*, the larger curve of the stomach. Despite absence of stomach acid, the women with pernicious anaemia had normal calcium absorption and normal serum levels of parathyroid hormone and 1,25-dihydroxy vitamin D. Gastric acid (seemingly) was not required for the absorption of dietary calcium. Thus, the loss of cancellous (honeycomb) bone had to be caused by some mechanism yet to be identified.

We may remember that *achlorhydic* people (individuals without sufficient stomach acid) have poor absorption and utilization of the B vitamins, maybe there's the rub....

HIGH FIBER DIETS

Vegetables and fruit are very high in fiber content. People who are predominantly vegetarian, and individuals who take large doses of high fiber supplements are at risk to get too much of an otherwise wholesome product. Excessive dietary fiber causes accelerated emptying of the colon, which results in mineral losses. "High fiber diets reduce calcium absorption. This is not further affected by [the levels of] stomach acid."[K100] Many cereals, such as rye, contain *phytic acid* which causes the formation of insoluble calcium salts, the *phytates*, and subsequent calcium loss.

In a British study on the importance of the speed of the intestinal transit of food, the authors concluded that "Increased fibre [sic] intake has been shown to reduce serum oestrogen [sic] concentrations. We hypothesized that fibre exerts this effect by decreasing the time available for reabsorption of oestrogens [sic] in the colon. We tested this in volunteers by measuring changes in serum oestrogen [sic] levels in response to manipulation of intestinal transit times with senna and loperamide, then comparing the results with changes caused by wheat bran.....*Senna* [a laxative] and *loperamide* [*Imodium*] caused the intended alterations in intestinal transit, whereas on wheat bran supplements there was a trend towards faster transit....[estrogen] fell with wheat bran (mean intake 19.8 g day(-1)) and with senna. No significant changes in serum oestrogens [sic] were seen with loperamide.... In conclusion, speeding up intestinal transit can lower serum oestrogen [sic] concentrations." [L071]

CHRONIC INFECTIONS, RENAL DYALISIS (KIDNEY MACHINE TREATMENTS)

When a person is undergoing prolonged dialysis or suffering from chronic, improperly treated infections, an abnormal protein, similar to the one found in the brains of Alzheimer's disease victims, is often formed. It is called *amyloid* ("Amy Lloyd"); it gets into bones and destroys them by coaxing white blood cells into a frenzy of "pack-man activities" madly chomping at previously useful bone. These proteins are ironically known as *AGE-modified protein*, not because they are caused by age, but because this is an acronym of their chemical name: *Advanced Glycation End-products (AGEs)*.[M290]

In laboratory tests, AGE-modified proteins make mouse bones lose calcium and prompt the bone eating *osteoclast* cells make pits in the outer layers of teeth, so when the normal bone gets modified with the AGEs that mimic age, it may show the fearsome consequences of osteoporosis.

SELF DESTRUCTIVE HABITS

CAFFEINE, SUGAR AND BONE LOSS

Sodas and other commonly used beverages are a constant drain on your calcium stores. Not only in the elderly, but even in young people, dietary indiscretions can cause problems. In a study of eighteen kids aged 13-18 years, they drank either a caffeine and sugar free soft drink, or a soft drink with caffeine or sugar. When caffeine was added, three hour urinary calcium excretion increased by 25% (from 6 mgr. to 20 mgr. per hour). When sugar was added to the caffeine drink, urinary calcium loss almost doubled (from 16 mgr. to 30 mgr. per hour). They found that *sodium, chloride* and *potassium* losses were also increased by caffeine. Phosphorus, found in most cola drinks, accelerates calcium and bone loss even more. Colas with caffeine and sugar added cause the greatest calcium and bone loss.

COLAS CONTAINING CAFFEINE, SUGAR AND PHOSPHORUS CAUSE SEVERE CALCIUM LOSS

The most disturbing feature is that the experimental dose used in this study was far less than the average teen's daily consumption of caffeine and sugar. After a hard physical workout, drinking soft drinks can cause calcium and potassium loss, and that in turn can cause sore muscles and delayed recovery time after exercise.

Really high protein diets and really high fiber diets, can cause bone loss also.[M060]

COFFEE

Should you really wake up and smell the coffee? It's OK, as long as you do not drink it....

Another unhealthy habit is the large, chronic intake of coffee: The excess fluid dilutes the minerals, the caffeine is a diuretic which encourages the loss of more minerals in the urine. In a study in health conscious California, at Rancho San Bernardo, the doctors from the Department of Family and Preventive Medicine at San Diego, who investigated the effect of coffee intake on health, tell us that: "There was a statistically significant graded association between increasing lifetime intake of caffeinated coffee and decreasing BMD at both the hip and spine, independent of age, obesity, parity [number of births], years since menopause, and the use of tobacco, alcohol, estrogen, thiazides, and calcium supplements. Bone density did not vary by lifetime coffee intake in women who reported drinking at least one glass of milk per day during most of their adult lives. Lifetime caffeinated coffee intake equivalent to two cups per day [much less than most people in the US drink] is associated with decreased bone density in older women who do not drink milk on a daily basis."[B030]

WHAT ABOUT DECAFFEINATED COFFEE

What is decaffeinated coffee? In the US, a coffee must have at least 97% of caffeine removed to qualify as decaffeinated. Coffee beans are decaffeinated before they are roasted, when the process can be done more cost effectively and with the least effect on the beans' flavor.

Caffeine is water soluble above 175°F, but water is generally not used by itself to decaffeinate coffee because it strips away too much of the essential flavor and aroma. Decaffeination usually involves the use of a decaffeinating agent. Coffee may be decaffeinated at the bean or at the solution level. In both methods, the agent is removed from the final product, but trace amounts may remain.

Various solvents are used to decaffeinate coffee. There are two main ways to decaffeinate with chemical solvents:

Direct contact method: The green (unroasted) beans are softened by steam, then repeatedly rinsed with one of the solvents which removes the caffeine from the beans. This is drained away, and the beans are steamed a second time for the remaining solvent to evaporate. They are air or vacuum dried. Manufacturers claim that virtually no solvent residue remains after roasting the beans.

Indirect contact method (water process): The green beans soak for several hours at almost boiling temperature. Gradually, the solution draws the caffeine, as well as other flavor elements and oils, from the beans. Then, it is treated with solvent, which absorbs the caffeine. The mixture is heated to evaporate the solvent and caffeine, after which the beans are replaced into the mixture, allowing them to regain most of the coffee oils and flavor elements. The solvent never touches the beans.

DECAFFEINATION AND CANCER? A CONCERN TO PEOPLE WHO ARE ALREADY WORRIED ABOUT TAKING ESTROGEN

How would you like to sweeten your coffee with paint stripper (***methylene chloride***)? You have probably seen what it does to the paint, penetrating, blistering, and lifting old finish. What could it do to your gut? It is touted to be safe by the decaffeination industry. It is converted by the body to carbon monoxide, which can lower the blood's ability to carry oxygen. Industrial "safety rules" accompanying paint stripper include the advice that individuals with cardiovascular or pulmonary health problems should check with their physician prior to the use of the paint stripper. Individuals experiencing severe symptoms such as shortness of breath or chest pains should obtain proper medical care immediately. I wonder what the repetitive intake of small amounts in beverages may do to us!

Methylene chloride has been shown to cause cancer in certain laboratory animal tests. Recent laboratory studies indicate, however, that the response is unique to animals tested and not relevant to humans (or so they report). Available human studies, moreover, do not provide the necessary information to determine whether methylene chloride causes cancer in humans.

ALCOHOL

For all manner of reasons, because we are too cold or too hot, or because we are depressed or happy, we have always found a good excuse to drink alcoholic beverages. Is this healthy?

> **ANYONE WHO DRINKS BEVERAGES CONTAINING MORE THAN ONE OR TWO OUNCES OF PURE ETHANOL IN 24 HOURS RISKS FREE RADICAL DAMAGE**

Alcoholic beverages have one thing in common, they contain the compound *ethanol* (the chemical name of the kind of alcohol in alcoholic beverages), which often induces the generation of damaged molecules, otherwise known as *free radicals* (discussed later in this book). These free radicals are dangerous to surrounding molecules and tissues, causing serious problems similar to a *biologic rusting*. Only relatively healthy adults are able to tolerate some drinking, and it is not long before even moderate drinking becomes more than they can detoxify. Anyone who drinks beverages containing more than one or two ounces of pure ethanol in 24 hours risks free radical damage. Even that apparently reasonable amount can be harmful on a regular basis, depending on how well the antioxidants are supplied. Two ounces of ethanol is the amount in either:

- beer — four eight-ounce glasses
- hard liquor — two to three shot glasses
- wine — four small glasses

Victims of chronic degenerative diseases should usually avoid the consumption of alcohol.

Alcoholism often causes a liver disease (*cirrhosis*) characterized by cellular destruction and hardening by growth of fibrous tissue, with decrease of function. This may reduce protein synthesis, the metabolism of many other substances, produce *ascites* (fluid in the abdomen), and even death.[M220]

In Spain, the rain may fall mainly on the plains, but alcohol weakens the bones of Spaniards as it does in the rest of the world. In a study conducted in Spain to evaluate the connection between *cirrhosis* (degeneration, scarring and death) of the liver, mostly due to alcoholism, and osteoporosis, it was found that in a group of 58 patients referred for liver transplant, 25 patients (43%) had osteoporosis, with lower bone mass measurements in the lumbar spine than in the femoral neck. Cirrhotic patients showed other chemical changes:

■ increased urinary *hydroxyproline* (a substance which is found in urine, and is a marker of the breakdown of bone *collagen*— gristle protein, discussed further in chapter II)
■ lower *osteocalcin* levels (low special bone protein)
■ lower serum 1,25-dihydroxyvitamin D (a type of vitamin D)
■ lower serum 25-hydroxyvitamin D (a type of vitamin D)
■ lower serum *parathyroid* hormone levels (a hormone of the small parathyroid glands, to the sides of the thyroid, which regulates the metabolism of calcium)
■ lower *testosterone* levels (male hormone)
■ reduced bone formation
■ significant disorders of bone mineral metabolism
■ significant decrease in bone mass, particularly in the lumbar spine

Across the Atlantic Ocean, a 1996 Canadian study of rats fed alcohol showed that (in rodents, at least), this habit can have deleterious effects on both adult and developing bone.[K070] The findings included:

■ decreased calcium content of maternal bone
■ delays in skeletal development
■ elevated serum parathyroid hormone levels
■ reduced mean fetal skeletal ossification
■ reduced mean fetal body weight

Not only calcium, but "magnesium (Mg) deficiency occurs frequently in chronic alcoholism and may contribute to the increased incidence of osteoporosis and cardiovascular disease seen in this population."[A020]

OSTEOPOROSIS IS PREVALENT IN THE ALCOHOLIC POPULATION

Osteoporosis is prevalent in the alcoholic population. Magnesium deficiency may contribute to increased bone loss by its effects on mineral homeostasis. In magnesium depletion, there is often hypocalcemia due to impaired parathyroid hormone (PTH) secretion, as well as renal and skeletal resistance to PTH action. Serum concentrations of 1,25-vitamin D are also low. These changes are seen with even mild degrees of magnesium deficiency and may contribute to the metabolic bone disease seen in chronic alcoholics.

TOBACCO

What I am going to say now is my personal feeling and opinion. It may be a little strong. SORRY!

Of all abhorrent habits I can think of, none is worse and more disgusting than the use of tobacco. There may be a natural need to drink, which may lead to the ingestion of alcohol to excess, there may be a need to correct physical or mental anguish which may lead to drugs. But there is no redeeming value to smoking! To use tobacco is voluntarily to create a state of illness, then to become dependent on the substance. It is dirty, unwholesome, it STINKS! And, to the unfortunate non-smoker, there is no escape.

THE HARMFUL EFFECTS OF SMOKING ARE INTERNATIONAL

The "Marlboro Man" may not have only suffered from cancer of the lung, but of problems with his bones. Cigarettes contain numerous poisonous chemicals:

- *cadmium*
- *nickel carbonyl*
- *nicotine*
- *pesticides*
- *radioactive plutonium*

Do smokers play Russian Roulette with their hormones? They certainly do! Morning serum steroid levels were determined in postmenopausal chronic smokers and nonsmokers. "Postmenopausal smokers...had significantly elevated levels of *cortisol, progesterone* [a female hormone, normally produced in the second half of the period and during pregnancy]..., *17-hydroxyprogesterone* [another female hormone]..., *androstenedione* [estrogenic hormone produced in the *adrenal* glands above the kidneys], and *testosterone* [male hormone] compared with nonsmokers.... The increases were most significant for cortisol...and 17-OHP.... *Estrone, estradiol, dihydrotestosterone*, and *dehydroepiandrosterone sulfate* [*DHEA*] did not differ between the groups.[F091]

Because the fact that smoking is associated with osteoporosis may be a surprising piece of information to many, I will enclose multiple quotes from various research centers so that the reader may see that the knowledge is not new, and abundantly documented.

In 1980, the combined incidences of vertebral and hip fractures necessitating hospitalization of women living in Knox County, Tennessee nearly doubled each five years after the age of 50. Among the reasons, it was obvious that personal habits [of the patients] such as drinking coffee to excess, and smoking were a factor. The Tennessee researchers advised that in the field of those habits "Intake of coffee and alcoholic beverages and use of cigarettes should be discontinued or minimized."[D020 J010]

> **TO PREVENT OSTEOPOROSIS, INTAKE OF COFFEE AND ALCOHOLIC BEVERAGES AND USE OF CIGARETTES SHOULD BE DISCONTINUED OR MINIMIZED!**

In a 1996 Swedish study evaluating the numbers of occurrences of second fractures in menopausal women who had already had one broken bone, and its relationship to smoking habits, concluded that "Both an early menopause and tobacco smoking were associated significantly with repeated fractures, while use of oral contraceptives had a protective effect against repeated fractures in the 1940 birth cohort."[J010] [emphasis added]

We tend to think of the Swiss as a nation of ruddy-faced mountaineers, strengthened by drinking milk and eating Swiss cheese, possessing a legendary skeleton, worthy of Robin Hood. But, they also have problems with osteoporosis: In a Swiss study on factors which increase and decrease the chances of becoming osteoporotic, the high-risk profile included the usually known factors plus the smoking of cigarettes. As expected, BMD was significantly different in these two subgroups of the population.

Osteoporosis was diagnosed in 72% of the high risk group and in only 17% to 19% of the low risk group.[B150]

The following report from London, England, may be enough to set your teeth on edge! In a 1983 retrospective study "two hundred eight white women, aged 60 to 69 years, had acquired 218 upper or lower full dentures. Each woman's smoking habits and current osteoporosis severity...were compared with the age at which she had acquired each full denture. Among osteoporotic women...who still had their natural teeth at age 50 years, 44% had required a new full denture before age 60, compared with 15% of non-osteoporotic women...Different denture requirements between these groups had not existed before age 50 but had continued after age 60. Fifty-two percent of smokers, 26% of nonsmokers, and only 8% of non-osteoporotic nonsmokers had required dentures since age 50. These observations strongly suggest that middle-aged women may be more likely to retain their teeth if they avoid smoking, and undertake a program effective in preventing progression of osteoporosis."[J030]

The British have done their share of observing: "Women and men who smoke are more slender than their non-smoking counterparts and have a bone density appropriate to their degree of slenderness. As a result, they are more likely to sustain a fracture than their non-smoking counterparts. The lower bone density found in smokers may arise because of less stress and strain imposed on the skeleton by a slim physique. Smokers have poorer oral hygiene and less teeth than their non-smoking counterparts. The relationship between smoking and tooth pathology remains unclear: smoking may either act via a direct mechanism based on the toxicity of tobacco smoke or indirectly through body weight (i.e., the effect on teeth is part of a wider effect on bone structure)."[J030]

If the previous study would suggest that "slimness" and eating habits are a cause of low BMD, rather than tobacco itself, an elegant French study, with a slight courtesy twist to the female gender (French cigarettes seem to be respectful of women), determines that smoking impacts on bone forming cells directly: "Smoking is a risk factor for osteoporosis. Nicotine and non-nicotine tobacco smoke components have been shown to depress osteoblast activity in a number of in vitro and animal studies...Overall, osteocalcin levels were significantly lower in smokers...than in nonsmokers...The difference between smokers and nonsmokers was significant in males...but not in females...These data suggest that smoking may induce osteoblast depression, either directly or via hormonal changes."[L040]

In a country where kangaroo and koala watching may be common activities, and Crocodile Dundee symbolizes the unspoiled outback, there still are bad lifestyle factors to contend with: "Epidemiologic evidence suggests that lifestyle factors, such as exercise, calcium intake, and tobacco consumption, have effects on bone density...BMD [bone mineral density] was significantly higher in men than in women (20% at all sites). There was an age-related decline in BMD at the femoral neck in both sexes and at the lumbar spine in women. Between the ages of 60 and 80, the decrease in BMD at the femoral neck among women was 18.9%, which is almost twice the decrease in BMD among men(10.1%). Tobacco consumption was associated with a reduction in BMD at both sites in both sexes (5-8%), and this effect was independent of calcium intake or body weight. Exsmokers [sic] had BMD intermediate between that of current smokers and never smokers, suggesting the influence of tobacco was partially reversible."[N050]

In another study in the "land down under", comparing twins, the researchers conducted a cross-sectional study of bone density at the lumbar spine and the femoral neck and shaft in 41 pairs of female twins, 27 to 73 years of age (mean, 49)...For every ten years of a standard number of packs per month of smoking, the bone density of the twin who smoked more heavily was...lower at the lumbar spine...the femoral neck...the femoral shaft (P = 0.04)...Smoking was associated with higher serum concentrations of follicle-stimulating hormone...and luteinizing hormone... and lower serum concentrations of parathyroid hormone...CONCLUSIONS. Women who smoke one pack of cigarettes each day throughout adulthood will, by the time of menopause, have an average deficit of 5 to 10 percent in bone density, which is sufficient to increase the risk of fracture."[H139]

TOBACCO, CANCER, GENETIC DISORDERS AND MUTATIONS

To understand the full and horrible implications of the following paragraph, we must remember that genetically engineered substances are held together by *vectors* (biologic magnets). Recently, in 1996, when the tobacco industry's public image was tainted by all types of law suits, and probably at its lowest, it started boasting that tobacco had some real redeeming values, and announced that it could be used to make such vectors or biologic magnets, to attach one particle of DNA to another in the manufacturing of genetically engineered substances. Since this really is a property of tobacco, the chance for man-made disaster is magnified, because such easily available "genetic glue" has the potential for unbridled and unexpected contribution to dangerous mutations and recombinations of genetic and viral particles and fragments already present in the human body.[S220]

An example of this is the binding of *tobacco mosaic virus* (*TMV*) [one of the earliest viruses to be discovered] to construct a *vector*, a "biologic wheel barrow" used as transport in genetic engineering, was accomplished in 1993, attaching particles of influenza virus *hemagglutinin* (*HA*), and one from human immunodeficiency virus type I (HIV-I) envelope protein, which suggests a potential for these processes happening spontaneously and uncontrolledly in the human body, with the catastrophic results we see every day.[H030]

Another study in Europe showed that certain segments of tobacco DNA had chains of links in its DNA, that were similar or the same as segments that induce malignancies, derived from other sources.[W070]

EATING DISORDERS, DIETS, AND OSTEOPOROSIS
ANOREXIA NERVOSA AND BULIMIA NERVOSA

"*Anorexia nervosa* and *bulimia nervosa* are prevalent illnesses affecting between 1% and 10% of adolescent and college-age women. Developmental, family dynamic, and biologic factors are all important in the cause of this disorder. Anorexia nervosa is diagnosed when a person refuses to maintain his or her body weight over a minimal normal weight for age and height, such as 15% below that expected, has an intense fear of gaining weight, has a disturbed body image, and, in women, has primary or secondary *amenorrhea*."[H020]

What is *bulimia nervosa* ?
- A feeling of lack of control over behavior during binges
- A minimum of 2 binge episodes a week for at least 3 months
- Persistent over concern with body shape and weight
- Recurrent episodes of binge eating
- Regular use of laxatives
- Regular use of diuretics

- Regular use of self-induced vomiting
- Strict dieting
- Vigorous exercise to prevent weight gain

"Patients with eating disorders are usually secretive and often come to the attention of physicians only at the insistence of others."[H020]

Medical complications include:

- **Bradycardia**—slow heart beat
- Dental erosion-damage to the outer surface of teeth due to constant acid flow to mouth
- **Edema** (swelling)
- **Esophagitis** (inflammation of the food pipe or **esophagus**)
- Fluid or **electrolyte** (sodium, potassium, etc.) imbalance
- Gastric dilation
- Gastritis
- **Gingivitis** (gum disease) in patients with bulimia nervosa
- **Hyperamylasemia**—too much **amylase**, a starch digesting enzyme
- **Hypotension** (low blood pressure)
- **hypothermia** (low body temperature)
- Infertility
- Osteoporosis
- Swollen **parotid** [salivary glands in the cheek] glands

Anorexia nervosa (AN) predisposes to osteoporosis through **hypothalamic dysfunction** (a disorder of the brain stem, above the pituitary gland), which may lead to elevated cortisol as well as diminished estrogen and progesterone. The osteoporosis associated with AN affects both trabecular and cortical bone, and increases the risk of osseous fracture. Fractures in this population may go unrecognized, because plain X-rays may be non-diagnostic for 6 weeks or more. Undiagnosed stress fractures may be identified by bone scan. Although moderate exercise in patients with anorexia nervosa-associated osteoporosis may be beneficial, strenuous exercise can be detrimental, with its potential risk of stress fractures and exacerbation of the underlying neurohormonal abnormalities. This risk for fracture may persist well after improvement in the patient's eating habits.[L010]

EXCESSIVELY HIGH FIBER DIETS, VEGETARIANISM AND VEGANISM

Are *veganism* and very strict *vegetarianism* eating disorders? This may apply more to *vegans* (who do not eat *any* food of animal source) than to *vegetarians* (who often eat cheese, eggs, and drink milk). I apologize to vegans and very strict vegetarians for my political incorrectness, but the answer may be a rotund Yes! If you consider this diet's impact on calcium metabolism, hormones and osteoporosis. You see, *Kiwis* (New Zealanders) suffer from osteoporosis too! In a 1993 New Zeland study of dietary habits in females, overweight and dietary fat intake did not influence circulating plasma female hormone (17 beta-estradiol) but a high dietary fiber intake reduced 17 beta-estradiol concentrations at various times of the menstrual cycle. They found that "...healthy New Zealand women of premenopausal age have lower 17 beta-oestradiol [sic] levels on high fibre [sic] diets than on low fibre [sic] diets. Because hypoestrogenism is a known risk factor for osteoporosis...high fibre [sic] intakes may influence bone mass adversely and be a risk factor for osteoporosis."[F010]

OBESITY AND OSTEOPOROSIS

Surprise, chubbies! Sometimes obesity, which usually contributes to various pathologies, is actually bliss, when it comes to osteoporosis (Obesity has a protective effect). Dieting, usually hailed as a positive thing to do, increases the incidence of osteoporosis. It is not fully understood why obesity has this effect, but thank God for small favors!

In a Swiss study on factors that increase and decrease the risk of getting osteoporosis, the only complete protector was severe obesity, where there was a drop to 1%.[B160]

This study evaluated 176 women aged 45-71 years, in whom only weight was significantly different. Comparison between groups revealed a significant effect of menopausal status and obesity on BMD and bone turnover. The results of this study suggested that even moderate obesity played a protective role on post-menopausal bone loss.[R040]

The bone density in pre-menopausal women was similar for both obese and non-obese women. For post-menopausal women, here is a table from the paper.

VARIABLES	NON-OBESE	OBESE
Mean weight of the group (kg)	57.2 kg	75.1 kg
Bone mineral density (g/cm^2)	0.974 +/- 0.14	1.056 +/- 0.12
Bone mass	34.4 +/- 8.15	41.2 +/- 8.6

Does nature discriminate between black and white. It surely does, and black wins when it comes to female body mass and the beneficial metabolism of the female hormone estrone: "Obesity offers protection against osteoporosis in older women. The mechanisms are not well understood, but relate in part to increased chemical conversion (*aromatization*) of...[male hormones produced in the adrenals to female hormones such as]...estrone in peripheral fat and muscle tissue. Two hundred and one white and 77 black women previously reported to be free of skeletal disease and to have normal bone mass had measurements of total body bone mineral (TBBM), fat mass (TBFM), and lean mass (TBLM) performed by dual energy x-ray absorptiometry. Serum [female hormone] estrone, [male hormone] androstenedione, and [DHEA} dihydroepiandrostenedione sulfate were measured on the same day. Body weight, body mass index, TBFM, and TBLM were all significantly higher in the black women. However, proportionately, there were no differences in body composition between the two groups. This suggests that the black women were not more obese despite their greater body mass index, and that future studies on the health impact of obesity in older black women should take this into consideration. Despite the greater TBFM and TBLM in the black women and no difference in serum androstenedione levels, the serum estrone level was not higher in the black women, and the higher bone mass in blacks was not related to serum estrone. In both ethnic groups, TBBM was significantly related to body weight....Both TBFM and TBLM were significantly related to TBBM in both ethnic groups. Serum estrone was significantly related to all measures of body mass in the white women, but to no measures of body mass in the black women, indicating apparent differences in the metabolism of estrone between older white and black women.[K091]

IMMOBILIZATION, SEDENTARY LIFE STYLE

General inactivity and immobilization have always been regarded as harmful to the bones. I remember early comments about these circumstances, coupled to degravitation, impacting on astronauts. What happens to extremities that are underused, mirrors the effects of general inactivity on aging bones. In a Finnish study involving men who had undergone surgical repair of *rotator cuff tears* of their shoulders, those who had regained function of the injured side, had no uneven increase of osteoporosis in their arms, but those who remained disabled had a remarkable decrease in bone mineral density in the unused arm.[K020]

ABUSING YOUR BODY WITH LAXATIVES

What goes in, must come out....Our population, especially the aged, suffer from an obsessive-compulsive love affair with the function of their bowels. As they eat badly and exercise poorly, they enrich the coffers of those who are in the business of selling bowel hygiene products. A group of South African doctors coined the name *Metabolic Madness* to describe a conglomerate of symptoms occurring in patients who often indulged in more than one aberrant habit, e.g., laxative and/or diuretic abuse, or bulimia: the clinical syndrome produced a myriad of confounding metabolic derangements.[M160]

> **ABUSE OF LAXATIVES, DIURETICS AND EATING DISORDERS**
> **= METABOLIC MADNESS**

Complications of "metabolic madness" are:
- Bone disease (osteomalacia, secondary hyperparathyroidism and osteoporosis)
- Cardiac failure
- Coma
- Confusion
- Convulsions
- *Hypocalcaemia* (low blood levels of calcium)
- *Hypokalaemia* (low blood levels of potassium)
- *Hypokalaemia* and *hypophosphataemia* acting together produced muscle damage
- *Hypomagnesaemia* (low blood levels of magnesium)
- *Hypophosphataemia* (low blood levels of phosphorus)
- Skeletal muscle weakness with or without paralysis or *rhabdomyolysis* (muscle damage)
- Urinary tract infections

After laxative withdrawal:

- **Chloruresis** (excessive elimination of **chloride**—a mineral)
- Edema
- **Hyper-reninaemia** (excessive blood levels of **renin**, a hormone)
- **Kaliuresis** (excessive elimination of *potassium*—a mineral)
- Kidney damage (*juxtaglomerular apparatus hyperplasia* as well as *medullary interstitial cell hyperplasia*—both are abnormalities in the intra-kidney cellular structure)
- Urinary *prostaglandin* (hormones related to inflammation and blood pressure) secretion persistently elevated
- Weight gain, followed by diuresis

COSMETICS, THE UNSUSPECTED OFFENDERS

Mirror, mirror on the wall, Who is the fairest of them all? We want to look beautiful, smell wonderfully, be elegant and groomed. Could our vanity make us good looking, but also ill? Because cosmetics are used in such large amounts, and by most of the population, knowledge of their potential chemical harm to the liver, where bone proteins are formed, is very important.

Cosmetics are substances used for modifications to the aesthetic appearance of the skin, hair, etc., not for the treatment of illness. Cosmetics are an unsuspected, yet dangerous element of chemical exposure in your life, for there are almost no restrictions to their composition. With the exception of color additives and a few prohibited ingredients, a cosmetic manufacturer may use almost any raw material as a cosmetic ingredient and market the product without an approval from FDA [Food and Drug Administration]. The Federal Food, Drug, and Cosmetic Act does require that color additives used in cosmetics must be tested for safety and be listed by the FDA for their intended uses.[U010]

The use of the following ingredients in cosmetics, all of them chemicals that need not be described in the context of this book, is either restricted or prohibited:

- **Bithionol**
- **Chlorofluorocarbon** propellants
- **Chloroform**
- **Halogenated salicyanilides**

- *Hexachlorophene*
- *Mercury compounds*
- *Methyl methacrylate monomer* in cosmetic nail products
- *Methylene chloride*
- *Vinyl chloride*
- *Zirconium complexes* in aerosol cosmetics

In addition, although not required by law or regulation cosmetic and fragrance manufacturers have voluntarily agreed to eliminate or to limit maximum use levels of certain ingredients that have been found to cause skin discoloration, redness and irritation, or other allergic reactions. Used on the skin, or in the mouth, they are easily absorbed through the membranes they touch— the skin (transdermal absorption) being the largest absorptive organ in the body: "Vanishing" creams vanish right into your system!

People are unaware how massive transdermal absorption really is: the only substance NOT absorbed through the skin is water. Interest in drug absorption through the skin was kindled when "prior to 1972, it was known that brain damage occurred in animals with prolonged blood levels of 2 microgram/ml *hexachlorophene* [*Phisohex*, a surgical skin cleanser], and that washing newborn babies with a standard 3% hexachlorophene liquid soap for 3-5 days resulted in significant blood levels of the compound. However, this knowledge was not disseminated widely enough to prevent the tragic deaths of infants after the use of baby powder contaminated with 6.6% hexachlorophene [1]. This incident highlighted the need for increased understanding of drug effects not only from the viewpoint of the skin as a target organ, but also of *percutaneous penetration* [entry via the skin] and resultant blood [and other tissue] levels...."[W051]

PETROLATUM, VASELINE, BABY OR MINERAL OIL

Since cosmetics are often made from white petroleum products, *petrolatum, Vaseline, baby or mineral oil*, etc., they are a constant source of toxic chemicals inviting such health hazards as lipid peroxidation, illness, viral growth, etc. The average person is totally unaware of the connection and the serious risk and sequelae involved. These products cause skin reactions and auto-immune diseases, often sharing symptoms with osteoporosis.[M200]

Recent studies on petroleum derivatives (*mineral hydrocarbon—MHC*) white oils and waxes have shown inflammatory effects in a specific strain of rat (*Fischer 344 - F-344*), but not in other rat strains or dogs. Some of the lesions include *mesenteric lymph node histiocytosis*, *liver granulomas*, and *inflammation of the mitral valve* (only seen with *paraffin waxes*). Human ingestion of MHC can result in noninflammatory *lipogranulomas* (*oil droplets*) in tissues which are regarded as clinically unimportant.[N020]

There are those who would want you to believe petroleum (Vaseline, baby oil) cosmetics are safe, but there is really only one article I have found that tells us so. It seems more like "damage control" than actual science. It is not based on new research, but on *observation*: "White mineral oils have a long history of safe use by humans in orally ingested and topically applied products. A re-evaluation of the use of certain mineral hydrocarbons in the preparation of food items by regulators in the UK, however, has prompted additional safety studies and a critical assessment of the toxicological effects of white mineral oils. As white mineral oils are present in many topically applied drug and non-drug products, it is of interest to review the toxicological effects of mineral oil produced by this route of exposure....On the basis of...[research]...findings and reports on negligible epidermal penetration...[entry through the skin]...of topically applied white mineral oils, there is no evidence of any hazard identified for topical exposure to white mineral oils at any dose in multiple species. This conclusion is supported by the long and uneventful human use of white mineral oils in drug and non-drug topically applied products."[N020] The interesting feature about this *defensive* article is that it was produced in 1996 by The Proctor & Gamble Company!

Despite all the denials, proof of harm to living creatures by these products abounds. In an experiment performed on rats in Sweden in 1995, experimental arthritis could be caused by injecting proteins (*rat type II collagen—RCII*) administered in *Freund's incomplete adjuvant oil* (*FIA*) or with only *FIA*. This is a substance used in virology, the main component of which is mineral oil![M280]

RETINOIC ACID (ACUTANE, RETIN-A)
Many years ago, a synthetic vitamin A was promoted for the treatment of acne. It caused numerous health problems, which also included malig-

nancies. It was eventually withdrawn from the market. But not for long! A pharmaceutical company pays a lot of money to develop and patent a product, and the Almighty Dollar rules. Cosmetic products do not undergo the rigorous evaluations that pharmaceuticals do, despite the fact that the skin is very absorptive, the largest absorptive organ in the body; and what gets put on the skin goes into the body. In fact, cosmetics have practically no controls as to safety.

There is widespread and unwitting use of the dangerous substance Acutane or retinoic acid in the osteoporotic age group, in the form of over the counter anti-wrinkling creams, and a prescription revitalizing cream called Renova, manufactured by Ortho Pharmaceuticals; therefore, it behooves us to talk quite a bit about this health hazard. Under normal circumstances, vitamin A, an essential food component, is converted within the body into two active forms, an *aldehyde* and an *acid* (contains the chemical group COOH) The aldehyde (*retinaldehyde*) is a light-sensitive molecule essential to vision: it converts electromagnetic energy of light into a chemical and eventually into an electrical signal from which the brain processes information. Lack of retinaldehyde causes blindness. Retinoic acid regulates tissues which are actively dividing. The acid (retinoic acid) is necessary for expression of many genes. It is vital for the proper functioning of practically all organs in the adult, and is essential for the developing embryo, in particular the emerging nervous system. While lack of retinoic acid leads to death of both adult and developing organisms, excessive retinoic acid is also catastrophic: accidental exposure of human embryos to retinoic acid, causes severe malformations, especially in *cerebellar* (a part of the nervous system which regulates balance) development....The effects of retinoic acid on the cerebellum resemble that of several genetic disorders, even suggesting the possibility that some genetic diseases may result from a hereditary disturbance in normal retinoic acid levels. The high vulnerability to retinoic acid entering from the outside of the body, reflects the critical dependence of the developing embryo to correct levels of retinoic acid. Dr. Dråger's work focuses on both aspects of vitamin A: on vision, and on the way by which endogenously (internally) synthesized retinoic acid influences formation of the nervous system; this includes the mechanisms through which disturbances in retinoic-acid cause malformations of the brain.[M071]

The reason to go this deeply into the subject, is that people in the menopausal and pre-menopausal ages often resort to anti-wrinkling creams, and in experiments performed in China on rats, the substance used to induce osteoporosis in these animals, was, believe it or not, the substance retinoic acid!

In a Chinese study the researchers were able to damage the ovaries and bones of rats by using the substance *retinoic acid*, the active principle in some *anti-wrinkle creams*!

Some newspaper stories tell the of the unbridled greed that endangers the victims of the many chemical industries. Articles by the Associated Press tell the story:

MANUFACTURER GETS FDA'S OK
TO SELL DRUG AS WRINKLE REDUCER
January 3, 1996

"WASHINGTON — Ortho Pharmaceutical Corp. has won permission to promote its acne drug as a wrinkle reducer.

"Tretinoin, sold under the brand name Retin-A, was approved in 1971 to treat severe acne. But it soon won wide popularity as a potent wrinkle remover — and a federal investigation into whether Ortho illegally marketed *tretinoin* for wrinkles.

"Although doctors can prescribe drugs for any purpose, companies cannot promote them without Food and Drug Administration approval.

"Ortho insisted it never did that, but last January paid a $7.5 million fine for shredding marketing documents sought in the probe.

"On Friday, the FDA said Ortho had proved that tretinoin does reduce fine wrinkles and brown spots, giving the company permission to sell a special cream version under the brand name Renova.

"Renova is different from Retin-A only because its more soothing cream formula is better suited for aging skin, Ortho said. It will be available next month.

"Studies indicate that after 24 weeks of using Renova, 30 percent of people had moderate improvement, 35 percent had minimal improvement and 35 percent saw no change.

"Renova does not eliminate wrinkles, reverse aging or repair the sun-damaged skin that leads to cancer, the FDA warned. The wrinkles gradually became more noticeable when patients stopped using the cream — but using Renova for more than a year has not been proved safe, the agency said."

STUDY: DRUG MAY PREVENT SKIN FROM WRINKLING IN SUNLIGHT

By MALCOLM RITTER AP Science Writer

Jan. 25, 1996

"NEW YORK (AP) - A drug spread on the skin to reduce wrinkles might also be able to prevent the effects of years of exposure to the sun, suggests a study released today.

"When applied to the skin of volunteers before they got a dose of ultraviolet light, the drug sharply reduced the production of skin enzymes that might promote wrinkling.

"The drug, tretinoin (pronounced treh-tin-OH-in), is the active ingredient in Renova, a prescription cream recently approved by the federal government for reducing fine wrinkles, brown spots and roughness of facial skin from chronic sun exposure.

"It's also the active ingredient in Retin-A, a prescription acne drug many dermatologists use to treat wrinkles. Retin-A and Renova are marketed by Ortho Pharmaceutical Corp.

"The research was funded by Ortho, a division of Johnson & Johnson, the Wall Street Journal reported today. That is not mentioned in the Nature report, but Nature editor Philip Campbell told the newspaper that the journal does not require scientists to disclose funding sources.

"The report was rigorously reviewed, and its findings should stand on their own," Campbell is quoted as saying.

"Dr. John Epstein, clinical professor of dermatology at the University of California at San Francisco, noted that it hasn't yet been shown whether tretinoin or a second drug used in the study actually prevent wrinkling.

"And Dr. David Bickers, chairman of the dermatology department at the Columbia University College of Physicians and Surgeons, cautioned that extrapolating from the short-term experiment to the long-term effects of sun exposure is "fraught with hazard."

"The other drug in the study, a steroid used in skin creams to reduce inflammation, worked about as well as tretinoin.

"Scientists studied the effect of ultraviolet B light, or UVB, the part of sunshine most effective in causing wrinkling, on volunteers' buttocks.

"Sun-induced wrinkling is thought to result from damage to the skin's collagen and elastin, which provide strength and elasticity. These substances can be damaged by certain enzymes created by skin cells.

"The new work showed that small doses of UVB stimulate production of the damaging enzymes. The researchers theorized that over decades, repeated assaults on the collagen and elastin by the enzymes could cause premature wrinkling.

"They also found that if tretinoin or the steroid was applied to the skin before the UVB dose was given, the amounts of enzymes produced after UVB exposure were sharply reduced. Tretinoin was also shown to suppress a genetic switch that turns on enzyme production.

"Epstein said it's not known whether the kind of damage caused by the enzymes actually leads to wrinkling.

"Dr. Sheldon Pinnell, chief of dermatology at Duke University, said recent studies suggest that ultraviolet light other than UVB may also contribute to wrinkling. The effect of tretinoin on that is not known, he said.

"Currently, to lower the risk of premature wrinkling from sun exposure, dermatologists recommend sunscreens, long sleeves, broad-brimmed hats and avoiding the midday sun.

"The study also found that a UVB dose equal to only two or three minutes of summer sunshine on unprotected skin can turn on production of the enzymes, dermatologist Dr. Barbara Gilchrest said.

"That suggests that just the "incidental exposures every single person gets while walking around" are enough to do harm, said Gilchrest, a professor at the Boston University School of Medicine.

"And if a person spends all day in the sun, even the best sunscreen could not keep out such a tiny dose of UVB, she said.

"Last April, Ortho agreed to pay a $5 million fine and $2.5 million in legal costs after admitting that its executives ordered workers to shred documents, effectively thwarting a federal investigation into whether it was illegally marketing Retin-A acne cream as a wrinkle remover.

"Under the plea bargain, Ortho could not be prosecuted for how it marketed the prescription drug.

"The agency began investigating Ortho following widespread publicity in 1988 - and in some cases, buying hysteria - that resulted when a small study said the drug appeared to reduce signs of aging."

RUBBING ALCOHOL

Does the alcohol soaked pad your lab personnel uses dissolve more than common skin oils? Our culture has a religious belief in "cleanliness" according to the tenets of the medical *Establishment*. Millions of times every day, before piercing the skin with a hypodermic needle, doctors, nurses and technicians engage in a ritual "purification" of the exposed skin with some kind of swabbing device and "denatured" alcohol, which we also call rubbing alcohol. Worse than that minor application, the elderly rub their aching legs or arms with this "rubbing" alcohol? Wait till you read the next few lines and you will cringe as I do when you watch this practice.

Rubbing alcohol can not be drunk, because it contains the substance *isopropyl* to "denature" it: that is why it is not burdened by high alcohol taxes. It is uncertain to me whether *rubbing alcohol* is better classified as a cosmetic or a drug, but, at any rate, the "denaturing" additive isopropyl is a highly toxic substance, and this toxicity, at least in rat studies, increases with the age of the living being treated, and "...[liver poison]-induced changes in *GSH* [an important antioxidant] were observed in *allyl* [*isopropyl*, the additive in rubbing alcohol] alcohol-treated old rats...."[R070] Since it affects the liver where proteins must be synthesized for proper bone formation, it may interfere with osseous building and repair in people who use a lot of rubbing alcohol. This sensitivity is quite specific, and worse than for other chemicals. Nervous system damage can also occur.

ANTIFREEZE

Even if you do not work in a garage, you are constantly exposed to *antifreeze*. The chemical family it belongs to is the *glycol* family, you usually see it featured under the name *poly-ethylene-glycol*, or *PEG*. It is an additive to many cosmetic products, and part of the so called *inert* or inactive ingredients of many medications, pills, tablets, etc. It even is included in many frozen products, such as ice cream.

"*Ethylene glycol* (*EG*) is the most representative of the glycols. It is a compound used as painting and plastic solvent, as antifreeze, and in dyes and synthetic fibers. It may also appear as a wine pollutant. Due to these various uses and conditions, EG can produce intoxication in men and animals...The pathologic effects are due to its metabolism resulting in the formation of *oxalic* and *glycolic* acids which are eliminated through the kidney causing renal failure. The toxic effects on the nervous system are not well known. In some circumstances, convulsions may occur. The changes in *neurons* [nerve cells] consist of neuronal degeneration."[C010][emphasis added]. Oxalic acids are known to bind and remove much calcium from the body.

THE TOXIC METAL LEAD IN HAIR CARE PRODUCTS

This product is a serious health hazard. The FDA tries to make light of it, but the opinions offered fail to explain how the results were arrived at:

"Lead acetate is used as a color additive in "progressive" hair dye products. These products are applied over a period of time to achieve a gradual coloring effect. In order to be approved for this use, a color additive petition was required to establish safety.

"The safety data submitted in support of this petition included results from trials on humans using the products. In the trials, people using the product under controlled conditions were monitored for the amount of lead in their bloodstream. No significant increase in blood levels of lead was seen in the trial subjects, and the lead was not shown to be absorbed into the body through such use. [The article does not state what criteria were used, who sponsored the study, and for how long the individuals were evaluated. The author's experience shows different results, which are not that reassuring].

"This data allowed FDA to determine that safe conditions of use could be established and a color additive regulation allowing the use of lead acetate in hair dyes was established. The regulation requires that specific labeling instructions appear on the product labels. These include cautions to use the product externally, not to use on cut or abraded skin, and to wash hands thoroughly after use. Consumers are advised to follow carefully all label directions.

"A new study published in the Journal of the American Pharmaceutical Association, raises the possibility of danger to children. The agency has not yet evaluated the new study, but will review it carefully to determine if the information warrants further attention or action. The data in hand, however, indicates that lead acetate containing hair dye products can be used safely. It is important, however, that consumers carefully follow the directions on the package and keep the products away from children.

"Consumers can determine if lead acetate is used in a particular hair dye product by reviewing the product ingredient declaration appearing on the label of the cosmetic in package form."[U010]

INSULTING YOUR BODY:
MEDICINES, DRUGS, AND OSTEOPOROSIS

DRUGS IN GENERAL

In 1995, a group of internists from Danbury, Connecticut, tells us that "Bone disease and the coincident risk of fracture and disability are well-documented with use of...glucocorticoids, thyroxine, ethanol, tobacco, anticonvulsants, neuroleptics, and chemotherapeutic agents. Physician awareness of these risks highlights the need for close monitoring of dosages and drug interactions and allows for intervention with nutritional support, antiresorptive agents, and proformation agents."[W080]

Many commercial forms of drugs contain PEG, titanium dioxide, and a host of other fillers and binders, which may cause calcium loss.

ASPIRIN IS PROBABLY GOOD FOR YOUR BONES, NSAIDS MAY ALSO BE

In a world where it is an almost universal practice to indulge in aspirin at the slightest provocation, it is important to know whether this can harm our bones. The news are actually good, for a change! In a study to evaluate the effect of *aspirin* on the bone masses of 12 growing dogs (who were first tortured by using a unilateral hind limb cast-fixation), and then were killed after 4 weeks, bone mineral content of the immobilized bone was studied. Aspirin treatment was associated with a 65 percent reduction in bone PGE, and a 13 percent bone mass sparing effect.[W030]

In the last decade, other pain killers, the NSAIDS have become quite popular. These also seem not to represent a problem as far as bone quality goes, at least to our present knowledge."...aspirin or nonsteroidal anti-inflammatory drug (NSAIDs) may inhibit bone loss and preserve bone mineral density (BMD) in vitro and in animal models....Regular use of aspirin or NSAIDs may have a modest beneficial effect on BMD in post-menopausal women. This effect persists after adjustment for obesity and the presence of osteoarthritis. However, among women who take aspirin or NSAIDs regularly, there is no clinically significant protective effect on the subsequent risk of fractures."[B050]

BLOOD PRESSURE MEDICATIONS

This group of medicines deserves extra attention because of the big media pressure that accompanies the issue. Does your blood pressure medication cause you to be unhealthy and break bones? Blood pressure is an important subject indirectly affecting the risk factors for fracture, because blood pressure medication can cause dizziness and falls, and high blood pressure is more often, than not, an indication of low calcium in blood. Some of the most obtuse arguments are used to induce "High Blood Pressure Phobia" in the elderly. Why? Because sales of blood pressure medications are a lucrative, steady business, and hapless older citizens (the bulk of the blood pressure market) are easy prey to manipulated information.

Just as the oil pressure in your car has to build up to satisfy the mechanical and lubrication demands, the blood pressure in the body had to fluctuate depending on the level of activity. An Olympic athlete has to be able to rev it up almost twofold to tolerate the effort of winning a race and bringing enough oxygen to his muscles.

The American media, representing the vested interests of the drug and medical industries, have millions of people toady to their lies and half truths. In pharmacies and grocery stores, at home and abroad, middle aged and older people spend valuable time in a bizarre ritual worthy of a description suiting the middle age quality of their pursuit: they wrap a broad band around their upper arm or insert their fingers in a quaint hood, and pump air into it until it torments their flesh, only to let the air go and then become transfixed watching the symbols on a bright display, often keeping records of such "divination" in some sacred book. They are measuring the pressure inside their arteries at all times of the day and at all levels of activity, expecting it to be "normal" (whatever that might mean), disappointed if it is otherwise. The values of "under 140/90" they are seeking, which they believe essential to well being, usually refer to "basal" readings (before getting out of bed, eating, drinking, talking or moving). That is how they were originally ascertained, many decades ago, only the meaning has been lost or adulterated with the passage of time.

Under physiologic conditions, blood pressure will rise in response to deficiency of oxygen, increased demand, upright position, caffeine, talking, excitement, weight gain, and rise it must to deliver enough oxygen. Just as women used to squeeze blood flow and breath out of their system to achieve a desired tiny waist thanks to unhealthy corsets, elderly people are running around zombified, with too little oxygen in their brains, but with "trophy" blood pressure numbers of a teenager, thanks to unwholesome drugs.

When researchers consider the patient's interest rather than the stock market performance of the companies that make the drugs, wonderful knowledge may surface. An excellent study of sensible guidelines in the treatment of hypertension in the elderly was done in Japan in 1995.[0030]

The doctors proposed important steps. They recommended lifestyle changes rather than drugs, and advised that "Antihypertensive therapy should be limited to patients in whom the merit of the treatment [was] obvious." The blood pressures considered in this study were in line with what I had learned in medical school, in the very early 60s:

> means "greater than"   < means "lesser than"

They considered blood pressure to be

■ "elevated"   Systolic BP is > 160..., diastolic BP is > 90...approximately by 10...

■ "normal"   Systolic BP < age + 100...for those aged 70 years and older.

They recommended that patients with mild hypertension (140-160/ 90-95 mmHg) associated with cardiovascular disease should be considered for antihypertensive drug therapy...

The goal of therapy for blood pressure? "The goal BP in elderly patients is higher than that in younger patients (BP reduction of 10-20 mmHg for systolic BP and 5-10 mmHg for diastolic BP). In general, 140-160/< 90 mmHg is recommended as the goal. However, lowering the BP below 150/85 should be done with caution...

"Rate of Lowering BP: Start with half the usual dose, observe at the same dose for at least four weeks, and reach the target BP over two months. Increasing the dose of antihypertensive drugs should be done very slowly."

Lifestyle modification recommended by the Japanese study:

- Calcium and magnesium by diet or supplementation
- Healthier diet
- Intake of fish (frequent)*
- Moderation of alcohol intake
- Potassium supplementation, with caution in patients with renal insufficiency
- Reduce saturated fatty acids
- Reduction of sodium intake (less than 10 g/salt a day). This is 2 teaspoonfuls, still a sizable amount! (only sea salt or other uncontaminated salt, please!)*
- Regular physical activity
- Smoking cessation
- Weight reduction (little or no commercially packaged and preserved foods, please)*

                                          * Commentaries are my own

You will notice, as I do, that they are really cautious in recommending any pharmacologic treatment: The Japanese researchers involved in this study tell it like it is; they are not as pressured as American researchers are to sell lethal potions for dirty money. So, their decisions are vastly different than what we see in the US, which can not be explained away by suggesting that Americans are biologically different from Japanese.

They emphasize that in aged individuals there are contraindications to many drugs:

Relative Contraindications

- **Alpha 1-blockers** are relatively contraindicated in elderly patients with hypertension
- **Beta-blockers** are relatively contraindicated in elderly patients with hypertension
- **Centrally acting agents** such as **reserpine**, **methyldopa** and **clonidine** are also relatively contraindicated

Absolute contraindications

Beta-blockers are contraindicated in patients with
- Arteriosclerosis obliterans
- Chronic obstructive pulmonary disease
- Congestive heart failure
- Diabetes mellitus (or glucose intolerance)
- Slow heart rate (***bradycardia***)

These conditions are often present in elderly subjects.

ORTHOSTATIC HYPOTENSION: A SPECIAL RISK IN OSTEOPOROTIC PATIENTS

The body is endowed with several "stabilizing sensors" that are part of a system of checks and balances for the numbers of the blood pressure. One of them is the pressure receptor (***baroreceptor***). It senses and adjusts the blood pressure according to the body's position: whether the body is lying down, or is upright. A higher pressure often protects the elderly from accidents: the pressure is supposed to rise when you are standing upright, because if it does not, the brain does not get enough oxygen and blood flow. Elderly people often have a faulty pressure receptor to measure increases and decreases due to postural changes (baroreceptor reflex), which poses additional problems to those suffering from osteoporosis: they are susceptible to a drop in blood pressure upon standing up suddenly (***alpha 1-blocker-induced orthostatic hypotension***) which causes dizzy spells. Orthostatic [related to upright posture] hypotension may cause falls and bone fractures in the elderly.

FLUID PILLS - LASIX -

People in the US, generally have poor diets, overloaded with contaminated salt, undersupplied in vitamin B6. For whatever reason, whether it may be fluid retention due to food, beta-blockers or other reasons, patients frequently reach for fluid pills. In a study of male patients who had hip fractures, in a large Australian (Melbourne) nursing home, vitamin D deficiency and hyperparathyroidism were frequent findings. Vitamin D deficiency was surprisingly frequent despite a climate in which vitamin D levels are thought to be ample. It was a provoking factor for increased risk of parathyroid problems. However, daily *furosemide* (*Lasix*) intake was an even more important factor for stressing the parathyroid hormone—PTH—in this population.[S210] Furosemide (Lasix) reduces the concentration of calcium in the cells.[R130]

In a more general evaluation of the relationship between drugs prescribed to 280 women with hip fractures (mean age 83 years) compared with those prescribed for 145 women controls (mean age 81 years), more fracture patients were taking fluid pills, and more of these fluid pills were either *loop or potassium sparing diuretics* in combination with another diuretic. More of the controls were on *nonsteroidal anti-inflammatory drugs* (*NSAIDS*). No significant differences were found for the heart medicines *digoxin*, *digitalis*, or *lanoxin*, blood pressure drugs, and those taking no drugs. In summary, hip fracture patients were slightly more likely to be taking diuretics and somewhat less likely to be taking NSAIDs than controls but there were no differences with respect to other drugs.[T010]

GLUCOCORTICOIDS , CORTICOSTEROIDS (CORTISONE, PREDNISONE)

It has often been said that when doctors don't know what a condition is, or how to treat it, they prescribe some cortisone derivative for good measure. This can be an extremely risky practice. *Glucocorticoids* such as *cortisone*, *prednisone*, etc., decrease calcium absorption, and increase fracture risk. In a recent study, oral calcium supplements plus 1,25-dihydroxyvitamin D decreased gluco-corticoid-associated bone loss. On the basis of these observations and other studies, oral calcium supplements should be used in all patients who are receiving these products. The specific disease for which the therapy is used (*rheumatoid arthritis*, *inflammatory bowel disease*, *asthma*) can be a determining factor in the occurrence and degree of bone loss.

Cortisone and cortisone-like substances can be wonderful medicines in the hands of conscientious, skilled physician, but can be a tool for man made disaster in other cases. These medicines are frequently used for osteoarthritis, rheumatoid arthritis,[H040] skin condition, asthma, allergies, etc. They are administered by mouth, injectable, and also creams. An often unsuspected source of whole body cortisone absorption, is the administration of inhaled corticosteroids.

How safe are the corticosteroids that are in nasal and bronchial sprays? It is quite common for asthmatics and persons suffering from allergies, to use inhalers which contain corticosteroids, *beclomethasone* and others. The hapless patients are usually convinced that such treatments are quite safe, and free of the common side effects of corticosteroids, but it is not so, not even at recommended doses. Whatever you inhale also goes to your general system. *Inhaled corticosteroids* have been widely used in asthma or allergic rhinitis for longer and longer periods. We now recognize that this therapy has serious consequences: adrenal failure, osteoporosis, growth retardation. The clinical consequences of long-term inhaled corticosteroids are not usually as intense as oral corticosteroids, but do present themselves.[L020] "...adrenal androgen levels in postmenopausal women are suppressed by short term high dose inhaled corticosteroids [beclomethasone dipropionate]. Such an effect, if sustained, may be a causative factor for long term bone loss."[S141]

Oral, injected or inhaled, even topically administered on mucous membranes and skin, these drugs may cause

■ Clinical features of *Cushing syndrome*
■ Complete suppression of endogenous (internally produced) adrenocorticotrophic hormone (*ACTH*) adrenal function (the hormonal) stimulation of natural cortisone
■ Osteoporosis
■ Primary testicular failure in the male

TRANQUILIZERS

In these days of foam padding and electronic wonders, we try to avoid even the slightest stress. We have lost our ability to cope and consider the most minor problem a terrible nuisance. We are the generation that does not reach to God, but to the shelf in the medicine cabinet. Northern Ireland, a country in turmoil, was the setting of an evaluation of the consequences of the use of sedatives and tranquilizers on osteoporotic fractures, probably due to an increase in falls. In a study in Belfast, long-acting sedatives did not appear to increase the risk of osteoporotic fractures, but *phenothiazine's* [a tranquilizer family] role in hip fracture could not be ruled out.[T010]

ANTACIDS
THE SOUR TRUTH ABOUT MEDICINES TO CONTROL ACID INDIGESTION

What are acid controllers? What is acid?

A reagent paper called *lithmus paper*, can be used to classify substances according to the changes in color they induce on this method, you detect *acid* (such as battery or stomach acid) and *alkaline* (such as baking soda) substances. Antacids are alkaline remedies for the stomach, neutralizers of acids, used for the fast relief of acid indigestion, heartburn, sour stomach and the upset stomach associated with these symptoms. They work by neutralizing excess stomach acid.

Antacids can be classified by whether they act directly or indirectly on the acid:
- *Direct antacids* unite directly with free acid in the stomach. This type of antacid includes, ammonium carbonate, potassium bicarbonate, lime water, magnesia and chalk
- *Remote antacids* act by being changed into *carbonates*. Carbonates increase the alkalinity of the blood
- There are drugs that act as both direct and remote antacids. Those include bicarbonates of sodium, potassium, magnesium and lithium

CALCIUM CARBONATE CONTAINING ANTACIDS
Calcium carbonate from antacid use and abuse may cause problems. Carbonates cause damage your health by contributing large amounts of unabsorbable calcium which induces an excess rebound acid secretion.

Among the lies, more lies, and half truths, dished up daily to the American public, is the recommendation to take TUMS as a calcium supplement. TUMS is highly un-bioavailable, it contains calcium carbonate which may be laboratory pure but is only poorly absorbable, especially after age 40. According to classic ways of thinking, it was believed that calcium carbonate requires much more stomach acid than most people can produce, to be properly digested. Even in South Africa they let the people know there may be problems through a package insert. [U101]

SIDE-EFFECTS AND SPECIAL PRECAUTIONS:

Enough calcium may be absorbed to cause systemic and renal effects in certain cases. The intake of calcium carbonate, like that of other calcium salts, may cause:

- Alkalosis
- Calcium salts may enhance the cardiac effects of digitalis glycosides
- Constipation
- Hypercalcaemia
- Nephrocalcinosis during chronic usage

KNOWN SYMPTOMS OF OVERDOSAGE AND PARTICULARS OF ITS TREATMENT:

Hypercalcaemia and alkalosis which may occur with excessive doses responds to withdrawal of the tablets.

From the internet we learn more about popular assumptions about calcium therapy. The site starts by reminding us that we are considered to be a nation of sheep, and that that is the reason why "our newspapers do the bidding of the large corporations:"

"TUMS TAPPED AS SAFE CALCIUM SUPPLEMENT"
(http://biz.yahoo.com/prnews/97/02/07/sbh_y0022_1.html)
SmithKline Beecham Consumer Healthcare

STUDY SAYS CONSUMERS CAN COUNT ON ITS PURITY

"PITTSBURGH, Feb. 7 /PRNewswire/ — TUMS, the calcium supplement and antacid, is a safe and pure form of calcium that consumers can use with confidence.

"TUMS's safety was recently reestablished by a study conducted by the University of California at Santa Cruz Department of Toxicology. The results of this testing proved that TUMS contains an extremely pure form of calcium.

"TUMS, which has been marketed in the United States for more than 60 years, contains an effective and natural form of calcium, and has also long complied with the United States federal guidelines for purity of ingredients set by the U.S. Pharmacopoeia. In addition, TUMS is the first calcium supplement product to be recommended by the National Osteoporosis Foundation.

"Calcium is an essential nutrient that plays a pivotal role during pregnancy, as well as throughout the lifetime of both men and women, by helping keep muscles, nerves and bones healthy. Calcium is also vital in the prevention and treatment of osteoporosis, a bone shattering disease that affects over 28 million Americans a year. Currently, less than half of all women get an adequate amount of daily calcium. According to the National Institutes of Health, the adult recommended daily allowance is 1,000 mgr. per day; for post-menopausal and pregnant women, the recommended level is 1,500 mgr. per day. For millions of Americans who do not consume enough calcium through diet, calcium supplements are essential to making up the difference.

"TUMS is manufactured and marketed by SmithKline Beecham Consumer Healthcare, and has been used safely in several major government and independent clinical trials researching calcium's medicinal benefits with post-menopausal women, pregnant women and children.

Of course, none of that information can be supported by honest data, but the constant pounding of TV advertising is a powerful force to be reckoned with.

ACID BLOCKERS: CIMETIDINE, TAGAMET AND OTHERS

If an alien would watch our TV advertisement, he could not help but think that we spend most of our lives devising ways to indulge in pepperoni, anchovies and green peppers without making "our heart burn" (heartburn), as a little boy in a popular ad for an acid blocker, likes to say. Estrogen is normally broken down in the body by a chemical process called *estradiol 2- hydroxylation*. Since Tagamet (*cimetidine*) inhibits this process, chronic Tagamet (*cimetidine*) use in males is associated with side effects such as enlarged breasts due to accumulation of unprocessed estrogen. This accumulation also occurs in women, but the elevation of estrogen does not result in increases of bone and calcium metabolism.[M170]

ALUMINUM CONTAINING ANTACIDS

Aluminum in the form of *antacid* medication, when taken in excess, may significantly increase urinary calcium loss. Aluminum antacids may mummify your brain with aluminum.[B182]

MEDICAL PROCEDURES

ORGAN TRANSPLANTATION

Ours is the first generation that has been programmed to undergo periodic fix-ups with spare body parts. Kidneys, hearts and livers are passed around like rebuilt alternators and repainted front ends. An often unrecognized cause for severe osteoporosis is having received an organ transplant. Those patients are at special risk for the development of osteoporosis, due to the nature of their illness, the nature of anti-rejection treatment, and other additional medical problems and treatments. "Osteoporosis following allogenic [foreign] organ transplantation represents an increasingly common medical and socioeconomic problem."[H110]

"The occurrence of osteoporosis is independent of the particular organ transplanted and has been frequently observed after heart, liver, kidney and bone marrow transplantation....28 to 74% of all *allograft* [foreign tissue] recipients have osteoporotic bone mineral density levels...and 17 to 65% have bone fracture after transplantation. These events are equally common in men and women."[U141]

"The observed high frequency of osteoporosis immediately after transplantation is caused by a particularly rapid loss of bone mineral density within the first few months."[U141] "Several risk factors contribute to this early loss of bone mass:...

■ Corticosteroid therapy (catabolic effects on bone)

■ Pretransplant bone disease

■ Immobilisation [sic] due to surgery

■ Immunosuppression with *cyclosporin* or *tacrolimus* [anti-tissue-rejection-drugs]

■ Hypogonadism [low function of sexual glands] in bone marrow
transplant recipients

■ Hyperparathyroidism in kidney transplant recipients

Therefore, it is important to start prophylaxis or treatment as soon as possible post-transplant- ation."[U141]

RADIATION

Commonly used as X-Rays, but in larger doses as cancer therapy, the invisible rays of death can work havoc on the bones.

A painful spinal syndrome, not unlike the osteoporosis of menopause, develops in people exposed to radiation. This was the finding in workers who took care of the demolition and clean-up of the Chernobyl power plant, and in workers at that location in earlier years.[R110] When the BMD was evaluated and compared between:

■ 1) Those who worked at the power plant in 1986 (55%)

■ 2) Those who worked there in 1987-1989

■ 3) Unexposed controls

They found that:
■ Bone mineral density in the lumbar vertebrae was significantly
lower in group 1 as compared to group 2 and lower in both groups
vs. unexposed controls

■ More than 5% osseous mineral loss was revealed in 73% of group 1
and in 43% of group 2

■ Analysis of spinal X-Rays in 45 workers showed a high incidence of
low grade osteoporosis without compression fractures of vertebral
bodies

■ Osteopenia or bone loss signs were found in 87% of group 1 examinees complaining of pain in the spine and in 73% of group 2 examinees

■ Signs of *osteochondrosis* and *spondylosis* were detected in 40% of
group 1 and in 47% of group 2 subjects

Hence, there was a higher incidence of osteopenia in the workers exposed to the higher levels of radiation. The higher detection rate in subjects exposed to higher radiation indicates a certain contribution of radiation factor to the development of the osteopenia syndrome in the Chernobyl "clean-up" workers.[R110]

WHAT IS QUALITY OF LIFE? YOUNG AT HEART AND YOUNG AT BONE

A very popular song tells us that "...this is the best part, you have a head start if you are among the very young at heart...." We all search for quality time and quality life, which is often hard to define, but we all have a feeling when life is and is not worth living. Nobody particularly enjoys being crippled or disabled, but the worst conditions of all are probably depression, pain and loneliness.

"...for about 10 years researchers have been oriented towards a working definition [of quality of life] identifying four fundamental dimensions:" [T030]

- cognitive conditions
- emotional conditions and social relations
- functional status
- physical symptoms

PAIN

The main assault on quality of life is pain. We should always remember that the only pain that is easy to take is the pain of others.

> THE ONLY PAIN THAT IS EASY TO TAKE IS THE PAIN OF OTHERS

FROM UNDERESTIMATION TO UNDERTREATMENT

Because "detection of the quality of life is a complex operation[,] physicians and nurses tend to underestimate the functional status and some physical symptoms (such as pain and dyspnea [shortness of breath] and to overestimate the degree of psychological discomfort (i.e., anxiety, depression and distress)....The logical consequence of an underevaluation is an undertreatment."[T030] More than half (52%) of people with pain are not given analgesic therapy according to the guidelines of the World Health Organization, because doctors who properly medicate pain patients are often delicensed by the incompetent members of state boards, and because the treatment is based more on the doctor's idea of what is going on, than by adequately investigating the patient's condition.

Although cancer pains may occasionally be properly attended to by the medical *Establishment*, all other pains are looked upon as a potential psychosomatic complaint, or the patient's request for proper analgesic prescriptions is often answered by an insult. Heartless, incompetent doctors and medical personnel engage in judgment to accuse them of being addicts. The patient has a greater chance of being ignored as to his or her pain, if the patient fits the following criteria:

■ being 70 years of age or older
■ being female
■ being treated where there are mostly ethnic minorities (Blacks and Hispanics)
■ remaining functional and active

"...the greater the cultural distance between two subjects, the greater the probability of reaching an erroneous judgment about what the other is feeling."[T030]

IS LOW BACK PAIN A RELIABLE INDICATOR OF THE LEVEL OF OSTEOPOROSIS?

We often think that we need some external evidence to believe somebody is in pain. Maybe we would tend to think that the greater the hunch on the back, the greater the patient's pain. Nothing could be further from the truth: Japanese studies showed that low back pain (*lumbago*), was not directly associated with fractures, but that fractures were distinctly associated with a markedly decreased bone mineral density, and that a threshold value for BMD, at which bone would easily break, could be determined. This value could be used to predict future fracture risk.[M020]

DEFORMITIES

As far as developing **deformities**,[D160] a study of women from 30 European centers revealed that these were affected by several factors [emphasis added]:

- Women who started their periods (**menarche**) late, age greater or equal to 16 years, had an increased risk of vertebral deformity.
- Increased menopausal age (greater than 52.5 years) was associated with a reduced risk of deformity.
- Use of the oral contraceptive pill was also protective, associated with a 25% reduction in risk of deformity, though the effect may be a result of the higher-dosage estrogen pills used in the past. There was a smaller protective effect associated with one or more years use of hormone replacement therapy.
- There was no apparent effect of parity or breast-feeding on the risk of deformity.
- Estrogen status is an important determinant of vertebral deformity.

KYPHOSIS

Are "hunch-backed" individuals usually in pain? What is the association among degree of kyphosis (forward curvature of the thoracic spine), the level of spinal osteoporosis (height loss and vertebral fractures), and chronic back pain and disability in older women?

"Older women with greater degrees of kyphosis are likely to have other manifestations of spinal osteoporosis, such as height loss, and thoracic fractures, and to suffer chronic upper and middle back pain." In a study including more than 6,000 women in Minneapolis, "...a 15 degree increase in kyphosis was associated with losing more than 4 cm [1 1/2 inches] of height...and having a vertebral fracture....Kyphosis was more strongly related to thoracic fractures than to lumbar fractures, and kyphosis was most prominent in women with multiple thoracic wedge fractures. Kyphosis was also associated with upper back pain...and middle back pain,...but it was not related to lower back pain....Women with greater degrees of kyphosis were only slightly more likely to report back-related disability...and poorer health status...."[E030]

HOW DOES KYPHOSIS AFFECT QUALITY OF LIFE: DID THE HUNCH-BACK OF NOTRE DAME GET THE PROPER MEDICATIONS?

A British study investigated the pain and disability experienced by 85 post-menopausal Caucasian women (average age 64), afflicted with spinal osteoporosis, exhibiting kyphosis and vertebral deformities.[R140] Their symptoms were related to the following variables:

■ Degree of kyphosis

■ Number of vertebral deformities

■ Severity of vertebral deformities

Persistent back pain was experienced by over 60% of the patients, mainly in both the lumbar and the thoracic spine. The severity of thoracic back pain was significantly related to the degree of their:

■ Kyphosis

■ Number of collapsed *thoracic* (trunk) vertebrae between *T4-T8*

■ Number of collapsed vertebrae in general

■ Summed score of the severity of collapse for all vertebrae

The women's secondary symptoms deriving from these problems were:

■ Difficulty obtaining suitable clothes was found in 42%

■ Disturbed sleep in 60% (Severity of osteoporosis was linked to seriousness of sleep disturbance.)

■ Moderate difficulties with functional activities in 47%

■ Severe difficulties with functional activities in 10%

PROBLEMS WITH DAILY ACTIVITIES

Patients with osteoporosis often have problems with daily activities such as:[L090]

■ Attending social events

■ Gardening

■ Preparing meals

■ Taking a shower

■ Visiting friends

■ Walking stairs

In addition, pain and disability may influence mood and lead to depression.

"The morbidity [illness] of osteoporosis is caused by fractures. Vertebral fractures lead to pain and disability and a decrease in quality of life."[L100] Questionnaires in this field usually consist of questions and visual analogues about such quality of life parameters as:

activities of daily living	leisure	pain and discomfort
general health perception	mobility	social activities
jobs around the house	mood	

FRACTURES

Broken bones in older people have become a world-wide epidemic. Fractures in general, occur in similar percentages among aged men and women, but because women live longer, the vast majority of osteoporotic fractures occur in elderly women: vertebral compression fractures, *Colles* fractures at the wrist, and hip fracture, and to a lesser extent fractures at other sites. "The reasons for this relate in part to the lower bone density of women at the time of maturity (peak bone density), and the accelerated bone loss that occurs after the menopause. Women live significantly longer than men, so that the prevalence of osteoporosis amongst elderly women is six-fold that of men. The age- and sex-specific incidence of osteoporotic fracture is rising in many countries, and if the current trends in the United Kingdom continue, then the number of hip fractures each year will more than double over the next 20 years."[K011]

One very puzzling finding is that "There is a marked *geographic distribution* in the incidence of hip fracture, and probably of other osteoporotic fractures. Indeed, the difference in incidence between communities is greater than the difference in incidence between sexes within communities. This suggests that the importance of gonadal [sex gland] insufficiency in women has been over-emphasized and that other factors, probably relating to life-style factors affecting peak bone density, account for ecological differences in incidence between communities and secular trends within communities."[K011]

WHO IS MORE PRONE TO FRACTURES DUE TO OSTEOPOROSIS?

Weak bone leads to fractures. Women experience more fractures than men, and whites have more fractures than blacks. When an injury occurs, what actually determines the likelihood of a break?

It is a question of structural quality, better addressed by the science of engineering, than medicine:

- Bone strength
- Intensity, direction, and duration of the applied force
- Scattering and redistribution (dissipation) of that force by soft tissue absorption
- Scattering and redistribution (dissipation) of that force by muscle contraction

Age increases the frequency of injuries. Energy dissipation diminishes with advancing age, as the muscle mass wanes. Reduction in bone mass and strength is the most important reason for the increased frequency of bone fractures in postmenopausal women and in the elderly. Many older people lack flexibility, so when they fall, they absorb a much greater shock than if they could cushion themselves effectively or right themselves quickly. As a result, hip fractures increase with age, mirroring the loss of agility that occurs for many elderly people..

Bone biopsies from some individuals with primary osteoporosis show high bone turnover rates; biopsies from others show low or intermediate rates of turnover.

WHICH FRACTURES OCCUR IN WHOM, AND WHEN?

Since each bone is built from different quantities of either trabecular or cortical bone, or a combination thereof, fractures occur at various body sites, according to which type of bone loss is involved. Accelerated loss of trabecular bone occurs most frequently in vertebrae of women aged 55 to 75. Slow loss of both cortical and trabecular mass occurring most frequently in older men and women, is linked to hip fractures.

Vertebral compression fractures occur more frequently in women than in men, and typically affect the *thoracic* (trunk) and *lumbar* (low back) vertebrae *T8-L3*. These fractures may develop during routine activities: bending, lifting, or rising from a chair or bed. The immediate symptom usually is severe, localized back pain, which lasts for several months. Some experience persistent pain due to altered spinal structure and movement. Some vertebral fractures do not cause pain.

Another problem, the loss of height of vertebrae (*vertebral compression*) may be gradual, without noticeable symptoms, and detected only upon radiographic examination. Loss of body height and/or *kyphosis* (hunchback, curving from back to front) may be the only signs of multiple vertebral fractures.

Skeletal problems also result in the *shortening of the thorax*, these may be accompanied by symptoms such as abdominal discomfort, debility, and, rarely, pulmonary dysfunction. Digestive symptoms such as getting full easily, bloating, and constipation may ensue.

HIP FRACTURES

These are very frequent in older and predominantly female patients. A woman's risk of hip fracture alone is equal to the combined risk of developing breast, uterine, and ovarian cancer. These result in additional, usually social, economic, and dependence problems, such as hospitalization for surgical repair, failure of the surgical procedure, depression. Most patients do not resume normal activity, and mortality within one year approaches a staggering 20%.

FRACTURES OF THE WRIST

These limit the use of the hand and forearm for periods from 4 to 8 weeks, but long-term disability for this is uncommon.

All fractures induce undesirable emotions:

- Depression
- Fear of additional falls and fractures
- Fear of loss of independent living

BROKEN BONES AND BACK PAIN

Could patient's back pain be more than a simple ache? Could it tell us that a bone has broken? "Back pain is a common symptom in post-menopausal women....However, acute back pain in post-menopausal women may be caused by vertebral fracture, and 'red flags' in the history and physical examination can help clinicians decide on the appropriate work-up....The diagnosis of existing vertebral fractures is critical because the probability of sustaining new spine and hip fractures is increased in women with one vertebral fracture, and the presence of multiple fractures puts the patient at risk for chronic debilitation....Evaluation of bone mineral density is a helpful guide to further management. Treatment may include calcium and vitamin D, hormone replacement therapy, bisphosphonates and/or calcitonin."[M180]

Vertebral osteoporosis fractures usually result from a decrease of bone mass, and deterioration of bone structure leading to loss of strength; the most common lesions are:
■ Biconcave deformities (the bone has a "scooped out" appearance on top and bottom, instead of the usual flat surfaces)
■ Wedge or crush fractures (the bone is crushed through the middle of the vertebral body, taking a wedge shape instead of the usual square shape)

New vertebral fractures are not always accompanied by pain, and disability does not correlate in a linear form with the number of vertebral fractures.

"Although falls are a major factor in the occurrence of femoral neck fractures, their type and frequency have not been studied in detail. A few case-reports have demonstrated that *bone insufficiency* can lead to spontaneous *femoral neck fractures* and that some falls occur as a result of acute pain preceding the fracture...; femoral neck fractures due to bone insufficiency have ranged from 3% to 24%."[M070]

Do people actually fall from a standing position as they break their hip? Some do:
■ 5.9% experienced acute pain before the fall
■ 9.8% reported trivial trauma before the break
■ 15.7 reported no trauma before the break
■ 45.5% had hip pain during the weeks preceding the fracture—more often than not only in the hip that was subsequently fractured

Spontaneous fracture (no fall) was preceded by the following symptoms in the hip:

- Gradually worsening pain
- Pain during the preceding weeks
- Pain in the inguinal or *crural* area
- Recent onset of pain, less than 3 months

Recommendations for virtually all asymptomatic post-menopausal women are moderate exercise and supplementation with calcium and vitamin D. In addition, most post-menopausal women without contraindications, would benefit from estrogen replacement therapy, primarily because of its cardiovascular benefits. In patients with contraindications or an aversion to hormone therapy, bone densitometry should be performed to determine risks before expensive non-hormonal treatment is initiated. Therapy with alendronate sodium (Fosamax®) or calcitonin (Calcimar, Miacalcin) is indicated by *Establishment* in women with developed osteoporosis, and may be appropriate for early post-menopausal women with osteopenia. Calcitonin is a good option in patients with disabling spinal bone pain. Slow-release sodium fluoride,[1010] although still considered experimental, may eventually be given for vertebral fracture in patients with mild to moderate disease. These are Establishment recommendations, not necessarily endorsed by me.

What is the experience of women who suffer post-menopausal vertebral fractures? As the women in a study done in Arizona described it, "the essential structure of the experience of post-menopausal spinal fractures was an abrupt descent into disease, disability, and deformity. Each informant described significant challenges to her ability to continue to function as a whole, independent person. Constant pain, loss of independent function, changes in physical appearance, feelings of isolation, a sense of vulnerability, and an uncertain future were the hallmarks of the experience."[P020]

What are the areas in which women with spinal fractures need assistance?
- Education
- Pain management
- Promotion of self-care ability
- Regaining or maintaining function
- Techniques to reduce stress and isolation

A study on the effects of exercise in osteoporotic women in an outpatient clinic (Medical School, University of Vienna) showed that sedentary post-menopausal women may benefit from regular long term therapeutic exercise in terms of subjective back complaints and slowed loss of bone mass.[P080 P081]

The purposes of physical therapy in the prevention and the rehabilitation of osteoporosis are to:
- Improve agility
- Improve mobility
- Improve physical skill
- Promote bone mass
- Relieve pain

Vertebral osteoporosis fractures usually result from a decrease of bone mass, and deterioration of bone structure, leading to loss of strength. The most common fractures are:
- Biconcave deformities
- Wedge or crush fractures

New vertebral fractures are not always accompanied by pain, and disability does not correlate in a linear form with the number of vertebral fractures.

Aging and osteoporosis have been associated with skeletal changes.[S140] Anomalies seen on X-Rays usually are:
- Abnormal vertebral body ratios (a number calculated by dividing the anterior to posterior height for each vertebra from T-4 through L-5)
- Kyphosis index determined by adding the anterior heights of each vertebral body, T-4 through T-12, and then dividing the total by the corresponding sum of the posterior heights of each vertebral body
- Lumbar lordosis (swayback)
- Sacral tilt or inclination
- Thoracic kyphosis (hunchback)

Back extensor strengthening exercises are highly recommended for management of back pain, especially back pain related to osteoporosis.

However, they must be balanced with other exercises, to avoid excessive increases in lumbar lordosis, They usually:

- Decrease thoracic kyphosis
- Increase lumbar lordosis
- Increase sacral tilt

Bone mineral density and physical activity score did not show any significant correlations with the radiographic factors. The results indicate that the stronger the back extensor, the smaller the thoracic kyphosis, and the larger the lumbar lordosis and sacral inclination. Back extensor strength is an important determinant of posture in healthy women. However, prescribing back extensor strengthening exercises, alone, may also increase lumbar lordosis, which is not desirable.

"Osteoporosis has obvious physical and functional consequences such as kyphosis, restricted range of motion, and pain. What are not so obvious are the psychosocial sequelae that result from this metabolic bone disease. Many patients in the initial phases of the disease express substantial anxiety, especially about the possibility of future fractures and physical deformity. As the disease progresses, depression can become profound for those who experience hip or multiple vertebral fractures. The effects of the chronicity of osteoporosis, its disabling and disfiguring aspects, and the chronic postural pain that develops as time passes challenge even the most stable individuals. In addition, osteoporosis has substantial impact on interpersonal relationships and social roles. The dependency created by this disease affects close relationships, because the patient with osteoporosis cannot reciprocate in social support. Today's older women find the restrictions of the disease socially devastating. These women, unlikely to work in the labor force, took pride in their roles of housekeeper and cook. Unfortunately, severe osteoporosis can force women to relinquish even these social roles, leaving them with no source of self-esteem or accomplishment. In all, osteoporosis is devastating both psychologically and socially."[G060]

FALSE HEALING OF FRACTURES

Some patients who have suffered compression fractures continue hurting after the fracture has apparently healed, (in fact, what has happened, is that the two halves have developed a false joint (*pseudoarthrosis*) at the level of the break). This joint is somewhat moveable and won't grow together, because a thickened membrane without adequate circulation prevents this. Surgical bone grafts joining both parts can correct this satisfactorily. Symptoms are dramatically improved immediately after operation and bony union can be confirmed by the doctors.[H060]

CHAPTER II

ANATOMY AND PHYSIOLOGY OF BONE

WHAT IS BONE?

The physical body is composed of many different tissues: muscle, skin, etc. *Bone* is the hardest tissue of the body. The architectural structure of bone tissue is made up of a framework of interlocking protein fibers, with calcium and phosphorous crystals embedded in it.

BONE PROTEINS

The proteins are:

■ *ostein,* which is rich in *collagen*, a gelatinous, gristle-like substance that derives its name from the Latin *colla*, glue, as in the word collate. It is the glue that holds and binds body cells and tissues together. This collagen is impregnated with minerals, largely calcium and phosphate.

■ *osteocalcin*, which is composed of several *non-collagen* proteins.

After this *connective tissue matrix* (support or holding plaster) has been laid down, mineralization with calcium salts occurs. The predominant structural form of calcium in human bone tissue is called *hydroxyapatite*. It is responsible for 67% of the total bone, weight, the remaining 33% being composed by collagenous fibers.

COMPONENTS RESPONSIBLE FOR STRUCTURE	STRUCTURAL CHARACTERISTICS OF BONE
mineral crystals	hardness strength and rigidity
collagen fibers	flexibility
magnesium, sodium, potassium,	"mortar" that bonds the calcium
citrate, fluoride? and other trace elements	phosphorous crystals

"Although it is known that collagen imparts mechanical strength to bone no detailed biochemical analysis has been made of osteoporotic bone collagen...yet, there are significant changes in the properties of the collagen...changes indicate...a higher turnover in the head region compared to the neck region of the femoral head [upper hip] and are consistent with the susceptibility of the neck region to fracture. Clearly, the collagen is altered in osteoporosis and these changes may play a role in the ...development...of the disease."[B008]

Normal collagen is composed of certain specific proteins. Alterations in the composition of collagen occur in other degenerative conditions, such as arteriosclerosis, and these changes are practically identical to *mutations* or changes induced in collagen by the action of *herpes* viruses (chicken-pox, small-pox, *herpes simplex* and *zoster*, *Epstein Barr*).[S161] It is interesting to think that there may be a direct virus and vaccine to osteoporosis, connection.

MINERAL AND PROTEIN COMPONENTS
- Calcium
- Magnesium
- Ostein, rich in collagen
- Osteocalcin and other non-collagen proteins
- Phosphate

The average adult skeleton contains 1,000-1,200 grams of calcium or 2.2-2.6 pounds. The hormone calcitonin from the thyroid gland triggers the deposition of calcium by the osteoblast bone cells while parathyroid hormone (parathormone) releases calcium from the osteoclast bone cells.

Between 2-4% of a person's skeleton is first dissolved and then rebuilt annually. This process is implemented by the osteoclast and osteoblast bone cells.

According to its structure and location, two major forms of *osseous* (bone) tissue exist:

- *Cortical* bone
- *Trabecular* or *medullary* bone

Compact *cortical* bone appears smooth and uniform, it forms the external envelope of the skeleton. *Trabecular* or *medullary* bone, small layers and tubes, forms plates that traverse the internal cavities of the skeleton. The proportions of cortical and trabecular bone vary at different sites, according to the bone's predominant function. Vertebral bodies contain predominantly trabecular bone, while the upper part of the thigh bone (*proximal femur*) contains predominantly cortical bone. The two forms of bone respond differently to metabolic changes, and their susceptibility to fracture differs.

HOW DOES BONE FORM?

Do not worry, there won't be a quiz about this! But, although the subject may seem complicated, it is important to learn a little about it, to understand why many of the compounds and molecules that take part in bone formation and structure can be used to develop and perform lab tests of great informational value. If technical details bore you, either skip this, or learn to make biology your friend.

Bone is not stationary: quite to the contrary, it undergoes continuous remodeling (turnover) throughout life. Like all other tissues, it is composed of units called *cells*, which produce *proteins* (similar to those which compose gristle, meat, etc.). Protein is made from smaller building blocks called *amino acids*. I first want to give a *mnemonic* (memory) rule to remember the names of the cells that form bone (*osteoblasts*) and break down bone (*osteoclasts*). When you form bone, you feel good, and have a *blast*, when it is reabsorbed, you may wind up in a *cast*. It is important to remember these names. Cells that aid the reabsorption or breakdown of already existing bone (*osteoclasts*) digest the surface of old, possibly fatigued bone to form *resorption cavities*; cells that form bone (*osteoblasts)* then reform the bone surfaces, filling the cavities with bone *connective tissue proteins*, most of which are *type I collagen* (a specific form of gristle). Normally, bone resorption and formation occur simultaneously, and in equilibrium. Several factors, mechanical and electrical forces, hormones, and local regulation, influence this remodeling. The complete process from resorption through formation takes about 100 days. About 10% of bone in the adult is replaced each year. The mechanical strength of this *fibrillar collagen* (proteins built like strands or fibers) is enhanced by *cross-linking* (a kind of braiding) of adjacent strands of a "binder" made from modified forms of the amino acid *lysine* (*pyridinoline* and *deoxypyridinoline*). These "cross-links" attach to the ends of this gristle, called *N-telopeptides*. When bone is resorbed, different structural and chemical forms of crosslinks are released, and eventually are found in the urine, both *free* (by themselves), and *peptide-bound* (attached to fragments of protein).

Peak bone mass is achieved at about 35 years of age. *Cortical* (smooth, compact outer layer of bone) bone peaks earlier than *trabecular* (honeycomb type structure) bone. Biology is oblivious of the constraints of political correctness—sex, race, nutrition, exercise, and overall health—all influence peak mass, which is approximately 30 % higher in men than in women and approximately 10 % higher in blacks than in whites. In each group, bone mass varies among individuals.

After reaching its peak, bone mass declines throughout life due to imbalances occurring in the processes of remodeling. Bones lose both mineral and organic matrix, but retain their basic organization. In women, bone mass decreases rapidly for 3 to 7 years after menopause. Bone loss also is enhanced in a variety of diseases.

WHAT CAUSES NORMAL BONE TO TURN INTO OSTEOPOROTIC BONE?

Although the percent of circulating calcium, compared to bone-bound calcium, is relatively minute, the body's *homeostatic* mechanism (the tendency to balance the values in the blood) will continuously cause the bones to release calcium into the bloodstream in order to maintain proper blood levels. So, while serum levels of calcium can test normal, in the absence of sufficient available dietary calcium, bone loss can be significant: this process is a primary cause of osteoporosis.

Osteoporosis manifests differently, according to any, or all, of the following:
- Which type of bone is involved
- Which cells are functioning improperly
- What chemistry is out of range
- What effect movement may have

Rapid bone turnover or reduced rates of bone formation have been documented in patients with primary osteoporosis.

For a long time, scientists believed that, in osteoporosis, the *amount* of bone was diminished, but that the *quality* of the bone was unaltered. However, novel methods of analysis have shown that, at the break site of osteoporotic fractures, there is:

- A marked change in the *molecular orientation or directional arrangement* of components (*proteoglycans*)[F020] of the non-collagenous bone matrix
- The *amount* of the non-collagenous bone matrix is unchanged

These results imply that the quality of the bone, as well as the quantity, may be generally affected in osteoporosis.

Considering the complex factors regulating normal bone metabolism, the existence of multiple causes for osteoporosis is not surprising. Among the many possible problems causing primary osteoporosis, research has primarily targeted two deficiencies, which are not the only ones:
- Estrogen
- Calcium

This belief is reinforced because rapid bone loss often accompanies menopause, and because premature osteoporosis follows the removal of both ovaries. Estrogen replacement prevents bone loss in both conditions. The following observations support a causal relationship between calcium deficiency and osteoporosis: Calcium deficiency in experimental animals causes osteoporosis; a low calcium intake is common among the elderly in the United States; and calcium supplementation reduces bone loss.

PRIMARY OSTEOPOROSIS FOLLOWS A DEFICIENCY OF ESTROGEN AND DEFICIENCY OF CALCIUM

IS ESTROGEN DEFICIENCY A LESS IMPORTANT FACTOR IN OSTEOPOROSIS, THAN THE DEFICIENCY OF CERTAIN ESTROGEN CONVERTING ENZYMES? THE 16-ALPHA FACTOR.

It may not be only the deficiency of estrogen, but an anomaly in the way the estrogen is converted or metabolized, that really matters. To burden the reader with a little more chemistry, a study published in Seoul, Korea, tells us that "Compared to non-osteopenic subjects, there were no significant differences in serum *estrone (E1)* and *estradiol (E2)* levels in patients with *osteopenia* (decreased bone mass). However, the urinary *16 alpha-hydroxyestrone [16 alpha- (OH)E1]* level (a breakdown product of estrogen we can call 16-alpha) was significantly lower in patients with spinal osteopenia [bone deficiency]. There were some other metabolic abnormalities also, making the researchers conclude that the activity of *estrogen 16 alpha-hydroxylase* (a specific enzyme) was decreased and/or the activity of *estrogen 2-hydroxylase* was enhanced in post-menopausal osteopenia."[L080]

NOT ALL BONE LOSS IS OSTEOPOROSIS

There are conditions of low skeletal mass and/or a fracture after minor injuries that often do not represent osteoporosis, but *metabolic bone disease*, such as:

- *Hyperparathyroidism* (imbalanced function of the *parathyroid glands*, small bodies to the side of the thyroid)
- *Hyperthyroidism* (imbalanced function of the *thyroid glands*, a master gland above the notch in the breast bone, below your neck)
- *Metastatic* disease (spread of malignancy)
- *Multiple myeloma*
- *Osteomalacia*
- *Paget's disease* of the bone
- *Secondary* osteoporosis (due to excessive *cortisone* intake, etc.)

Blood or urine tests, and a good medical history may help distinguish between these conditions. A proper diagnosis is very important to start a successful line of therapy.

NOT ALL BONE DISEASES AND PAINS ARE OSTEOPOROSIS

It is important to be aware that other conditions may cause symptoms similar to osteoporosis, and that these, too, must be treated. I have often seen suffering patients, whose neuromuscular and joint conditions, were being ignored and untreated because their physician blamed every symptom on osteoporosis. Some of these conditions are:

- Ankylosing spondylitis
- Arthritis and Bowel Disease
- Behcet's disease
- Carpal tunnel syndrome (CTS)
- Gout
- Lumbar Disc Problems
- Metabolic osteopenia and bone disease
- Systemic Lupus Erythematosus

ANKYLOSING SPONDYLITIS

It primarily affects the spine or back. The joints and ligaments that normally permit the spine to move become inflamed and stiff. The bones of the spine may grow together, causing the spine to become rigid and inflexible. Other joints such as the hips, shoulders, knees, or ankles also may become involved.

ARTHRITIS AND BOWEL DISEASE

Arthritis means inflammation of joints. Inflammation is a body process that can result in pain, swelling, warmth, redness, and stiffness. Sometimes, inflammation can also affect the bowel. When it does, the process is called *inflammatory bowel disease (IBD)*.

BEHCET'S DISEASE

It is a condition that affects the inner lining of the mouth and genitals, and the small blood vessels throughout the body. There is no cure for it, but the symptoms usually can be controlled.

CARPAL TUNNEL SYNDROME (CTS)

This is a condition that can cause pain, tingling, numbness, and weakness in the fingers and thumb, due to pressure on the median nerve.

GOUT

It is an acute arthritis resulting from deposition of crystals of *sodium urate* in the peripheral joints and tendons. It is usually recurrent, and may become chronic and deforming.

LUMBAR DISC PROBLEMS

Since osteoporosis is often accompanied by *lumbar disc problems* (a narrowing or damage to the gelatinous discs that are located between each two vertebrae), a glimpse into this condition may be of interest. Surgical therapies are the best known. Considering that surgery is traumatic and often ineffective in alleviating pain, massage, traction and other non-invasive therapies may be considered.

METABOLIC OSTEOPENIA AND BONE DISEASE

■ Corticosteroid induced osteopenia
1. chronic glucocorticoid therapy
2. overproduction of adrenal corticosteroids

- ***Osteitis fibrosa***: increase in mineral and matrix resorption resulting from parathyroid hormone excess
- ***Osteomalacia***: inadequate mineralization of bone matrix
- ***Phosphate wasting*** syndromes
- Vitamin D deficiencies

NEUROMUSCULAR AND DISCOGENIC BACK PAIN:
One of the most common health problems in the United States, yet its cause is generally undiagnosed, excepting when a patient is lucky enough to go to an acupuncturist, chiropractor, or osteopath, or when someone concerned performs a CAT scan or MRI.

People with discogenic problems are often subjected to not always successful back surgeries. In the last ten years, micro surgeries using fiberoptic instruments have been used. Other new treatments include a novel, *avant garde*, "replacement disc" (kinematic disc prosthesis model (SB Charite); this is considered "the best disc replacement compromise, and is the basis of the evolution of the prosthetic concept at the dawning of the year 2000." However, it is very important to know whether the back pain is due only to disc, or also to osteoporosis, because surgery will often fail unless the quality of the bone is improved."[L060]

SYSTEMIC LUPUS ERYTHEMATOSUS
A whole-body (systemic) autoimmune disorder producing a chronic inflammatory disease affecting all organ systems.

CHAPTER III

DIAGNOSTIC
PROCEDURES

HOW IS OSTEOPOROSIS DIAGNOSED?

It is easy to look at the typical osteoporotic female, elderly, frail, hunch-backed, maybe walking with a walker, and realize that she suffers from osteoporosis. But in somebody less obviously ill, the deficient bone mass must be determined by one process or another. Sophisticated machines are now available to measure bone mass and diagnose osteoporosis quickly, painlessly and safely, before severe problems arise. Unfortunately, physicians are usually not deeply concerned with early detection and prevention, and all too often it is only the occurrence of a bone fracture that alerts the physician to the presence of osteoporosis.

If you are not sure about the status of your bones, excellent tests are available to evaluate the likelihood of developing osteoporosis. The tests also allow physicians to diagnose osteoporosis in the early stages before the bone loss is so severe that fractures occur. These tests include the:

- *Computerized axial tomography* (also called a *CAT scan*), which can measure bone density in the spine. The CAT scan uses higher x-ray dosages and is a more expensive test
- *Conventional x-ray*, which picks up osteoporosis only when 30 percent or more of the bone mass is lost
- *Dual photon densitometer*, which measures the spine, hip, or other bones
- *Single photon densitometer*, which measures the density of the forearm

You may choose to have a bone density test done if you are trying to decide whether or not to use *HRT* (*hormone replacement therapy*) — I use the memory aid "*HeaRT*". If the tests show accelerated bone loss for your age group, you should seriously consider the use of HRT unless other major health issues contraindicate the use of hormones.

Another test for osteoporosis involves collecting a 24 hour urine sample. The laboratory then determines the proportion of two substances normally present in urine: calcium and *creatinine*. A high calcium ratio indicates increased calcium excretion and accelerated bone loss.

The National Osteoporosis Foundation can provide you with information that will help you understand osteoporosis and bone density testing. You'll learn methods available to measure bone density, who should have the tests, and what test results mean. As of Jan. 1995, Medicare reimbursement rates for Bone Mineral Density Tests have been increased (on a national average) from $68 to $124. You can learn ways to judge your own risk of developing osteoporosis and steps you can take right now to preserve and protect your bone health. The National Osteoporosis Foundation is usually glad to inform and educate: 1150 17th Street, NW, Suite 500, Washington DC 20036-4603 (IL Dept. on Aging/Network News).

RADIOLOGIC TESTS FOR OSTEOPOROSIS

BONE DENSITY SCANNING

Several non-invasive methods are available to evaluate the thickness of the outer and inner layers of the bone, and to compare them to desirable values. These vary widely in cost, availability, and radiation dose.

> "YOU CAN TAKE A NORMAL PATIENT AND AN ABNORMAL X-RAY TECHNICIAN, AND GIVE THE PATIENT OSTEOPOROSIS AT WILL."

STANDARD X-RAYS

Standard X-Rays of the spine are widely available and less expensive than other, more sophisticated tests, but they are very low sensitivity indicators of bone loss, since bone density must be decreased by at least 20 to 30% before the reduction can be appreciated, and it is a subjective appreciation of the film by the naked eye which makes the diagnosis. We may remember Dr. Resnick's humorous "rule," as quoted by Dr. Richardson on the www: "You can take a normal patient, and an abnormal X-ray technician, and give the patient *osteoporosis* at will."

Characteristic abnormalities on standard X-Rays are often sufficient for establishing the diagnosis of osteoporosis. If the spine film is not diagnostic but clinical suspicion is high, a variety of other procedures may be indicated. These include:

- *Compton scattering*
- *Dual-energy x-ray absorptiometry (DXA)*
- *Neutron activation*
- *Photodensitometry*

- **Radiogrammetry** for measurement of cortical thickness
- **Singh Index** of femoral trabecular pattern
- **Single and dual photon absorptiometry**
- **Single and dual energy computed tomography**
- **Ultrasound**

The doctor's choice among these techniques will depend on their availability, cost, and further studies of their discriminatory capabilities and sensitivity.There are four main types of bone density scanning machines, but it is widely accepted that a procedure called **dual-energy x-ray absorptiometry (DXA)** offers the greatest reliability, safety, precision, and convenience. Two other techniques, **radiographic absorptiometry** and **ultrasound**, are now under investigation.

"DEXA" MACHINE
It's never been easy for doctors to determine how weak or strong bones are, but now they have discovered a new way to determine bone density accurately. They use a piece of equipment known as a "DEXA" machine. A narrow beam of X-ray scans through the sine, hips and arms and can detect even the most minor of changes in bone density. Doctors say the results could help identify osteoporosis — or brittle bone disease — before it reaches an advanced stage.

Bone loss and wasting is not equal in all bones. Which bone proved to be the best to measure of genuine age-related decrease in bone density? Researchers doing a study on 674 elderly living in a rural community of Nangai Village, Akita Prefecture, compared the reliability and consistency of DXA measurements of several bony areas: the lumbar spine and three areas of the upper thigh (proximal femur) and found that BMDs in the proximal femur [upper thigh] were the best and most reliable bone areas.[S230]

When talking about the reliability (and lack thereof) of DXA or DEXA, Dr. Ed White who is working with the "Osteoporosis Initiative", tells us that: "...there are some incredibly fancy computerized x-ray (very low dose—equal to the amount of passive radiation one receives spending one day in the mountains) machines, called Dual Energy X-ray Absorptiometry (DXA) machines that measure bone density at different sites of the body. They are 'accurate' and consistent when used absolutely correctly but there are so many technical pitfalls in their use and interpretation of their images that one can easily start depending on information which has been 'contaminated' by lack of attention to detail."[W060]

As this chapter is edited, October 1997, we learn that an FDA Panel Gave a **Bone Ultrasound** Device a unanimous recommendation for approval. The **Sahara Ultrasound Device** is manufactured by Hologic. It is portable, more economical than DEXA, and measures the density of the heel bone in about one minute.[M120]

An invasive analysis, **histomorphometry**, is usually performed on a bone biopsy from the **iliac crest**, the prominent part of the hip, bone mass can be evaluated and **osteomalacia** and certain forms of secondary osteoporosis can be excluded. Bone biopsy is safe but requires specialized equipment and expert analysis which is not widely available.

The interest in DEXA testing has grown remarkably. "When Evanston Hospital opened a bone density screening site at a department store in an upscale CHICAGO MALL, THIS SPRING, it offered — perhaps as a nod to its new location — an introductory half price sale on axial dual x-ray absorbtiometry: $150 instead of the usual $299."[O020] The machines were soon booked a month ahead. Portable DEXA machines that test extremities only can be placed in a van and charges may be no higher than $40.

TBMAS

A novel device, Trabecular Bone Morphology and Analysis System (TBMAS) permits studies of bone 3D structure, as important to its function as its mineral content. Trabecular bone from the spine has an intrinsic "spring-like" macro-sructure which provides an efficient means to absorb energy and withstand external impact during loading, as states at the following website: [http://www.emba.uvm.edu/VSGC//ugrad/tbmas/tbmas.htm]

The mechanial properties of trabecular bone are being studied with the support of a grant from the Whitaker Foundation ("Predicting the Mechanical Behavior of Trabecular Bone: Application to Aging and Osteoporosis") to provide an improved characterization of the mechanical behavior of normal and osteoporotic trabecular bone in terms of both

1. traditional denistometric measures of bone quality (bulk density, mineral content) and
2. non-traditional measures of bone structure (morphology).

The significant findings from these studies include:
- the weight-bearing skeleton exhibits more structural anisotropy (irregularity) than trabecular bone from the non-weight bearing skelton;
- ash density (apparent dry density x mineral fraction) is the most sensitive measure of the bulk physical properties of trabecular bone;

A "trabecular conectivity index," TCI, has been formulated to measure trabecular fracture risk, and an iterative boundary condition method has been developed to stimulate experimental compressive mechanical test conditions (described in the following sections).

A very promising software has been refined over the past several years to
- display and pre-process 3D images of bone structure
- compute physical and structural indices based upon bone architecture studies

TBMAS allows the user to specify the viewing direction, and the starting and ending locations within the specimen, and compute flat and 3D structural indices.

TESTS FOR BIOCHEMICAL MARKERS OF BONE METABOLISM: LABORATORY BLOOD AND URINE TESTS

BIOCHEMICAL MARKERS

Certain biological substances derived from the metabolism of bone, are present and measurable in urine and blood (***biochemical markers*** of bone resorption), and indicate the rate at which bone is being broken down. These can be used for diagnosis, and also to assess the impact of treatment. Biochemical markers are useful to follow the status of bone metabolism in patients with osteoporosis, although bone densitometry is the only way to measure actual bone mass, estimate fracture risk, and diagnose osteoporosis, and measure the end result of treatment. But bone densitometry cannot be repeated at close enough intervals to make early adjustments in therapy because of its precision error. Response to treatment by densitometry might not be evident for six months at the earliest and often not until two years. It is within this time frame that biochemical markers are useful. Through them one might determine if the desired biochemical effect of treatment has occurred.

ALKPHASE-B® (BONE ALKALINE PHOSPHATASE)

Alkphase-B® is a new blood test for measuring **bone alkaline phosphatase**. Bone alkaline phosphatase is an enzyme found on the surface of osteoblasts, the cells responsible for bone formation. Its levels adequately parallel bone formation. *Alkphase-B®* is a **monoclonal antibody** test (antibodies derived from a group of daughter cells which originate from one mother cell) which improves the specificity and sensitivity of alkaline phosphatase testing. Bone alkaline phosphatase levels have an advantage over some of the other biochemical markers of bone metabolism such as **urinary N-telopeptide crosslinks, free urinary pyridinoline** and **serum osteocalcin** (see below). Blood levels of bone alkaline phosphatase tend to be more stable throughout the day.

Alkaline phosphatase is present in humans in several variants or **isoenzymes** (similar enzymes): liver/bone/kidney, intestinal, and placental. Bone and liver enzymes are difficult to distinguish. Former techniques which have been developed are cumbersome, and lack precision and sensitivity. It has been possible to measure bone alkaline phosphatase in the past by separating it from other isoenzymes through **electrophoresis** (a process that separates chemicals by running an electric current through a liquid), but the new test is more efficient, specific, and reproducible. To the joy of tired lab technicians, it is reported to compare favorably with the best and most tedious of the electrophoretic techniques, and to be better than most of them. Unfortunately this test does not discriminate between normal and low levels very well. However it does a good job in discriminating between normal and high levels, and is well quantified in this range. Bone alkaline phosphatase levels have the advantage of being stable throughout the day, makes testing much easier. One does not have to collect a blood specimen at any particular time of the day, and no fasting is required.

- *High levels* of bone alkaline phosphatase are seen in several clinical disorders other than osteoporosis, including Paget's disease, osteosarcoma, hyperparathyroidism, and hyperthyroidism.
- *Low levels* might be anticipated in certain forms of osteoporosis, but unfortunately the test does not discriminate very well between normal and low levels of the enzyme.

In women, superimposed upon this age-related bone loss, is an accelerated post-menopausal bone loss due to increased bone resorption. As a result of estrogen deficiency the number and activity of osteoclasts is increased. This accelerated bone loss persists for five to ten years, after which bone loss usually proceeds at the expected age-related rate.

Techniques also are available to measure bone *formation*. During bone formation newly synthesized osteocalcin (bone protein), as well as the enzyme bone alkaline phosphatase are released into the blood stream by osteoblasts. These can be accurately measured. A collagen precursor called *procollagen peptide* is also released, and likewise can be measured.

NTX TEST AND PYRILINKS

This may sound really technical, but you may skip the hard parts.

During bone resorption, *collagen* (*gristle*) is broken down (*degraded*). Fragments containing *cross-links* are released into the blood. These fragments, which include amino acid sequences (strings of amino acids which make up a protein molecule) of *N-telopeptide* (the attached portion of bone collagen), are further degraded, releasing free molecules of *pyridinoline* and *deoxypyridinoline*. Tests measuring these markers, are used to identify patients experiencing rapid bone loss, as well as to monitor the effect of treatment. Two such tests have recently been approved by the FDA. They are enumerated and then clearly explained below.

- NTX
  Tests for *pyridinoline*

- Pyrilinks
  Tests for *pyridinoline* and *deoxypiridinoline* still attached to the *N-telopeptides* of bone collagen

PYRILINKS®

Each substance introduced into cells (*antigen*) can induce the production of a binding chemical which can fit the antigen as a key fits a lock. We call these binders *antibodies*, as they can be effectively used to perform laboratory tests. Antibodies generated by cells which derive from one parent cell are called *monoclonal antibodies* (as one cell cloned).

You may remember the strength of bone collagen derives from the substances which tie together the collagen fibrils, *pyridinoline,* and *deoxypyridinoline crosslinks*. Bone resorption releases these crosslinks into the circulation, either as free forms or attached to small segments of collagen called N-telopeptides. These are eventually excreted into the urine. This particular test measures free pyridinoline in the urine. However, pyridinoline is present in other forms of collagen (tendon, cartilage, ligaments, fascia, and blood vessels), not just the type I collagen of bone, so it may give false positives.

The FDA has recently approved a monoclonal antibody test called *Pyrilinks®*, to detect the substance pyridinoline in urine. This test was developed to identify individuals with elevated rates of bone resorption such as those observed in many women after menopause.

ADVANTAGES OF THIS TEST
Pyrilinks can be used to gauge a person's response to medications. When bone breakdown is very active, the test results become elevated. As bone resorption decreases when hormones arrest the process of osteoporosis, high levels of pyridinoline fall in response to treatment.

Bone resorption ——> releases - crosslinks ——> into circulation and urine
— —> measurable by **PYRILINKS®**

DISADVANTAGES OF THIS TEST
There are disadvantages to any of the urinary crosslink measurements:

■   Mean levels of urinary crosslinks are higher than normal in all conditions which are associated with high rates of bone turnover:
1. Early menopause
2. Hyperthyroidism
3. Hyperparathyroidism
4. Paget's disease
■   Widely varied results are produced, depending on the time of day

PYRILINKS®-D
The *Pyrilinks®-D* urinary assay provides a quantitative measure of the excretion of *deoxypyridinoline collagen crosslinks*, (substances left behind by the breakdown process of the body, an indicator of bone resorption). It is also a monoclonal antibody test that demonstrates specificity for deoxypyridinoline, which is bone specific.

The actual amount of bone present or left behind, can only be measured clinically by bone densitometry (see DEXA), but what is actually happening to bone at a given point of time can only be measured by biochemical markers. The measurement of specific degradation products such as deoxypyridinoline provides quantitative data on the rate of bone breakdown. Anti-resorptive therapy should decrease the rate of breakdown, and hence the quantity of deoxypyridinoline detectable in the urine.

OSTEOMARK® - THE NTX TEST

It is based on the measurement of certain chemicals which are a residue of bone breakdown. As previously stated, bone is cyclically broken down and rebuilt as part of a normal remodeling process. Osteoclasts reabsorb the organic matrix of bone which consists mainly of type I collagen (a substance we can compare to gristle). Made from chains of certain molecules, these strands are cross-linked or braided for strength and resilience with the chemicals pyridinoline and deoxypyridinoline. These cross-links attach to the ends of the collagen chains, in regions known as N-telopeptides. When bone is reabsorbed, free cross-links, and cross-links which are still attached to N-telopeptides, are released into the blood, and eventually excreted in the urine. Measuring these fragments of bone resorption gives an estimate of bone turnover, specifically bone resorption.

The FDA has recently cleared the first commercial laboratory test to measure this: The NTx Test. This test measures cross-links which are still attached to the N-telopeptides ends of collagen. This is probably the most specific test of accelerated bone loss now available. It can be used not only to measure the rate of bone loss, but also to monitor effects of therapy, lower test results indicating that treatment is working towards reducing bone loss. NTx testing is currently available at many local clinical laboratories.

N-telopeptide cross-links (fragments left when bone resorption occurs) are measured by **ELISA** (**Electro Immuno Absorbency**, a genetically engineered antibody test). **Ostex®** purports that their test is more specific than tests which measure free cross-links. Free cross-links are common to bone, cartilage, and other connective tissues. N-telopeptides are specific to bone. Therefore the attached N-telopeptides in the NTx test should confer specificity not found in other collagen cross-link tests.

An advantage to the NTx Test is that it can distinguish between individuals with normal bone resorption and those with low bone resorption. It may help physicians select the best treatment for osteoporosis, and also to evaluate whether or not that treatment is working. However, a disadvantage of NTx is that the level of the bone breakdown products being measured, N-telopeptide crosslinks, varies considerably throughout the day. This makes it more difficult to compare tests on the same person before and after treatment.

Bone density measurement by DEXA scan can then be repeated in a year or so to confirm whether the ultimate goal of treatment has been met— namely the achievement of a higher bone density with its concomitant decrease in the risk of fracture. Norland Laboratories DEXA measures forearm bone mass, thus making it possible to follow a patient on treatment, with confidence. Larger spine and hip scanners measure combined spine and hip mass, but are much more expensive.

CHAPTER IV

TRADITIONAL TREATMENT OF OSTEOPOROSIS

THE TREATMENT OF THE PATIENT WITH OSTEOPOROSIS

How can osteoporosis be prevented and treated? There are standard ways preferred by the medical *Establishment*. There also are alternatives. I will first discuss the standard methods, their advantages and disadvantages. The latter part of the book (Chapter IV) will be dedicated to the *Alternative methods*.

STANDARD OR ESTABLISHMENT MEDICAL APPROACHES

These will be enumerated and addressed in detail despite the fact that alternatives are the main subject of this book. <u>The public should know, not only the benefits, but also the many dangers and risks inherent to *Establishment* treatments</u>. Some medical approaches are better and safer than others, and risk vs. benefit must always be considered.

Patients, physicians and other health professionals should be well informed about the different approaches to the problem of osteoporosis, and always emphasize measures which have been proven to retard or halt it before irreversible structural defects occur:

- Additional nutrition
- Calcium
- Exercise
- Hormone replacement therapy (*HRT*) (estrogen, estrogen with progestin)

EXERCISE AND CALCIUM BALANCE

Moderate, appropriate exercise IMPROVES FUNCTION, BALANCE, and PROBABLY BONE STRENGTH. *Immobilization* produces a rapid decrease in bone mass, well documented in individuals placed on *bed rest* and in individuals with *paraplegia* and *quadriplegia*. Under these circumstances, the rate of bone loss may be rapid, partly related to an increase in bone resorption and a decrease in bone formation. Increased calcium intake under these conditions may increase the risk of:

- Abnormal locations of calcium deposits (*ectopic calcification*)
- Abnormal bone formation (*ectopic ossification*)
- Increased blood calcium (*hypercalcemia*)
- Kidney stones (*nephrolithiasis*)

As result of a recent study by military physicians in Beaumont, Texas, moderate exercise and supplementation with calcium and vitamin D are recommended for virtually all asymptomatic post-menopausal women.[1010]

MEDICATIONS

The reader will find that most medications receive rather extensive coverage. The reason for this is that the patients need to be well informed before making a decision to take certain drugs. These drugs have been dealt with in detail, especially their side effects., in the corresponding chapters.

ANTIRESORPTIVE THERAPY FOR WOMEN

It is the *Establishment's* opinion that estrogen supplementation or replacement should always be considered in peri-menopausal to 5-year post-menopausal women, and probably in older women as well. At the level of our current knowledge (January 1999), I share this opinion, although with certain differences in the choice of products. The prevalent opinion is that the decision whether or not to employ estrogens depends upon balancing the probable benefits against the possible risks and side-effects. Combined replacement with *progestin* is now touted by the *Establishment* as "essential for any woman who has an intact uterus", in order to offset the alleged increased risk of uterine cancer with unopposed estrogen. Continuous-combined, monthly cyclical, or long cyclical regimens, all are options. Doctors agree that periodic pelvic and breast examinations, including mammography, [God forbid!—see further on] should be performed as required. From their point of view, the use of estrogens along with other antiresorptive agents has not been well studied. They say that there may be clinical situations where combination therapy should be considered, and there are no reported contraindications. We do not agree with this, and more information is found under the appropriate headings.

ESTROGEN REPLACEMENT

In addition, most post-menopausal women who do not have conditions which could represent contraindications, would benefit from estrogen replacement therapy, primarily because of its cardiovascular benefits. They advise that in patients with contraindications to estrogen or an aversion to hormone therapy, bone densitometry should be performed to determine the grade of risk of fracture or deformity before expensive non-hormonal treatment is initiated. They are of the opinion that therapy with *alendronate sodium* (*Fosamax*®) or *calcitonin* (*Calcimar*®, *Miacalcin*®), described in more detail under the pharmaceutical approaches to osteoporosis, is clearly indicated in women with established osteoporosis and may be appropriate for early post-menopausal women with bone thinning (*osteopenia*). Calcitonin is a good option in patients with disabling spinal bone pain. Slow-release *sodium fluoride*, still considered experimental, is eyed with favor by some *Establishment* therapists, but is an absolute non-option in my vocabulary.

TAKE HEART AGAINST HURT WITH HRT

WHAT IS ESTROGEN?

Estrogen is a female hormone that is primarily produced during the first half of the menstrual cycle. Its levels in the body, their waxing and waning, time certain events in the cycle: their increase helps mature the ovum. They decline at the end of the menstrual cycle; this, in combination with the cessation of *progesterone* secretion, brings on menstrual bleeding. Some women have menstrual cycles that do not include the production of an egg cell: (*pre-ovulatory* or *nonovulatory* cycles), and in these, estrogen alone is the primary determinant for the onset of menstruation. Estrogen levels also affect the release of pituitary hormones—the *pituitary gonado- tropins*).

THE MANY TYPES OF ESTROGEN

Estrogens, according to their source, can be:
- Natural (manufactured in the body)
    - Ovarian
    - Adrenal
- Synthetic

NATURAL ESTROGENS

They exist *naturally* in various related molecular forms:
- *Estradiol*
- *Estriol*
- *Estrone*

The primary source of *natural* estrogen in normal adult women who have regular menstrual cycles, is the *ovarian follicle* (where the egg cell forms). It secretes *estradiol* (a form of estrogen which exists predominantly *inside* the cells, and binds the strongest to the receptor), in smaller and larger amounts that depend on the time of the menstrual cycle. This is converted primarily to **estrone** (another estrogenic hormone), which circulates in roughly equal proportion to estradiol, and to small amounts of **estriol** (another estrogenic variant).

Which are secondary sources of *natural* estrogen? A hormone of the *adrenal cortex*, the outer layer of the adrenal glands above the kidneys, **androstenedione**, results into most of the non-ovarian estrogen, as **estrone** (**sulfate ester**).

SYNTHETIC ESTROGENS
Ethinyl estradiol and **nonsteroidal estrogen** are higher in potency than naturally-occurring estrogens, when taken orally (by mouth).

Where are changes and breakdown of estrogens processed?
- A well functioning liver is essential to the proper metabolism (transformation) and inactivation of hormones.
- The human proteins **globulin** and **albumin**, act as binders and carriers.
- A certain proportion of the estrogen is excreted into the bile, then reabsorbed from the intestine and returned to the liver through the portal venous system.
- Their elimination is through the kidneys.

To understand certain of estrogen's influences on various parts of the body and biologic functions, we must remember that hereditary information, such as "blue eyes" or "curly hair" is transmitted by **genes**, particles of **nucleic acids**. Estrogens influence or activate a limited number of these genes, by binding to a special cellular location, the **nuclear estrogen receptor**, a DNA-binding protein which is found in **estrogen-responsive tissues**. Activated estrogen receptors bind to elements that have a hormone-response, which leads to certain effects such as breast development or body weight distribution. *Estrogen receptors* exist in the:
- Bone of women
- Breast
- Hypothalamus
- Liver
- Pituitary
- Reproductive tract

FUNCTIONS OF ESTROGENS

- Affect menstrual cycle
- Affect ovulation
- Affect pituitary gonadotropins
- Affect pregnancy
- Antioxidant
- Cause growth and development of the fallopian tubes
- Cause growth and development of the uterus
- Cause growth and development of the vagina
- Contribute to the shaping of the skeleton
- Contribute to puberal growth spurt (initiate changes in the epiphyses of the long bones at puberty)
- Contribute to the maintenance of tone and elasticity of urogenital structures
- Darken the pigmentation of nipples and genitals
- enlarge the breast (in conjunction with pituitary hormones and progesterone)
- Help develop and maintain the female reproductive system
- Help develop and maintain secondary sex characteristics (axillary and pubic hair)
- Termination of puberal growth spurt (terminate changes in the epiphyses of the long bones at puberty)

Most effects are well recognized, but the very interesting and important fact that estrogens are potent *antioxidants* is less well known. In fact, estradiol is almost as effective an antioxidant as vitamin E (*alpha-tocopherol*) "in terms of fatty acid peroxidation but is far more effective than alpha-tocopherol in terms of cholesterol peroxidation."[A100]

ESTROGENS ARE POTENT ANTIOXIDANTS

WHAT ARE THE EFFECTS OF LOWERED ESTROGEN PRODUCTION?

They have been previously described. This is simply a summary and reminder.

The lack of sex hormones affects not only the bones, but also the muscles:

the body tends to sag and lose tone after menopause. This may affect pelvic, as well as facial and arm muscles. The loss of pelvic muscle tone can affect not only looks, but also sexual pleasure, even the ability to hold urine. Facial drooping can appear fairly rapidly within a year or two of menopause. Other tissues, such as the breasts, lose their tone and droop more. The lack of estrogen is probably also responsible for the increase in low back and pelvic pain that women experience around this time.

A menopausal woman's physical appearance after menopause may change from an hourglass figure to a pear shape, as the distribution of weight on the body changes. The waist and upper back get thicker, the hips and breasts tend to lose some of their fat. Many women find that they gain weight more easily (10 to 15 pounds in the first years following menopause) no matter how diligently they diet or how much they exercise. It has been estimated that the lack of female hormonal support, plus the slowing of metabolism are probably responsible for these changes. Careful attention to diet and regular exercise can help, but may not entirely correct these physical changes.

HOW DO YOU KNOW THAT YOUR ESTROGEN LEVELS ARE LOW?

- You can go to you doctor, and run expensive laboratory tests in blood or urine.
- You can go to friendly labs which do not require a prescription to run the tests.
- You can have a conscientious doctor run a hormone level on your Papp smear, often at no additional cost.
- My favorite test? Does love making feel like a sandpaper massage? You can check the moisture of your vagina, which should be, at least, as moist as the inside of your lower lip. A dry vagina is a sign of dry bones. Vaginal lubrication signals bone regeneration to me.

WHAT IS HORMONE REPLACEMENT THERAPY

Medical studies show that hormonal therapy after menopause, not only helps prevent osteoporosis but also protects women against further bone loss. Hormones that may work very effectively are
- DHEA (dehydro-epi-androsterone)
- Estrogen
- Human growth hormone (HGH)

- Parathyroid hormone (PTH)
- Progesterone?
- Testosterone

Most people hear the word hormone and only think of estrogen, maybe progesterone, but this is not the only approach. Yet, it is the most prevalent in use. The other hormones are discussed in the section on treatments the *Establishment* chooses to ignore.

WHAT IS ESTROGEN REPLACEMENT THERAPY?

Estrogen replacement therapy (*ERT*) is the administration of estrogen to estrogen-deficient females, it is considered highly effective for preventing osteoporosis: this hormone prevents bone resorption and retards or halts postmenopausal bone loss. It is generally accepted that a substantial reduction in hip, wrist and vertebral fractures is noticed in women who begin estrogen replacement within a few years of menopause. Even when estrogens are started as late as 6 years after menopause, they do prevent further loss of bone mass, but do not restore it to premenopausal levels.

HOW DO WE PROVE ERT IS EFFECTIVE?

To demonstrate the impact of estrogen on the bones, a study performed in Czechoslovakia[Z020] evaluated the effects of the removal of both ovaries (*bilateral oophorectomy*), and subsequent estrogen supplementation in women who were close to menopause, but still menstruating at the time of surgery. Researchers measured the blood levels of substances related to bone growth and maturation, including the women's secretion of *certain hormones* (before and after surgery):

- Calcitonin
- Parathyroid hormone (PTH)
- Plasma insulin growth factor-I

and the serum levels of
- Magnesium
- Phosphorous
- Vitamin D3

before and after surgery.

Some values were altered, others were not, but therapy with transdermal (skin patch) estrogen substitution (100 micrograms/day for 6 weeks) returned the values listed below, to the preoperative range.

CHANGED VALUES	UNCHANGED VALUES
decrease of PTH	calcitonin secretion
increase of calcium	serum 1,25(OH)2 vitamin D3
increase of IGF-I	serum magnesium
increase of phosphorous	

HOW EFFECTIVE IS ESTROGEN REPLACEMENT THERAPY (ERT)

Many efficacy studies were done, but almost exclusively in white women. Therefore, the recommendations on estrogen therapy for osteoporosis pertain more specifically to that group.

WHO SHOULD RECEIVE ERT?

Menopausal women—particularly those in the categories with higher risk for osteoporosis—should receive ERT. Doctors say that cyclic estrogen therapy should also be given to women whose ovaries were surgically removed before age 50, or those who have had a natural menopause, where there are no specific contraindications, if they understand the risks and agree to regular medical evaluations. IMHO (in my humble opinion), I would add that one would want to be sure the women are really deficient in the hormone before initiating therapy. I am a devotee of the concept that "if it works, don't fix it."

PHARMACEUTICAL ESTROGEN THERAPIES: RESULTS AND DOSAGE

Do you want to keep from shrinking? Take HeaRT! Maybe you need seriously to consider HRT (HeaRT— hormone replacement therapy). Using **Premarin®** (conjugated estrogens from **PREgnant MARe urINe**) has prevented osteoporosis from occurring in later life in 90% of postmenopausal women who had no pre-existing osteoporosis, and this effect occurs with even very small doses (0.3 to 0.625mg daily). In one study done in Scotland by Dr. Robert Lindsay, women on ERT (estrogen replacement therapy) maintained their normal stature, while control women had a significant loss of height. A study comparing vertebral fracture rate in postmenopausal women treated with various combinations of estrogen, calcium, and sodium fluoride demonstrated that those utilizing **ERT** had the lowest rate of vertebral fractures. Wrist fractures and hip fractures were also reduced in various studies. A higher dosage of estrogen is usually utilized if osteoporosis has already developed, normally 1.25 to 2.5 mgr. per day. Estrogen from horse urine, Premarin, is available in:

- Injections
- Oral tablets
- Transdermal patches
- Vaginal creams

Other, non-prescription estrogens, from plant or ovarian source are also available. These will be dealt with further, under "Alternatives".

Estrogen appears to protect the bones through several mechanisms:

- Facilitates calcium absorption from the intestinal tract
- Increases calcitonin (a thyroid calcium regulating hormone) production: this stimulates bone formation
- Increases parathyroid hormone production—PTH: (this facilitates calcium absorption)
- May even have a stimulatory effect on osteoblasts (the cells that build up new bone)
- Reduces the elimination of urinary calcium
- Reduces the elimination of the amino acid **hydroxy-proline**, which suggests it inhibits osteoclast function (the action of cells that break down bone tissue)

From all points of view, estrogen appears to be *critical* to bone remodeling; therefore, it may well be the most essential component of prevention for osteoporosis.

**ESTROGEN IS CRITICAL TO BONE REMODELING;
IT IS THE MOST ESSENTIAL ELEMENT OF PREVENTION OF OSTEOPOROSIS**

Does calcium protect bones without added estrogen? Sorry, despite the wishful thinking of many, it does not. In a Japanese study at the Osaka University,[N080] postmenopausal and elderly women were treated either with **calcium lactate** (a chelated form of calcium, bound to a protein) alone or with calcium and **estriol**. The test was done for 10 months. At the end, when *before* and *after* measurements of bone density in the lumbar vertebrae were compared with each other, there was no doubt that only the group receiving the additional estrogen did well. Half of the "calcium alone" groups actually lost bone mass!

WHEN NOT TO USE ESTROGEN MEDICATIONS?

The "bible" of pharmaceutical drugs and drug uses, the Physician's Desk Reference (PDR) advises against using estrogens in patients who have:

- Active blood clotting disorders
- Known or suspected pregnancy (estrogens may harm the unborn)
- Known or suspected estrogen-dependent malignant tumors
- Known or suspected cancer of the breast
- Undiagnosed abnormal vaginal bleeding

The ability of female hormones to stimulate cell division in certain target organs such as the breast, endometrium, prostate and the ovary, may lead to accumulation of random genetic errors in any of those cells, that ultimately produce the malignant forms (*neoplastic phenotype*).[S070]

Studies on the capacity of estrogens to increase the incidence rate of uterine cancer have diverse and conflicting results:

> "The reported endometrial cancer risk among unopposed estrogen users is about 2- to 12-fold greater than in non-users, and appears dependent on duration of treatment and on estrogen dose. Most studies show no significant increased risk associated with use of estrogens for less than one year. The greatest risk appears associated with prolonged use—with increased risks of 15- to 24-fold for five to ten years or more. In three studies, persistence of risk was demonstrated for 8 to over 15 years after cessation of estrogen treatment. In one study a significant decrease in the incidence of endometrial cancer occurred six months after estrogen withdrawal. Concurrent progestin therapy may offset this risk but the overall health impact in postmenopausal women is not known."[P051]

As far as breast cancer is concerned:

> "While the majority of studies have not shown an increased risk of breast cancer in women who have ever used estrogen replacement therapy, some have reported a moderately increased risk (relative risks of 1.3-2.0) in those taking higher doses or those taking lower doses for prolonged periods of time, especially in excess of 10 years. Other studies have not shown this relationship."[P051]

RISKS AND PROBLEMS CAUSED BY PHARMACEUTICAL ESTROGENS

If the dosages of estrogen are excessive, or if people have an unusual sensitivity to the substance, the following symptoms may occur:

- Abdominal cramps, bloating
- Abnormal laboratory tests
- Abnormal withdrawal bleeding or flow
- Aggravation of *porphyria* (a disorder of the metabolism of *porphyrins*—derivatives of hemoglobin)
- Birth defects when used in pregnancy
- Blood pressure increases
- Breakthrough bleeding, spotting
- Breast lumps or cysts
- Changes in cervical secretions
- Changes in libido (sex drive)
- Changes in vaginal bleeding pattern
- *Chloasma* or *melasma* (*mask of pregnancy*), brown spots on the face, upper lip, mid line of abdomen, more noticeable in people with darker skin pigment, and may persist when drug is discontinued.
- *Chorea* (St. Vitus's dance)
- Decreased quantity and quality of nursing mothers' milk
- Dizziness
- Edema (swelling)
- Elevation of blood calcium — in patients who have breast cancer and bone metastases
- *Erythema multiforme*
- *Erythema nodosum*
- Fluid Retention
- Gallbladder Disease (2 to 4 fold increase in gallbladder surgery)
- Headaches
- Heart attacks
- *Hemorrhagic eruption*
- *Hirsutism* (increased body hair)
- Increase in the size of *uterine fibroids* (tumors of the womb—usually benign)
- Increased incidence of cancer of the uterus (very small increase)
- Increased blood clotting
- Increased cancer of the breast (very small increase)

- Intolerance to contact lenses
- Jaundice
- Liver dysfunction
- Loss of scalp hair
- Mental depression
- Migraines
- Nausea, vomiting
- Pancreatitis in patients with familial lipid disorders
- Pulmonary embolism (blood clots in the lungs)
- Reduced carbohydrate tolerance
- Steepening of corneal curvature
- Strokes, clots in the brain or eyes
- Swelling of breasts
- Tenderness of breasts
- Thrombophlebitis (blood clots in varicose veins)
- Triglyceride elevation in patients with familial lipid disorders
- Vaginal *candidiasis* (yeast infections)
- Weight changes

UNTIL THE TWELFTH OF NEVER?

The question of how long to stay on HRT or ERT is an important one for many women. Although the research data on this issue are not yet definitive, women who want to protect their bones from developing osteoporosis should consider using ERT at least ten years, possibly for life. The consensus usually is that, ideally, estrogen should be started within three years of the last menstrual period. In my opinion, estrogen should only be supplemented if it is deficient, no matter what the date, so this could be before, during, or long after menopause. Women already showing accelerated bone loss and considered at high risk for osteoporosis should probably make a lifetime commitment to ERT.

It is generally accepted opinion that the longer you use ERT, the more protection your bones will have, and as soon as you stop using it, your bones will begin to show signs of calcium loss and bone aging. It is never too late to begin estrogen therapy. Women in their 80s and 90s who had pre-existing osteoporosis showed some benefit after starting estrogen therapy. According to one recent study, supplemental hormones, benefited women

15 years after initial diagnosis of osteoporosis. In another study, estrogen therapy increased vertebral bone mass and bone density at the femoral head. Interestingly, the best response was in women farthest away from menopause, and who had the lowest bone mass.

From all points of view, estrogen appears to be *critical* to bone remodeling; therefore, it may well be the most essential component of prevention for osteoporosis.

> ### THE LONGER YOU USE ERT, THE MORE PROTECTION YOUR BONES WILL HAVE

It is generally accepted opinion that the longer you use ERT, the more protection your bones will have, and as soon as you stop using it, your bones will begin to show signs of calcium loss and bone aging. It is never too late to begin estrogen therapy. Women in their 80s and 90s who had pre-existing osteoporosis showed some benefit after starting estrogen therapy. According to one recent study, supplemental hormones, benefited women 15 years after initial diagnosis of osteoporosis. In another study, estrogen therapy increased vertebral bone mass and bone density at the femoral head. Interestingly, the best response was in women farthest away from menopause who had the lowest bone mass.

> ### AS SOON AS YOU STOP USING ERT, YOUR BONES
> ### WILL BEGIN TO SHOW SIGNS OF CALCIUM LOSS AND BONE AGING

Doctors are often puzzled about the factors that make people more or less compliant with a therapy,[P060] in this case, that of hormone replacement. The variables are factors linked to lifestyle and health behavior: in a study done in Sweden, compliance or lack thereof were clearly represented in certain population groups:

NO HRT OR ONLY SHORT-TERM	LONG TERM HRT
higher number of children	high level of education
earlier age at first birth	heavy physical exercise
lower prevalence of hysterectomy	high intake of food fibers
lower prevalence of oophorectomy	climacteric symptoms

ERT MAY HELP MORE THAN JUST YOUR BONES

There are additional benefits in using HRT:

- Regeneration of muscle firmness
- Regeneration of muscle tone
- Relief from mild symptoms of incontinence and prolapse of the bladder and uterus
- Relief from generalized muscle aches and pains
- Relief from generalized joint aches and pains

Muscle weakness does not just affect playing tennis or practicing aerobics. Good muscle strength is necessary for the firmness of our limbs and back, as well as the support tissues for other organs. Muscle weakness is particularly pronounced in the pelvic area of women with low estrogen levels, and urinary incontinence or uterine, bladder or urethral prolapse may result. HRT helps restore muscle tone and may relieve mild symptoms of incontinence and prolapse. However, women with severe cases may still require more drastic therapy, such as surgery. As mentioned earlier, muscle pain may accompany joint pain, particularly in the low back. HRT may help here too.

Age often results in thin skin which bruises or injures with great ease. Although estrogen supplementation will not restore skin to its youthful appearance, it can have a significant impact on skin quality. Women on estrogen therapy usually have thicker, moister and firmer skin. ERT improves subcutaneous fat deposition, which makes the skin tighter, and collagen turnover, which thickens and firms up the skin. Estrogen also increases fluid retention in the skin, making it look moister and plumper. However, to improve skin condition estrogen should be started soon after entering menopause because it cannot completely reverse any significant skin damage that has already occurred.

Facial and body hair are considered to be unattractive and often torment women who are up in years. ERT does not have quite as much dramatic effect on body hair, but it will balance the male hormone (**androgen**) levels. As a result, unwanted hair on the chin, the chest and the abdomen will stop growing. Once a woman has started ERT, these hairs can be pulled out and will not regrow as fast (or not at all), as long as estrogen therapy continues.

HORMONE REPLACEMENT THERAPY

There is much controversy on this issue: A recent advertisement from Eli Lilly, a pharmaceutical laboratory "Dedicated to Postmenopausal Health", remarks that "If estrogen is the answer, why are there so many questions?"[R000]

Medical studies show that hormonal therapy after menopause not only helps prevent osteoporosis but also protects women against further bone loss. It has been reported that a Danish study done in 1991 showed that a combination of estrogen and another hormone, a *progestogen*, given no later than three years after the onset of menopause, completely prevented bone loss in 18 women. Does this mean that the *progesterone* was necessary? NO! Replacement of estrogen alone gives almost identical results, without the added side effects of the very undesirable progesterone, including its potential for increases in breast cancer. In contrast, untreated women suffered significant bone loss.

Actions are said to speak louder than words. Acceptance of ERT is high among female physicians, who are "...twice as likely as women in the general population to use hormone replacement therapy, but [who]...tend to steer clear of hormones if they have a personal or family history of breast cancer...."[B141] In a study of 1,500 postmenopausal doctors, about 50% of them admitted to the use of hormone replacement, whereas only 10% of the general population do so. The percentage was even higher in women who had undergone hysterectomies and oophorectomies. The researchers found that those women who had used birth control pills were more likely to also use HRT. They were surprised, however, that the doctors were not steered to hormone use by a family history of cardiovascular disease, despite the well known benefits of hormone therapy in preventing these diseases. Female physicians also had healthier life styles than non-medical females.

OTHER BENEFITS OF ERT

Another plus for ERT might be, that according to information released in 1994 by V.W. Henderson, A. Paganini-Hill, C.K. Emanuel, M.E. Dunn, and J.G. Buckwalter at the Alzheimer's Disease Research Center at the University of Southern California, "estrogen replacement in women after menopause is associated with a reduced risk of developing Alzheimer's Disease."[A081] In the past few years we have seen more and more statements along this line, each researcher claiming the priority of discovery, when in fact this had been included in a patent issued as far back as 1984, issued to Dr. Chaovanee Aroonsakul from Illinois.

BREAST AND OTHER GYNECOLOGIC CANCER SURVIVORS, A NEED TO RETHINK ERT?

"'The major concern of most physicians in prescribing estrogen replacement therapy [ERT] to women with a history of breast cancer is that metastatic, quiescent cancer may be activated, that the fire of breast cancer might be ignited by the fuel of estrogen,' said Dr. Wendy Brewster, a fellow in gynecologic oncology at the University of California, Irvine School of Medicine.

"But results of several studies, including one recently completed at U.C. Irvine, suggest that estrogen replacement does not adversely affect long term outcome in cancer survivors. In many cases ERT may actually reduce recurrence and confer a survival benefit."[G071] Even in other gynecologic cancers, survival rates did not seem to suffer due to hormonal therapy.

The researchers were concerned that, with increased longevity, thirty million American women were going to spend forty years or more in the postmenopause. The worry is even greater because certain chemotherapeutic approaches result in permanent ovarian failure at an earlier age, adding more women to this large cohort.

The outgoing president of the North American Menopause Society, Dr. Wolf Utian stated that it was premature to give any advice, but Drs. Brewster and Schwartz believed that the studies were significant enough to let patients weigh the potential risks vs. benefits of ERT in their condition, and make informed decisions.[G071]

ASSESSING SOME RISK VS. BENEFIT RATIOS

Despite the findings described in the preceding paragraphs—findings which are just recently and scarcely published—there is considerable controversy about the indications for estrogen and/or estrogen/progestin use in primary prevention, even among the *Establishment*. In assessing whether a woman should receive estrogen replacement, several factors are often considered by doctors:

CORONARY HEART DISEASE RISK FACTORS

- Blood pressure
- Cholesterol
- Family history
- Smoking status
- Weight

OSTEOPOROSIS RISK FACTORS

- Body build
- Bone mineral density
- Physical activity level
- Race

INCREASED RISK FACTORS FOR BREAST CANCER

- Early menarche (beginning of menstrual periods before age 12)
- Late menopause (after age 50)
- Late parity (first baby after age 30)
- Personal and family history

PATIENT DESIRE FOR QUALITY-OF-LIFE BENEFITS

- Decreased *vasomotor* symptoms (flushing)
- Genitourinary tract symptoms

PATIENT TOLERANCE FOR SIDE EFFECTS

- Breast tenderness
- *Endometrial* (lining of uterus) bleeding

PATIENT WILLINGNESS TO PARTICIPATE IN FOLLOW-UP

- Endometrial sampling
- Mammography

It is the consensus of most *Establishment* opinions that In order to prevent irreversible bone loss, it may be desirable to begin estrogen replacement soon after the onset of menopause. I agree with this opinion. An absolute upper age limit for estrogen replacement has not been established. The use of progestin or careful endometrial monitoring is recommended by doctors for women with intact **uteri** [plural for uterus in Latin]. I believe that progestin is practically never an option.

Establishment also recommends pelvic examinations, endometrial examinations, if there is abnormal vaginal bleeding, and breast examinations. I have no quarrel with these procedures, unless they become an invitation for unnecessary surgeries or other abuses of women.

MAMMOGRAMS: A NOTE OF CAUTION, OR SOUNDING RED ALERT?

Do the mammograms you are so frequently reminded of cause the breast cancers you dread? The media, displaying a visible enthusiasm fueled by large profits, portray mammograms as a wonderful, lifesaving tool. Whereas until a few years ago a patient could benefit from an innocuous test which read the breast's temperature, a **thermogram**, now women of all ages and descriptions subject themselves to ionizing radiation in cumulative amounts worthy of a Hiroshima nightmare. Although doctors do not address any potential risk of harm from this procedure (and who would scare off potential customers at what each test brings in, in dollars and cents), risks have been known for quite a while. In fact, I remember that I always told my patients that mammograms were never and option because in the very early days of mammography I had read that each subsequent mammogram increased the incidence of breast cancer about 5%. Common sense would have it that radiation on a potentially cancerous cell could do nothing but unleash a malignant process. Facts and statistics bear this out:

**DO THE MAMMOGRAMS SO FREQUENTLY RECOMMENDED
CAUSE THE BREAST CANCERS YOU DREAD?**

In a study done in Hawaii in 1997,[M051] the researchers "...investigated the association between mammography utilization and breast cancer incidence in Hawaii with the hypothesis that geographic areas with high mammography use have higher breast cancer incidence than geographic areas with low mammography use. Insurance claims for mammograms received during 1992 and 1993 were combined with breast cancer incidence data from the Hawaii Tumor Registry and data from the 1990 Census ZIP File. The claims data were obtained from four private and three public health plans and covered approximately 85% of women 40 years of age and older. Age-specific breast cancer incidence rates for the 79 ZIP code areas were regressed on mammography rates and selected aggregate demographic variables using multiple linear regression. An estimated 42% of women 40 years of age and older had received at least 1 mammogram during 1992 and 1993, with the highest rate (45%) in women ages 50-64 years old. Overall, 23% of the variation in age-specific breast cancer incidence could be predicted by mammography utilization, 23% by increasing age, and 4% by higher education. The relationship between mammography use and breast cancer incidence was strongest for women 50-64 years old and for localized disease."[M051] *Establishment* tried to talk themselves out of being concerned about the "...magnitude of the association between breast cancer incidence and mammography utilization [by comparing those values]...to the increase in breast cancer rates observed in Hawaii during the mid-1980s...[pretending those numbers upheld that... "the sharp increase in breast cancer incidence was attributable to screening and early detection....[but even they had to admit that]...the long-term 1% increase in breast cancer incidence requires alternate explanations."[M051]

90-RAD. IS THE LEVEL OF RADIATION TO THE BREAST ABOVE WHICH THE INCIDENCE OF CANCER MAY BE INCREASE[D].[H071]

Another study evaluated the benefit vs. risk of screening for breast cancer, including both mammographic and clinical examinations, "...are analyzed [sic] by means of a ***probabilistic*** [based on probabilities] model. The model, applied to previously unpublished data provided by the HIP (Health Insurance Plan of Greater New York) breast cancer screening project, permits more precise...figuring...by age than previous analysis[,] and allows for incorporation of ***oncogenic*** [cancer causing] risks *due to mammography*. It is assumed that, from the tenth year of screening onward, radiation induces 6 cases of breast cancer per year per million women screened per rad...delivered to the breast tissue per exam. The predicted pattern of breast cancer cases and deaths is commensurate with that actually observed in the first nine years of the HIP study. In extrapolation to lifetime experience, the model predicts an ultimate decrease in the probability of dying of breast cancer only for women over age fifty at initial screening and an increase in life expectancy for the entire screened group, at an exposure level of three rads per exam. Had radiation dosage been one rad., or less per exam, which is within the range now possible with modern equipment and procedures, the radiation risk would not offset even a modest benefit such as is predicted for the younger women, either in number of deaths or years of life expectancy."[D090]

The medical press releases would never tell about the need of avoiding or limiting levels in radiation, but fact is that "Tens of thousands of mammograms are performed daily in the United States. Accumulated radiation biologic data suggest that approximately 90-*rad*. [a measurement of radiation received] *is the level of radiation to the breast above which the incidence of cancer may be increase[d]*.[H071] [emphasis added]

In fact, studies on radiation risks were done for prolonged periods of time on women who had had breasts exposed to radiation for other reasons, such as the treatment of an inflammatory condition of the breasts after giving birth (***post-partum mastitis***).

In a 1977 article published by the National Cancer Institute, they tell us that "Breast cancer has been studied by mail survey up to 34 years in 571 of 606 women treated with x-rays for acute postpartum mastitis. The incidence of **neoplasms** [malignant tumors] was compared with that of three non-irradiated [sic] control groups—nonirradiated [sic] sisters of the treated women, women with acute postpartum mastitis not treated with X-rays, and their non-irradiated [sic] sisters. For the irradiated group, with mean dose of 247 rads to both breasts, the overall relative risk of breast cancer was 2.2 for years 10-34 post irradiation and 3.6 for years 20-34. The dose response for malignant and benign breast neoplasms was compatible with a linear fit. For comparable total doses, [giving the radiation in smaller increments] ***fractionation of exposure*** did not reduce carcinogenic action. Women over age 30 years at radiation treatment had as great an excess risk of breast cancer as did younger women. The overall excess risk of developing breast cancer was about 8-10 cases per million women per rad. per year, an increase of about 0.5% per rad.."[S111] If my mathematical talents don't fail me, this would come out to 5% per 10 rads, 50% per 100 rads, 123.5 % for 247 rads! DOUBLE!!! I hope that the readers of this book will consider this information an eye-opener. Recent articles (end of 1997), precisely deal with the concern that the US has double the amount of breast cancer of other countries.

In fact, America's honeymoon with mammograms has been a little disconcerting to me, ever since in the mid seventies. At that time "The number and types of breast lesions treated surgically at the Flower and Fifth Avenue Hospitals during the period from November 1974 through February 1976, increased sharply in monthly incidence as compared with the period from January 1973 through October 1974. This increase was attributable to public awareness of breast cancer because of the publicity given to its occurrence in the wives of the President and Vice-President. However, *the consequent increase in mammography and breast surgery was not accompanied by any improvement in the stage characteristics of the breast cancers treated.* The proportion of prognostically [sic] unfavorable stage II cases with involvement of four or more axillary nodes was undiminished, while the proportion of stage 0 and stage I cases was not increased among breast cancers diagnosed since Nov 1, 1974."[B171]

THE CONCERNS ABOUT THE ESTROGEN-CANCER CONNECTION

There is much confusion underlying this often hyped up subject. It is worth stressing that even something as apparently random and disorderly as cancer develops according to a programmed logic; it has first to be *induced*, then *promoted.*

Induction is accomplished by the genetic messages of certain abnormal particles called *oncogenes*, which are to the tumor as the seed is to the plant. These oncogenes are sometimes:

- Inherited,
- Acquired
    - Biologic materials
    - Vaccines
    - Genetically engineered products
    - Transfusions
    - Blood products

> CANCER PRODUCING PARTICLES CAN BE INTRODUCED THROUGH VACCINES, BLOOD PRODUCTS, AND OTHER BIOLOGIC PRODUCTS.

Promotion is accomplished by activators such as:
- Hormones (estrogen is only one of them, and *not all cancers are hormone dependent.*)
- Malnutrition
- Pesticides
- Pollutants
- Toxins

WHAT SUGGESTS THAT A CONNECTION EXISTS BETWEEN CANCER AND FEMALE HORMONES?

Some cancers are activated by certain hormones, or are treatable by others. The occurrence of most **hormone independent** adult cancers rises continuously with age, but **hormone responsive** cancers of the breast, the ovary and the lining of the uterus rise with age until menopause, and then level off. Some medical researchers believe that this may indicate that the main causes for these cancers occur in the pre-menopausal period. The use of HRT constitutes the other major setting in which exogenous (not produced in the body) steroid hormones are widely used in essentially healthy women, and has had a remarkable impact on cancer incidence and mortality. The cells of the uterine lining divide faster in menopausal women on ERT, than in those not on medication—just as fast as during the **follicular phase** of the menstrual cycle: so, for the whole month they actually multiply twice as much in the treated woman as compared to the younger person.

Yet, as a whole, estrogen-associated endometrial cancer is rare, usually noticed at an early stage and seldom fatal when managed appropriately. The bulk of evidence suggests that estrogen use is not associated with an increased risk of breast cancer, but may activate an existing one. It has often been postulated that adding a **progestogen** probably reduces the risk of endometrial cancer, but this is not fully proven. There is little information about the safety of long-term combined estrogen and progestogen treatment in post-menopausal women, and it has been suspected that this kind of hormonal cocktail may actually increase the incidence of breast cancer. Younger patients receiving progestogens in oral contraceptives experienced an increased risk of hypertension and cardiovascular disease. Another disadvantage is that some progestogens may blunt or eliminate the favorable effects that estrogen has on blood levels of lipoproteins (fats).

The *Establishment* is quite adamant in its profession of concern about cancer-estrogen connections. Extensive warnings are prominently displayed in the PDR.[P051]

"1. ESTROGENS HAVE BEEN REPORTED TO INCREASE THE RISK OF ENDOMETRIAL CARCINOMA IN POST-MENOPAUSAL WOMEN."
[emphasis supplied]

In a column surrounded by a frame of asterisks, *not* identical to the ones I have placed here, it states:

****

"Studies of women who received diethylstilbestrol (DES) during pregnancy have shown that female offspring have an increased risk of vaginal adenosis, squamous cell dysplasia of the uterine cervix, and clear cell vaginal cancer later in life; male offspring have an increased risk of urogenital abnormalities and possibly testicular cancer later in life. The 1985 DES Task Force concluded that use of DES during pregnancy is associated with a subsequent increased risk of breast cancer in the mothers, although a causal relationship remains unproven and the observed level of excess risk is similar to that for a number of other breast cancer risk factors."

****

In a study on over 600 women in Cuomo, Italy, the researchers determined that the problem of cancer of the breast could not be clearly ruled out, but that there was a very definitive increase on thickening or density of the breast tissue, which was detectable on X-Ray. "Hormone replacement therapy (HRT) in post-menopausal or ovariectomized women reduces mortality due to cardiovascular diseases, lowers morbidity [illness] due to osteoporosis[,] and improves *vaso vagal* [neuro-circulatory—hot flashes] symptoms. Long-term therapy, however, increase[s] the risk of side-effects. HRT may decrease mammographic sensitivity, markedly increasing glandular density. Enlargement of pre-existing *cysts* [sacks full of liquid] and *fibroadenomas* [benign fibrous glandular solid tumors] has also been reported after HRT. The correlation between HRT and breast cancer is highly controversial."[D031] [emphasis added]

They further stated that "The statistical analysis [of bone mineral density—BMD] showed a significant difference between the HRT group and the control group only for the lumbar spine. Mammographic changes...were shown in 150 of 550 HRT patients. Increased breast density was the most frequent finding. Benign lesions arising *de novo* [as a new finding], or increasing in size and/or number were observed in 41 of 150 patients (27.3%) in the HRT group...3 breast carcinomas were detected, versus 1 breast cancer only in the control group [which was only 100 women, 1/3 of the other group]. HRT had a marked positive effect on bone mineral content (BMC) at 2 years' follow-up, but [and here is a classical example of how scientific language is manipulated if the results of a study are not exactly what is expected] it remains debated if it *reduces* [???] breast cancer risk."[D031] [emphasis added]

Who might *not* be a good candidate for estrogen therapy?[A021]

Contraindications for estrogen replacement include the presence of:
- Active liver disease
- Cancer of the breast (recently under review)
- Chronic impaired liver function
- Cysts of the breast and/or ovaries
- Endometrial (uterine) cancer (recently under review)
- Recent blood vessel obstruction and clots
- Unexplained vaginal bleeding

Conditions that may be less stringent contraindications are:
- ***Endometriosis***
- Familial ***hyperlipidemia***
- Gallbladder disease
- High Blood Pressure
- Migraine headaches
- Seizures
- Thrombophlebitis
- Uterine fibroids

WHERE IS THE REAL CLEAR AND PRESENT DANGER?

It is a matter of the ***risk vs. benefit ratio***. To a one, women who are low in estrogen are *always* progressively going to lose bone mass, a serious problem, probably much more serious than the potential for any malignancy connection. The *Establishment* agrees that it is especially important to use estrogen, (with or without progestogen) therapy for conditions that confer a high risk of osteoporosis, such as the occurrence of premature menopause. When I made this statement, I had not yet found this one, by Dr. Gordan, written seventeen years ago!

> **"DEAD WRONG —
> ESTROGENS, OSTEOPOROSIS CANCER AND PUBLIC POLICY"**[G080]

"Practicing physicians must constantly decide what is the best treatment for each patient. Their decisions are often influenced by prominent professors and by a climate of opinion created by the press and regulatory agencies. If these are wrong, because of pressure from 'consumer advocates', wrong interpretations, or the risks of litigation, physicians may be forced into making inactive decisions which can cause more harm than the treatment under attack. My attention was drawn to this problem by recent actions of the press and the FDA discouraging the use of estrogens because of a putative risk of endometrial cancer. Even if the danger were real, and I consider the evidence faulty, doctors would have to balance risks against benefits. We have 2,718 deaths each year, constant for ten years, from endometrial cancer and at least 50,000 female deaths because of preventable osteoporotic hip fractures. Recent data establish that the doses of estrogen needed to prevent post-menopausal bone loss are lower than those associated with any cancer."[G080]

Summing up:

ESTROGEN REPLACEMENT THERAPY REDUCES BONE LOSS AND FRACTURES

HOW DO YOU FEEL ABOUT INGESTING THE SEDIMENT OF A MARE'S URINE?

We believe we live in an "Age of Reason", and have often scoffed at so called "primitive" cultures which attributed magic properties to animal claws or excrement; but what do we do? We place our faith in pharmacologic estrogens produced by the drug industry, usually extracted from the urine of pregnant mares. You can prove the veracity of my words by scratching the sugar coating of a pill, and smelling it). The effects of *conjugated estrogens* are similar to those of internal or endogenous estrogens. They protect the bones even at low doses, such as 0.625 mgr. of *conjugated equine estrogen*, (25 micrograms of *mestranol* and 2 mgr. of *estradiol valerate* daily. They are soluble in water and are well absorbed from the gastrointestinal tract. In responsive tissues (female genital organs, breasts, hypothalamus, pituitary), estrogens penetrate deep into the cell, and are transported into the cell's core or *nucleus*. There they can bind to specialized sites called estrogen receptors, and, by switching genes on and off, can control the formation of specific forms of *RNA* (the genetic material in the cell body), and certain proteins.

The horror story of how the urine of pregnant mares is harvested and sold for high profits was never told until "Inside Edition", a television journalistic program, had the guts to defy corporate opposition, mostly due to the courageous support of actress and animal lover Mary Tyler Moore.

Commercial preparations may differ by mode of administration, dosage, variants of the hormone, so called "inert ingredients", etc. The main thing to remember is that they all contain estrogenic substances, and therefore the benefits and side effects are similar.

Medicines not only contain the *active principle* (the specific drug), but also other multiple chemicals euphemistically (substituting an innocuous for a dangerous word) called *inert* ingredients. They constitute the bulk of the pill, and the color. These ingredients are seldom inert, and often are more toxic and problematic than the medication itself. As though the potential side effects of the estrogen in Estrace (estradiol tablets, USP, 2 mgr.), were not sufficiently noisome, this two mgr. pill also contains the coloring agent *FD&C Yellow No. 5* (*tartrazine*) which may cause allergic-type reactions (including bronchial asthma) in sensitive individuals. Although the overall incidence of FD&C Yellow No. 5 sensitivity in the general population is low, it is frequently seen in patients who also have aspirin hypersensitivity.

SOURCES OF ESTROGENS

Estrogens can be:
- Pharmaceutical
     from natural sources
     synthetic
- Natural derived from animals in a whole form and
- Natural derived from plants

Source: (University of Iowa, Last Modified: February 27, 1997

(librarian@vh.org.http://indy.radiology.uiowa.eu/Providers/ClinGuide/PreventionPractice/AImmunProph/46.html)

**TAKING ESTROGENS IN MENOPAUSE HAS IMPORTANT BENEFITS,
BUT ALSO SOME RISKS.**

Estrogen supplementation after menopause can reduce the risk of osteoporosis, with an added benefit in the prevention (35% reduction in relative risk) of coronary heart disease, which nowadays causes approximately 30% of deaths of women over 50 years of age. A recent *meta-analysis* (a review of information after the events happened) found a 25% decrease in the relative risk of suffering a hip fracture for women over the age of 50 years who have ever used estrogen. There are additional benefits to estrogen supplementation:

■ Decrease of vasomotor symptoms (hot flushes or flashes)
■ Improvement of genitourinary symptoms (vaginal dryness, urgency, incontinence, frequency)

On the down side, there may be significant negative health outcomes. Women with intact uteri who use estrogen for 10 to 20 years are reported to have (depending on whose study) a two to eight-fold increase in the incidence of endometrial cancer. This does not represent a worry to women who have had hysterectomies. Controversy surrounds the question of whether women taking estrogen supplementation are at increased risk for breast cancer. It is reported not to be affected by short-term estrogen use (less than 5 years), but may be increased by approximately 25% with usage (over 10 years).

COMMON PHARMACEUTICAL PREPARATIONS OF FEMALE HORMONES

ESTRACE® (ESTRADIOL VAGINAL CREAM, USP, 0.01%) is used in the treatment of vulval and vaginal atrophy in menopausal women with or without osteoporosis.

Its main medical indications are for:
■ Hypoestrogenism (low estrogen) due to
    hypogonadism (low glandular performance)
    castration (removal of the ovaries) or
    primary ovarian failure.
■ Prevention of osteoporosis
■ Vasomotor symptoms (hot flushes)
■ Vulval and vaginal atrophy

* The female offspring of women who received DES during pregnancy have an increased risk of *clear cell vaginal cancer* later in life, *squamous cell dysplasia of the cervix*, and *vaginal adenosis*; males have an increased risk of genital and urinary abnormalities, possibly *testicular cancer* later in life. Some of these changes are benign, others are followed by malignancy.

** Because estrogens may cause some degree of fluid retention, conditions which might be exacerbated by this factor, such as asthma, epilepsy, migraine, and cardiac or renal dysfunction, require careful observation.

ESTRACE (ESTRADIOL TABLETS, USP)

ESTRACE® (*ESTRADIOL TABLETS, USP*) for oral administration contains 0.5, 1 or 2 mgr. of *micronized* (divided into extra small particles) estradiol per tablet. And, of course, the multiple chemicals that are masqueraded by the words "inert or inactive ingredients".

ESTRACE® Tablets, 0.5 mgr., contain the following "inactive" ingredients: *acacia, dibasic calcium phosphate, FD&C Blue No. 1 (aluminum lake), FD&C Yellow No. 5 (tartrazine) (aluminum lake), lactose anhydrous, magnesium stearate, colloidal silicon dioxide*, starch (corn), and talc.

ESTRACE® Tablets, 1 mgr., contain the following "inactive" ingredients: acacia, *D&C Red No. 27 (aluminum lake)*, dibasic calcium phosphate, FD&C Blue No. 1 (aluminum lake), lactose anhydrous, magnesium stearate, colloidal silicon dioxide, starch (corn), and talc.

ESTRACE® Tablets, 2 mgr., contain the following "inactive" ingredients: acacia, dibasic calcium phosphate, lactose anhydrous, magnesium stearate, colloidal silicon dioxide, starch (corn), and talc.

Tartrazine is an industrial color which can cause asthmatic attacks.

ESTRATAB® (ESTERIFIED ESTROGENS TABLETS)

A mixture of estrogenic substances, principally estrone, of the type excreted by pregnant mares.

It has the same problems, risks, side effects and benefits as all the other estrogenic preparations.

PREMARIN® (CONJUGATED ESTROGENS TABLETS, USP)
EQUINE SOURCE

For oral administration: a mixture of estrogens obtained exclusively from natural sources, the average composition of material derived from pregnant mares' urine. It contains the following varieties of estrogen

- 17 alpha-dihydroequilenin
- 17 alpha-dihydroequilin
- 17 alpha-estradiol
- Equilenin
- Equilin
- Estrone

PROGESTERONE, MUCH ADO ABOUT FALSE PROMISES

THE BIG LIE: PROGESTINS (PROGESTERONE)
Q. WHO benefits from PROGESTERONE therapy?
A. The manufacturer

Are you in the market for getting the following symptoms . . .?

- Bloating
- Breast tenderness and swelling
- Depression
- Irritability
- Nausea
- Pregnancy symptoms
- Pulmonary embolism
- Tenderness
- Thrombophlebitis
- Unpredictable vaginal bleeding
- Weight gain

If you are, just make sure to take a progestin type drug. Progesterone, now romanced both by the *Establishment* and by the alternative practitioners and devotees, is the hormone of pregnancy, and induces the body to mimic this condition. So that the public understands the absurdity of using this therapy, it must be considered that some women go through their menstruating years without any progesterone—they just are infertile. It makes no sense (at least in this author's opinion) to give this substance to a woman after menopause, since estrogen by itself provides all the hormonal support that is needed; and the side effects of progesterone are highly undesirable.

> **ESTROGEN BY ITSELF PROVIDES ALL THE HORMONAL SUPPORT THAT IS NEEDED; AND THE SIDE EFFECTS OF PROGESTERONE ARE HIGHLY UNDESIRABLE**

Except for the hypothetical prevention of a purported increase in uterine cancers in those women who have not yet been assaulted by a hysterectomy, it has absolutely *no* indication. The most common side effects of progestin are:

- Impairment of glucose tolerance
- Immunosuppression
- Increase of cell division in breast epithelial tissue
- Problems with lipoprotein metabolism
  (lowering HDL and raising LDL)

PROGESTERONE - NATURE'S IMMUNOSUPPRESSANT

Not only does progesterone create unpleasant hormonal side effects, it also suppresses the so important immune system.[S110] It has always been postulated that the body fights against foreign tissues or bacteria through the activation of specific immune processes which are necessary to fend off certain illnesses. When tissue is grafted from one creature to another, such as kidneys or livers, they are usually rejected by the recipient of the transplant *(graft-versus-host* interactions: in a kidney transplant, for example, the kidney would be the graft, the patient, the host) unless an *immunosuppressant* drug is given, to prevent rejection. Most immunosuppressants are pharmaceutical drugs or viruses which interfere with these natural processes. Immune suppressants are also given when people suffer from some connective tissue diseases (Drugs such as Cyclosporine). *Opportunistic infections* (such as we see in AIDS), can prosper in individuals who are immunosuppressed.

It has long been known that progesterone is the substance which helps the body adjust to the pregnancy and prevent fetal rejection.

While an enzyme from the *pokeweed* plant (*pokeweed mitogen*) normally activates white blood cells, progesterone decreases this phenomenon, as well as other immune substances normally present in the body: *sialic acid* and *sialil-transferase* .[S110]

If the body is in good immune condition, foreign tissues, such as a skin graft, are rejected. If the body is immunosuppressed, a graft survives. So pronounced is the immune suppression of progesterone, that experiments performed to see if it helps skin grafts survive, showed that it prolonged, significantly, the survival of hamster-rat and mice-mice skin grafts. "The duration of immune response suppression could be correlated to progesterone concentration...[Other hormones such as] pregnenolone, estradiol, or cortisol were not effective in prolonging skin graft survival."[K090] This held true, at least, under these research parameters.

Drs. Pavia and P.K. Siiteri who in 1978 studied the effects of certain hormones in preventing fetal rejection, have concluded that sex hormones are such powerful immunosuppressants, that they "...may be important in preventing graft rejection or *graft-versus-host* interaction which may arise as a consequence of fetal engraftment during pregnancy."[P050]

DO CERTAIN HORMONES ACTIVATE CANCER CELLS?

As early as 1976, researchers knew that certain corticosteroids and sex hormones, including estrogen and progesterone, activated the formation of tissue centers of cancer, although in this particular study they did not create the original cancer centers. This must be borne in mind when using these hormones, so that people who have an existing cancer do not use them.[S050]

MORE BAD NEWS ABOUT CORTISONE AND PROGESTERONE

Another evidence for immunosuppression by cortisol and progesterone, was found in a study utilizing another type of steroid called CHP[,] as a control.[M030] In this 1975 study significant numbers of mice receiving a single large injection of cortisol or progesterone succumbed to progressive tumor growth under the experimental conditions used. The experimental model described provides a simple method of assessing the possible immunosuppressive effects of naturally occurring and synthetic agents on viral-induced tumor growth.

One study on mice in the early and mid seventies, another set of involuntary victims fallen prey to pharmaceutical and medical greed, revealed yet another facet of the immunosuppressive effects of progesterone, namely that experimental tumors rapidly caused the death of animals which received progesterone. "...significant numbers of mice receiving a single large injection of cortisol or progesterone succumbed to progressive tumor growth..."[M040]

As early as 1975, several American researchers determined that cortisol and progesterone, caused progressive tumor growth which killed test animals under the experimental conditions used in their experiments.[M040]

A few other tumors did not seem equally vulnerable to all hormones. Foreskin is notorious for its strong immunity, having been a source for the anti-viral *interferon* because of its high content of this substance, long before the genetically engineered preparations became available. In a study that evaluated the effect of hormones on a cat-virus induced malignancy on human foreskin cells, it was noticed that gluco-corticoid hormones, dexamethasone, hydrocortisone, cortisol acetate, and prednisolone significantly enhanced [the] growth of tumors, but that the female hormones [used in this study] did not do the same.[S050]

Concern about the bad effects of progesterone on the immune system gave rise to a "pooh-pooh" and disclaimer article in 1981, which without adding any new information to the matter, dismissed proper research by a stroke of the keyboard, in favor of a more politically correct and financially profitable view.[B080]

A widely publicized article has in recent months caused a great deal of concern among individuals interested in responsible promotion of family planning. The article contains a long series of factual errors, distortions and biased quotations. This commentary presents evidence, based on current knowledge, that Depo-Provera is a satisfactory contraceptive with several advantages and some disadvantages, and poses no more unresolved problems than oral contraceptives. There is no evidence that, at contraceptive doses, it increases the risk of cancer, impairs bone mineralization, "shocks" the hypothalamus, damages the liver or the immune system, or causes premature aging. Studies to date have not shown damaging effects on infants exposed to the drug in utero or via breast milk. To most women, disruption of the menstrual cycle, the major side effect, is not a health hazard. Finally, women in various parts of the world have shown to be quite capable of choosing for themselves whether or not the advantages of the drug can overcome the disadvantage of almost certain menstrual disturbance.

Another study of immune disruption by the use of progesterone dates back to 1980, when an experiment showed that it could act just like pharmaceutical drugs in mice, protecting grafted tissues against rejection.[K090]

The immuno-suppressive effects of hormones are more or less noticeable, depending on the stage of the disease or condition evaluated. The break-up of white blood cells through activated cells or *natural killer cells*, a process known as *cell-mediated lympholysis* (*CML*), is necessary to the proper functioning of the immune system and destruction of foreign tissue. Progesterone and estradiol added to cultures of white blood cells, before exposing them to malignancy, block the generation of aggressive white blood cells necessary to destroy cancerous tissue; cortisol, on the other hand, is only partially inhibiting. However, these hormones added at a later phase, when cells have already been activated, do not bother the process. Testosterone does not impair these immune processes.[P050]

EFFECTS OF HORMONES ON THE
FORMATION OF DEFENSIVE CELLS

	progesterone	estradiol	cortisol	testosterone
added *before* exposure of body cells to cancer cells	inhibits formation of defensive cells[S130]	inhibits formation of defensive cells	partially inhibits formation of defensive cells	does not inhibit formation of defensive cells
added *after* exposure of body cells to cancer cells	does not inhibit formation of defensive cells	does not inhibit formation of defensive cells		does not inhibit formation of defensive cells

The people who have vested interests in the manufacture and distribution of certain drugs, fear truth. In a 1981 "analysis" of the debate on a progesterone product (*Depo-Provera®*, a hormonal contraceptive found to cause innumerable side effects), the interested parties went into real panic and vehemently denied, but did not refute the information that was emerging. They stated that "A widely publicized article has in recent months caused a great deal of concern among individuals interested in responsible promotion of family planning. The article contains a long series of factual errors, distortions and biased quotations. This commentary presents evidence, based on current knowledge, that Depo-Provera® is a satisfactory contraceptive with several advantages and some disadvantages, and poses no more unresolved problems than oral contraceptives. There is no evidence that, at contraceptive doses, it increases the risk of cancer, impairs bone mineralization, "shocks" the hypothalamus, damages the liver or the immune system, or causes premature aging. Studies to date have not shown damaging effects on infants exposed to the drug *in utero* (in the womb) or via breast milk. To most women, disruption of the menstrual cycle, the major side effect, is not a health hazard. Finally, women in various parts of the world have shown to be quite capable of choosing for themselves whether or not the advantages of the drug can overcome the disadvantage of almost certain menstrual disturbance."[B080]

The authors did not present any valid evidence to support these claims.

Other studies did nothing but increase the evidence that progesterone was not safe. In 1980 it was published that sustained release progesterone-collagen combinations significantly prolonged the survival of hamster-rat and mice-mice skin grafts. The duration of immune response suppression could be correlated to the level of progesterone in the collagen matrix. Collagen sponges containing pregnenolone, estradiol, or cortisol were not effective in prolonging skin graft survival.[K090]

PROGESTIN MEDICATION IS THE WAY TO ASSAULT WOMEN WHO HAVE NOT YET BEEN ASSAULTED BY A HYSTERECTOMY

When one analyzes the studies that deal with progesterone and progestins, and their use in osteoporosis, which are available through a computer search, one can not help but be amazed at the bizarre design of these studies. Normally, the subjects tested and the controls, are selected to be as similar as possible, and the treatments to be comparable. In this field, though, nothing such happens, subcutaneous estrogen plus testosterone is compared against oral estrogen plus progesterone, women who have been subject to the removal of their ovaries are compared to women who are naturally menopausal. In this fashion, conclusions mean little or nothing. It is as though a deliberate effort has been made not to compare the two real variables, plain estrogen to combined therapy, and combined daily therapy to alternating, cyclic combined therapies. It seems that industry does not want anyone to know...

Q. WHY GIVE PROGESTERONE TO A POST-MENOPAUSAL WOMAN?

A. IT MAKES MONEY

If estrogens can be a source of riches, why not sell two drugs instead of one? After all, 4000 women a day are reaching menopause, as the baby boomers become older. The interest in connecting progesterone with osteoporosis grows as the years go by, and more women are out to be cheated into turning good money into poor medicine. The figures of a "Medline" search of the two key words *osteoporosis* and *progesterone* show the following figures:

Medline Years	Citations Retrieved
1994-97	77
1990-93	74
1985-89	57
1980-84	12
1975-79	8
1966-74	5

ESTROGEN-PROGESTIN COMBINATION THERAPY

It has been stated with more emphasis than certainty, that the concomitant use of progestin with estrogen decreases the risk of endometrial cancer in women who still have a uterus (to a level comparable to that of women not taking estrogen). Progestin use, however, also seems to decrease the cardiovascular benefits of estrogen, although the risk of coronary heart disease is probably still reduced by combination therapy.

But, how firm is the concept of reduced cancer risk? A 1997 article, reporting on a study done in the Bronx, N.Y., tells us that, in the opinion of the scientists who carried it out, "Hormone replacement therapy (HRT) provides relief of menopausal symptoms, reverses atrophic urogenital changes, prevents osteoporosis, and produces favorable lipoprotein effects. Continuous combined HRT using 2.5 mg of medroxyprogesterone was designed to increase patient compliance by eliminating withdrawal bleeding while at the same time retaining the beneficial effects of HRT. There are limited long-term data, however, regarding the safety [or, as I would say, lack thereof] of continuous combined HRT. *Of concern are reports of endometrial carcinoma arising in women receiving continuous HRT with low-dose progestin.* Eight cases of women who developed endometrial carcinoma while on this regimen are presented. The possible increased risk of endometrial cancer associated with this regimen may be related to inadequate progestin dose, prior use of unopposed estrogen, poor patient compliance, use of less effective progestins, less efficient reversal of hyperplasia, and the use of progestin continuously."[C101]

ADDING PROGESTIN IS NOT PROTECTIVE AGAINST BREAST CANCER AND MAY ACTUALLY INCREASE ITS RISK

Therapy using a cyclic combination of estrogen and progestin can produce menstrual-like vaginal bleeding, a side effect which some women find unacceptable.

PREMPRO®
Pharmaceutical preferences swell and wane with the expiration of patent terms. Whereas until the last two decades estrogen or estrogen-testosterone combinations were the hormones favored for post menopausal osteoporosis prevention and treatment, today's push is for estrogens plus progestins.[R030] These are new and patentable products.

The public is very confused already about the use of estrogen, and is now even more confused about estrogen-progestin combinations. There is much marketing hype for such illogical and unnecessary combinations. Despite the constant endorsements of such unholy mixes, even staunch *Establishment* institutions such as the American College of Physicians, (ACP), state a position which is not in line with the industry's hyping of combined products:

> "All women, regardless of race, should consider preventive hormone therapy. **Women who have had a hysterectomy are likely to benefit from estrogen therapy. There is no reason to add a progestin**

to the hormone regimen in such women. Women who have coronary heart disease or who are at increased risk for coronary heart disease are likely to benefit from hormone therapy. If such women have a uterus, a progestin should be added to the estrogen therapy unless careful endometrial monitoring is performed. The risks of hormone therapy may outweigh its benefits in women who are at increased risk for breast cancer. For other women, the best course of action is not clear." [Emphasis added]

From my point of view there is NO good reason to use progestins for menopause or osteoporosis.

Prempro® is a combination of estrogen plus progestin to be used daily, and containing *Premarin*® 0.625mg (conjugated estrogens) and *Cycrin*® 2.5mg (*medroxyprogesterone*). The cost of this combination product is less than the two medications prescribed separately. The manufacturer, Wyeth-Ayerst, also provides a very readable pamphlet for patients contemplating HRT, called "Hormone Replacement Therapy and Your Health", which supports the *Establishment's* point of view. There is a section on "Menopause and Osteoporosis", and a questionnaire on osteoporosis risk factors.

Why is there such a combination? Allegedly, it is to prevent undesirable menstrual bleeding. The enthusiasts of this type of product claim that daily estrogen has an advantage over cyclic estrogen in the prevention and treatment of osteoporosis, in that the antiresorptive (bone protective) effect of estrogen is continuous rather than intermittent. They also say that daily progestin, given concomitantly with estrogen, has an advantage over cyclic progestin in that it does not promote menstrual periods. Actually, a disadvantage of this regimen is the *irregular* nature of the bleeding, which may lead to greater difficulty in determining what the reason for irregular bleeding might be. We have been advised by the *Establishment* that their records show an increase of malignancies of the uterus with hormone therapy. They neglect evidence that progesterone activates human bone cancer (*osteosarcoma*) cells. It has been overemphasized that using progesterone is safer because it allegedly decreases this increase. Even if this were so, it would be offset by a minimal increase in breast cancers. After learning more about these hormones, the reader must decide whether it makes any sense to give it to women who have had hysterectomies, or to any women at all.

OSTEOPOROSIS AS A SOCIAL AND FINANCIAL PROBLEM

Osteoporosis is a medical, social and economical problem for developed countries. Prevention remains the only realistic approach to reduce the burden related to this disorder. Primary prevention of osteoporosis is based on efforts to reach a maximal peak bone mass at the end of the growth period and, subsequently, at the time of menopause.

In comparing several of the available options, researchers in Belgium consider that a systematic screening of asymptomatic postmenopausal women followed by the induction of hormonal replacement therapy in high risk subjects appears to be an interesting cost/benefit strategy in terms of reasonable attribution of health resources. They reach this decision after comparing it to nasal administration of calcitonin and bisphosphonates, and *experimental estrogen receptor modulators*, not on the market yet.

OTHER THERAPIES TO STRENGTHEN BONES

Other drugs have been used besides HRT to prevent bone loss and to protect against the development of osteoporosis. Some therapies have been found more effective than others.

Estrogen plays an important role in the growth and maturation of bone, as well as in the regulation of bone turnover in the adult skeleton. Bone growth does not take place in the already hardened bone shaft or heads, but in areas between the end of the shaft and the neck of the heads. These areas are known as the *epiphyseal growth plates*.[v010] During periods of accelerated bone growth estrogen is needed for proper closure of epiphyseal growth plates both in females and in males, which terminates longitudinal growth about age 18. Even in young skeletons, estrogen deficiency leads to increased osteoclast formation and enhanced bone resorption. In menopause, estrogen deficiency induces cancellous as well as cortical bone loss. Highly increased bone resorption in cancellous bone (the bone portion that looks like a bee hive) leads to general bone loss and destruction of local architecture because of *penetrative resorption* (dissolving bone mass deeply into the bone), and *microfractures* (small breaks in the structural, tiny scales, that make up the bone).

In cortical bone the first response of estrogen withdrawal is enhanced endocortical (inner lining of the "crust" or cortex of the bone) resorption.

Later, also intracortical (middle lining of the crust) porosity increases. These lead to decreased bone mass, disturbed architecture and reduced bone strength. At cellular level, estrogen inhibits differentiation of osteoclasts thus decreasing their number and reducing the amount of active remodeling units. This effect is probably achieved by substances known as *cytokines*, substances intimately interconnected with the immune system, also known as *interleukins*, *IL-1* and *IL-6* being the strongest candidates. It is believed that the effects of estrogen on osteoblasts is either direct or due to a balancing act between bone formation to resorption.

Estrogen may be protective against further bone loss, but is not a rebuilder; its effects on bone remodeling are slightly different than expected.[V021] Treatment reduces:
- Bone turnover
- Erosion depth
- Resorption cavity size
- Wall width

In a UK study of conventional hormone replacement therapy it was shown that beneficial skeletal effects are not from the rebuilding of bone, but from suppression of bone turnover and a reduction in the size of resorption cavities.

Several agents and modalities of treatment are currently under investigation, but their efficacy and/or safety have not been established, or are highly questionable. These include:
- *"ADFR"* (a complex system of several drugs)
- *Sodium fluoride*
- *The 1-34 fragment of parathyroid*,
- *Thiazides* (fluid pills that reduce calcium elimination and loss)
- *Weakly androgenic anabolic steroids*

NON-ESTROGEN DRUGS DESIGNED TO TREAT OSTEOPOROSIS

BISPHOSPHONATES: FOSAMAX® (ALENDRONATE)

Fosamax® (*alendronate*) has recently been approved by the FDA for the treatment of osteoporosis in post-menopausal women. Like other bisphosphonates this drug is an antiresorptive agent, allowing bone formation to catch up with bone breakdown in the bone remodeling process.

Alendronate is prescribed at a dose of 10 mgr. daily, taken with a glass of water on an empty stomach, with no food, drink, or medication for at least one half hour (30 mins.) afterwards. The reason for this is that Fosamax®, like other bisphosphonates, is very poorly absorbed. These dosing restrictions may be a problem for some individuals. The duration of efficacy of treatment is estimated to be at least 3 years, but clinical research currently in progress may extend these recommendations. The pharmaceutical companies state that it is important to provide adequate calcium and vitamin D supplementation while giving bisphosphonates.

The medical diagnosis of osteoporosis, before the use of alendronate, can best be established by DEXA, the method of bone mass measurement currently most favored. Although the drug has not been approved for use in men or pre-menopausal women with osteoporosis, many physicians will consider these situations to be acceptable "off-label" indications for the drug.

The drug's alleged principal skeletal effect is to increase spinal bone mass 7-10% over three years, and to increase hip bone mass 5-8% over the same period. This is said to result in fracture reduction of 30-40%. This increase of bone should have a life-time effect, delaying the age to fracture threshold.

"Taking alendronate either 60 or 30 minutes before a standardized breakfast reduced bioavailability by 40% relative to the 2-hour wait. Taking alendronate either concurrently with or 2 hours after breakfast drastically (> 85%) impaired availability. Black coffee or orange juice alone, when taken with the drug, also reduced bioavailability (approximately 60%). Increasing gastric pH (decreasing acidity), by infusion of *ranitidine* [*Zantac* —an antacid] was associated with a doubling of alendronate bioavailability."[G040] (emphasis added)

Adverse reactions are said to be minimal. However the manufacturers recommend that the drug should be used with caution in individuals with upper gastrointestinal problems such as heartburn. To avoid esophageal symptoms of this kind, it is recommended that one not lie down within a half an hour of taking the drug. Individuals who are on non-steroidal anti-inflammatory agents (NSAIDS) may generally continue to take them. They also discourage individuals with severe renal disease are discouraged from taking the drug, as higher than desired levels of it might accumulate in the body. The effect of this is not yet known.

Fosamax® (alendronate) is manufactured by Merck and Co, Inc. The company has prepared a package insert which it recommends should be read before taking the drug.

Adequate calcium and vitamin D are also required to be taken in conjunction with this drug.

ETIDRONATE (DIDRONEL®):

Didronel® (*etidronate*), has been used for many years, although the FDA has not approved *etidronate* for the treatment of osteoporosis in either males or females. The dose is 400 mgr. daily for 14 successive days each quarter. Prescribing information states it is best to discontinue calcium supplementation during this 14 day period. Etidronate is recommended to be taken on an empty stomach, with no food two hours before or two hours after the medication. The duration of efficacy of treatment is at least 4-5 years, but clinical research currently in progress may alter these recommendations. There is considerable debate among the experts whether patients doing well on Didronel® should automatically be switched over to Fosamax®. The cost of Didronel® is less than one third that of Fosamax®, certainly a factor for some patients.

Do they work for immobility induced osteoporosis? Some experimental bisphosphonates do.

In a Russian study in which unscrupulous scientists abused laboratory rats to prove drug benefits, in order to increase the value of stock market certificates of drug companies, the little critters were immobilized to study the effects of a drug of the family of the bisphosphonates. The design was to evaluate the effects of the substance in preventing osteoporosis which developed due to immobility (*hypokinesia*).

"The agent prevented osteoporosis and did not affect the epiphyseal growth plate. The agent modified significantly the bone cell count: osteoblasts decreased and osteoclasts increased...It is assumed that the agent modifies the relation between bone formation and bone resorption. Its osteotropic effect manifests as *inhibition of bone resorption.*"[S120] [emphasis added]

The manufacturers recommend that calcium and vitamin D should always be supplemented when the drugs **calcitonin** or the **bisphosphonates** are used.

CALCITONINS

WHAT ARE CALCITONINS?

They are thyroid hormones naturally occurring in the body, intimately linked with female functioning and skeletal preservation. "Plasma-calcitonin levels, measured with an established and reliable...technique, were significantly higher throughout normal pregnancy and lactation than in normal[,] non-pregnant women, and were not immediately influenced by the acute stimulation of breast-feeding. Thus, more calcitonin circulates at times of physiologically increased calcium need. It is suggested that an important function of calcitonin is the protection of the healthy maternal skeleton from excessive resorption by opposing the resorptive action of 1,25-dihydroxy-cholecalciferol on bone."[S212]

CALCITONIN-SALMON (CALCIMAR®, MIACALCIN®)

Another treatment, a pharmaceutical option different from the bisphosphonates is **calcitonin-salmon.** Bisphosphonates and calcitonin are generally not given together. The dose of calcitonin injected under the skin (**subcutaneously**) is 50-100 international units (**IUs**) daily to 50-100 **IUs** every other day. Since calcitonin-salmon may also reduce pain, especially bone pain, it may be preferable to give the medication daily under certain circumstances. Calcitonin may also be given as a nasal spray (**intranasally - Miacalcin® Nasal Spray**). According to manufacturer's instructions, nasal calcitonin is not indicated during the first five years of menopause. The duration of treatment for both routes is at least 2-3 years. Both forms of calcitonin may be given cyclically. Doctors say that it is important to provide adequate calcium and vitamin D supplementation while giving calcitonin.

Establishment medical doctors agree that calcitonin-salmon should be considered in preference to the bisphosphonates:

■ When osteoporosis pain management is a desired supplemental benefit

■ When the dosing constraints of the bisphosphonates are a problem

■ When treating patients with severe renal disease for whom bisphosphonates are contraindicated

■ When treating patients with certain upper gastrointestinal conditions
caused or aggravated by the bisphosphonates

The patients should consider that any foreign protein placed directly into
the body, in an undigested form, such as by a hypodermic needle, will give
rise to antibodies and produce an allergic state. I question the wisdom of
injecting a foreign protein (fish) into a population that has not yet developed fish allergies, but has already been made allergic to beef, eggs, chick-
en, etc., by the irrational practice called vaccination and by the use of other
biologic products such as *INSULIN*. If the reader would think that this
concern represents unjustified paranoia, please consider the results of a
German study at the University of Heidelberg.

Salmon calcitonin (SCT), which differs in 14 of the 32 amino acids from
human calcitonin, has found a wider distribution world wide, although
antibody formation against SCT has been reported in more than 70% of
the patients on continuous SCT treatment. The clinical significance of
these antibodies has been discussed controversially, because the occurrence of antibodies is not always associated with the development
of...resistance [to the drug]....The formation of neutralizing antibodies
against calcitonin is common after treatment with salmon but a rare phenomenon after treatment with human calcitonin."[G083]

ORAL CALCITONIN?

LONDON — May 13, 1997 — Positive results on an ongoing
double-blind European Phase II/III Macritonin(TM) clinical trials were announced today show the *oral formulation of salmon
calcitonin* is a effective in the treatment of osteoporosis.

".... Macritonin(TM) was developed by Cortecs International,
the United Kingdom based pharmaceutical company. Calcitonin
is a well tolerated treatment for osteoporosis presently given by
injection and (in some countries) intranasally.

The trial analyzes [sic] included data from 212 women aged between 55 and 77 years who had osteoporosis diagnosed by measurement of bone mineral density. Treatment in the trial is planned to continue for two years, during which the effects of Macritonin™ on bone mineral density will also be evaluated. There are three UK centers in the trial. The fourth and lead centre [sic] is the Centre [sic] for Clinical and Basic Research at Ballerup in Denmark which is among the World's foremost institutions for research in bone disease.

CrossLaps™ [cross links in the US] is the term for a group of chemicals which are excreted in the urine when bone is broken down. A large European study (EPIDOS) showed that high levels of CrossLaps™ excretion correlate with increased risk of fractures.

Results of treatment with 400iu and 800iu Macritonin™, when combined, showed a statistically significant reduction in the excretion of CrossLaps™ in the urine compared to the placebo control group who were receiving concomitant administration of vitamin D and calcium."

EVISTA® (RALOXIFEN)

Chemically related to Tamoxifen, a highly toxic substance used in the treatment of breast cancer patients, it is more ado about an unwholesome chemical with many side effects. I'd just forget it!

ANDROGENS (MALE HORMONES) — TESTOSTERONE (TEST TOASTER ON), THE SEXY HORMONE

The male anabolic hormone *testosterone* might also be considered as a therapeutic approach. Osteoporosis is an "off-label" indication for testosterone (It has not been specifically approved by the FDA for treating osteoporosis.) The expert opinion is that the age of the patient should be considered in making the determination, and that contraindications include carcinoma of the male breast, and known or suspected carcinoma of the prostate. An injection of 200 mgr. every 3-4 weeks should be sufficient.

What is a very effective hormonal treatment for osteoporotic men?[A060] Fine English gentlemen can also fall prey to osteoporosis, but they can be much improved by the use of male hormones. In a therapeutic trial of regular moderate androgen supplementation in men with established osteoporosis, 23 men, aged 34-73 years (with vertebral crush fractures and back pain, in whom secondary causes of osteoporosis had been excluded) were treated with bi-monthly intramuscular injections of 250 mg testosterone esters (Sustanon 250(R)) for six months. In all, 21 men completed the study period. "Mean bone mineral density at the lumbar spine increased from 0.799 g/cm(2) to 0.839 g/cm(2) during treatment..., a rise of 5% in...[six]...months. Bone mineral density at the hip did not change. As an added benefit, testosterone markedly improves potency in a large percentage of patients."[K060] Females may also benefit of small doses of male hormone: combinations of estrogen and testosterone were very popular in the sixties and early seventies, and still available from Upjohn Laboratories as *Depo Testadiol*. It does not only address the osteoporosis, it increases sex drive!

A medical team from Torrance, California, strongly endorses male hormones for their beneficial effects in the elderly. "Androgens have important biological effects on accessory sexual organs and have a broad range of effects on metabolic processes. Male hormones have been shown to have important organizational and activational effects on...[the looks, behavior and intelligence of]...experimental animals.... The effects of testosterone on sexual drive are well established in humans, although the threshold for such activity appears to be lower than that required for many of the other and organic effects of testosterone. There are suggestive data to link fetal androgen levels to cognitive [intelligence] and behavioral activities in children and adults, but the behavioral activities may be modified by social and other learning processes. Androgen levels fall in older men at a time when impaired sexual function, osteopenia [bone loss], and decreased muscle mass can be identified. The relative importance of androgen deficiency in these disorders requires further study, since they are likely to be multifactorial in pathogenesis [causation]. Replacement therapy of elderly men who have lowered testosterone levels has been proposed to decrease bone and muscle loss as well as to improve sexual function and general well-being. Careful studies will be required to assess the risk-to-reward ratio of such treatment, since theoretically [one may fear]...adverse effects on prostate and cardiovascular diseases. While conservation in management has its virtues, we should be reminded that several decades ago estrogen replacement of postmenopausal women was highly criticized until data supporting its favorable therapeutic ratio were demonstrated."[S231]

Unfortunately, the Medical Establishment thinks it is more important to toady to fads and hysteria in professional sports, than to care for the sick: testosterone, previously available by simple prescription has joined the ranks of "dangerous" drugs, in the undeserved company of scoundrels such as heroin and cocaine. The athletes get their drugs on the black market, the elderly suffer.

WHAT PROBLEMS MAY TESTOSTERONE CAUSE?

Bearded women are not the beauty ideal of our times. Women medicated with male hormones, may be at risk for various *virilization* problems, the development of male traits, such as:

- Acne
- *Clitoromegaly* (enlarged clitoris)
- Deepening of the voice
- *Hirsutism* (increase of body hair)
- Menstrual irregularities
- *Policythemia* (an abnormal increase in red blood cells)

Discontinuation of drug therapy at the time of evidence of mild masculinization, the development of male characteristics in a female (*virilism*) is necessary to prevent irreversible virilization. Such virilization is common following androgen use at high doses and is not prevented by concomitant use of estrogens. *Androgens* (male hormones) may alter serum cholesterol concentration, so caution should be used when administering these drugs to patients with a history of myocardial infarction or coronary artery disease.

DELATESTRYL (TESTOSTERONE ENANTHATE INJECTION)

DELATESTRYL® (*Testosterone Enanthate* Injection) provides testosterone enanthate, a derivative of the *endogenous* or internally produced male hormone (*androgen*) testosterone, for intramuscular administration. Endogenous (internally produced) androgens are responsible for the normal growth and development of the male sex organs, maintenance of secondary sex characteristics, and certain metabolic functions:

- Alterations in body musculature
- Decreased protein *catabolism* (breakdown)
- Decreased urinary excretion of calcium
- Development of male hair distribution (beard, pubic, chest, and axillary)

- Fat distribution
- Growth and maturation of penis and scrotum
- Growth and maturation of seminal vesicles
- Growth and maturation of prostate
- Improved nitrogen balance (only when there is sufficient intake of protein)
- Increased protein *anabolism* (build up)
- Laryngeal enlargement
- Retention of nitrogen
- Retention of phosphorus
- Retention of potassium
- Retention of sodium
- Vocal chord thickening

PARATHYROID HORMONE

We know that the parathyroid glands produces parathyroid hormone, which is essential to bone formation. Can this hormone be used therapeutically in osteoporosis? In a research study done in California at the well known Roche laboratories, the researchers found that a partly natural *(semi-synthetic) parathyroid hormone* was very effective in restoring bone, even more so than the natural one; it increased trabecular and cortical bone in rats that had lost bone after having their ovaries removed.V040 An event in 1997, when a young Danish mother was arrested for leaving a baby on the sidewalk as is customary in their non-violent and clean country, showed that their morays are very different from ours, but they too face old age with osteoporosis. In a study done on rats who had had their ovaries removed, they compared the effectiveness of *parathyroid hormone (PTH),* estrogen, and the bisphosphonate *Risedronate®* (NE-58095) therapies on improving femoral neck bone strength. The latter two substances had some minimal effect, but PTH produced significant increases in structure and strength. Concurrent treatment with PTH plus estrogen or PTH plus Risedronate also significantly increased the femoral neck bone strength, but neither showed any advantage over treatment with PTH alone.[S170] [emphasis added] As usual, the score is:

nature: 1	pharmaceuticals: 0

If you are interested in some slightly complicated chemical and biological trivia, you can learn that the activation of osteoclasts by parathyroid hormone (PTH) is mediated by PTH stimulation of osteoblasts, and is dependent on a PTH-induced rise of the activity of the enzyme in protein kinase C. It is interesting that other hormonal secretions, such as insulin reduce the ability of PTH to activate protein kinase C in osteoblasts.[M071]

TRANSDERMAL DEVICES (SKIN PATCHES)

DO YOU WANT TO SOAK UP A GROWTH ACCELERATOR FOR SPROUTS?

The *Establishment* believes that *transdermal* estrogen (the application of a patch containing this substance to the naked skin), can be used in order to diminish some of the more common side-effects and complications of other modes of therapy, and in order to enhance the efficacy of estrogen in some patients, particularly smokers. *Transdermal devices* (*skin patches*) often are made from certain plastic substances, such as *ethylene vinyl acetate copolymers* (*EVAc*). Some chemicals, such as *ethyl acetate* and *ethanol* (grain alcohol), are added to help more intensive delivery of the medications they carry). The bad news is that EVAc are growth accelerators, often used commercially to enhance the growth of alfalfa sprouts in water culture. The unknown effects of such a compound on the body, and its potential for the acceleration of growth of malignant cells must not be underestimated.[F100]

SPECIAL MEASURES FOR DRUG-INDUCED OSTEOPOROSIS

Inappropriate treatments with can give rise to Drug-Induced Osteoporosis— the most common are:

- Exogenous Thyroid-Induced Osteoporosis
- Steroid-Induced Osteoporosis

Special attention and treatments are often recommended.

EXOGENOUS THYROID-INDUCED OSTEOPOROSIS

"Recent studies indicate that patients who have been treated with excessive doses of thyroid hormone over long periods of time may be at increased risk for developing osteoporosis. This may be due not only to too much thyroid, but also to an imbalance between the **anabolic** and **catabolic** endocrine hormones."[L050]

Both anabolic and catabolic hormones include **steroids**. Steroids are not just something that athletes take for enhanced muscle development and performance, but the word defines a chemical structure common to those drugs, also to cortisone.

- **Anabolic** hormones are those that help to rebuild the body and would include DHEA, estrogens, progesterone and the male hormone, testosterone
- **Catabolic** hormones are those that help to break down dead tissues and rid the body of metabolic waste. These would include thyroid hormone and hydrocortisone

anabolic hormones	catabolic hormones
DHEA	thyroid
estrogen	hydrocortisone
progesterone	
testosterone	

A physician who is trying to balance a person's thyroid function must also look at all of the other hormones and other aspects of the person's lifestyle, including diet, nutritional supplements, exercise patterns, and stress coping mechanisms. The nutrients that are especially important to a proper functioning thyroid are the mineral iodine and the amino acid tyrosine to make thyroid hormone in the thyroid gland (T4). This thyroid is inactive and requires the minerals iron, selenium, zinc, and copper to convert the inactive T4 to the active T3.[S040]

Thyroid function can be tested in many ways, even in ways that require no blood specimens or laboratory fees. The sudden honeymoon with the **TSH** thyroid function test which measures a pituitary hormone which induces thyroid hormone production in the thyroid gland (recently patented), as compared to the usually used thyroid tests of yesteryear (not any longer patented), is probably induced not only by its practicality, but by the financial benefits that can be derived by using it.

CORTICOSTEROID-INDUCED OSTEOPOROSIS

Most people are already aware of the many health risks inherent in taking the often miraculous yet very dangerous corticosteroid drug, **cortisone**, **prednisone**, or other cortisone-like preparations—especially when such intake is prolonged.[K050] Their serious side effects are:

- Atherosclerosis
- Infection
- Osteoporosis
  - * bone mass density (BMD) loss of up to 15% in the first year of medication
  - * decreased gastrointestinal uptake of calcium
  - * diminished osteoblast activity with decreased bone formation.
  - * excessive loss of calcium via urine
  - * *secondary hyperparathyroidism* with increased bone resorption (a condition which involves a disorderly production of *parathyroid hormone* by the *parathyroid glands*, (located on both sides of the thyroid)

In one retrospective study performed in Connecticut, reviewing cases previously treated with cortisone, and control or placebo (sugar pill) cases, infections, osteoporosis and tuberculosis all occurred more frequently in the steroid than in the placebo group.[C110]

Certain exams can be done to verify risks when a person is taking cortisone: one may ask his or her doctor, or go directly to a cooperative lab, to run some of the tests that can be used to show that osteoporotic alterations are being induced by the intake of cortisone:

- 24 hour urinary calcium
- Serum 25-hydroxyvitamin D level

The logic measure would be to never take these substances, but this is not always practical: some people may not be able to discontinue them (which is very dangerous to do unless it is decreased stepwise under proper medical direction). Medical experts are of the opinion that the most effective way of avoiding their side effects is simply to avoid the overuse of glucocorticoids.

So, the *establishment* approach is usually as follows:

If the urinary calcium loss is high (above 300mg/24hrs) and the patient can not get off the corticosteroid drug for medical reasons, doctors may prescribe a diuretic or fluid pill, **hydrochlorothiazide** (accompanied by potassium) which decreases calcium loss through the kidneys. If urinary calcium is low (below 100mg/24hrs), doctors may recommend optimizing calcium and vitamin D intake, even pharmacological doses of vitamin D (50,000 IU 1-3 times weekly), or **1,25-dihydroxy-vitamin D (Rocaltrol®)** at doses of 0.25 μγρ..γ daily or every other day. These treatments carry the added risk of inducing excessive blood calcium (**hypercalcemia**) and/or excessive urinary calcium (**hypercalcuria**). They are especially risky in patients at prolonged bed rest. Summing up, therapies to prevent side effects from the administration of corticosteroid drugs include

- Calcitonin
- Calcium
- Diuretics (fluid pills) - *thiazide*
- Estrogens
- Etidronate
- Vitamin D

All of these may add problems as they diminish calcium loss.

WHAT ARE THE DIRECTIONS FOR FUTURE RESEARCH BY THE ESTABLISHMENT?

The *Establishment* and pharmaceutical interests in medicine choose to ignore the safe, effective directions which have already been found to be successful, and prefer to lay out a plan for maximum Research and Development (R&D) money, and financial gains to the chemical companies.

According to the internet information at "Osteoporosis Online from Southeast Texas", future research in osteoporosis should approach the currently unanswered basic research questions concerning the development and maintenance of bone as a tissue. They recommend clinical and epidemiological research to further explore and extend the current potential for practical prevention and treatment of the disease, a deeper knowledge of factors controlling bone cell activity and regulation of bone mineral and matrix formation and remodeling.

"Current therapeutic approaches to postmenopausal bone loss or established osteoporosis vary widely among the different regions of the world. Because no treatment of osteoporosis has unequivocally demonstrated full prevention of the appearance or the recurrence of axial or peripheral fractures so far, many investigational compounds are being developed.

"*Anabolic steroids* act mainly as inhibitors of bone resorption with very few, if any, effects on bone formation. Because of the high occurrence of signs of virilization [the development of male characteristics, such as facial hair] and the weak effects on bone structure, the risk/benefit ratio in osteoporosis should be considered at least problematic.

"If ongoing large-scale trials confirm the expected benefits of *estrogen antagonist/agonists* on the skeleton and confirm no cardiovascular risk to postmenopausal women with optimal uterine safety, these substances are likely to become the most prominent alternative to hormonal replacement therapy after the menopause.

"Additional studies are requested to evaluate the potential benefit of *growth hormone* or *insulin-like growth factors* in treatment of osteoporosis.

"*Ipriflavone* acts predominantly as an inhibitor of bone resorption. To confirm the efficacy of ipriflavone on the prevention of vertebral fractures and its effects on bone mineral density in women with postmenopausal established osteoporosis, a large multi-centric European study is being conducted. Treatment with *parathyroid peptides* induces a significant gain in bone mass, mainly in the axial skeleton. Long-term studies that compare peptides, doses, and regimes are needed to better understand the exact position of parathyroid peptides as treatment of osteoporosis.

"Prolonged administration of *strontium* to postmenopausal osteoporotic women resulted in a decoupling between bone resorption and formation that yielded a significant increase in the lumbar spine bone mineral density of treated subjects. In the view of these promising results and of the excellent tolerance of strontium during preliminary trials, additional investigations of this compound in prevention and treatment of osteoporosis should be promptly initiated.

"Several other compounds have been punctually suggested for treatment of osteoporosis or are at very early stages of development. Finally, besides pharmacologic approaches to the treatment of osteoporosis, hip fractures may also be reduced by the use of *hip protectors*."[R031]

Are there any other novel treatments in the making? In a Polish study which aimed at determining the therapeutic effect of *synthetic human calcitonin* (*SHC*), treatment with calcitonin resulted in a positive analgesic effect. The functional capacity and mobility of the patients increased as pain decreased. The researchers were satisfied that "SHC appears to have a significant analgesic effect in treatment of primary osteoporosis."[K040]

ANTIRESORPTIVE THERAPY FOR MEN

No drugs are currently approved by the FDA for a treatment indication of osteoporosis in men. That does not mean that others may not be used by resourceful physicians, as an "off label" prescription.

VITAMIN D

Vitamin D is absolutely essential for the maintenance of a healthy skeleton. Without vitamin D, children develop rickets and adults exacerbate their osteoporosis and develop osteomalacia. D_3 stimulates intestinal calcium absorption and mobilizes stem cells to mobilize calcium stores from bone. Other benefits include protection against[H120]

- Cancers of the breast, prostate, and colon
- Cardiac arrhythmias
- Chemotherapy-induced hair loss
- Diabetes mellitus type I
- Hypertension
- Leukemias and myeloproliferative disorders
- Rheumatoid and psoriatic arthritis
- Seizure disorders
- Skin diseases like psoriasis and ichthyosis
- Skin rejuvenation

For further information on vitamin D, see the section on vitamins.

DOES YOUR VITAMIN D GET LOST IN BABY OIL

Mineral oil used internally as a laxative, or similar products often used on the skin surface in the form of baby oil or cosmetics, bind vitamin D in the gut and reduce its absorption.

FORMATION OF THE VITAMIN

Vitamin D (**Calciferol**) is a generic name for several fat-soluble vitamin variants, related to each other, all of which are **sterols** (cholesterol-like) substances. There are:

1. - early stage or **pro-vitamin Ds**

■   **D2**, or **activated ergo-calciferol**, is the major synthetic form of provitamin D

■   **D3**, or **cholecalciferol**, is found in animals, mainly in fish liver oils

These are converted in the liver and kidneys to major circulating

2. - *Active forms of vitamin D*

■   *25-hydroxycholecalciferol*

■   *1,25-dihydroxylcholecalciferol*

FORMATION ON THE SKIN

Vitamin D is also known as the "sunshine" vitamin because it is actually manufactured in the human skin exposed to the ultraviolet light in the sun's rays. The sunlight interacts with a cholesterol derivative, **7-dehydrocholesterol**, to form the pro-vitamin D cholecalciferol, which is then transferred to the liver or kidneys and converted to **active vitamin D**. Wintertime, clouds, smog, and darkly pigmented skin reduce the body's production of the "sunshine" vitamin.

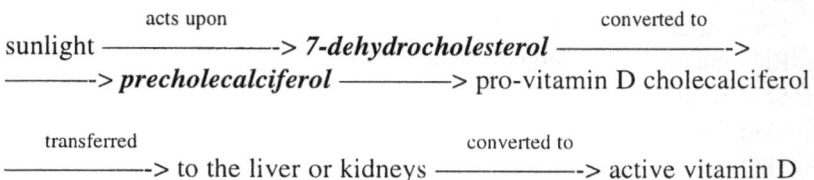

	acts upon		converted to

sunlight ————————-> **7-dehydrocholesterol** ———————->
————-> **precholecalciferol** ————-> pro-vitamin D cholecalciferol

            transferred   converted to
————————-> to the liver or kidneys ————————-> active vitamin D

SUNSHINE ALMOST ALWAYS MAKES ME HIGH....

It takes the ultraviolet (UV) frequencies of the sunshine, and also its warmth, to manufacture wholesome amounts of natural vitamin D. All vertebrates, including humans, obtain most of their daily vitamin D requirement from casual exposure to sunlight...[where]...the solar ultraviolet B photons (290-315 nm) penetrate into the skin where they cause the breakdown by light (*photolysis*) of *7-dehydrocholesterol* to *precholecalciferol*. Once formed, precholecalciferol undergoes a thermally induced rearrangement of its double bonds to form *cholecalciferol*."[H130]

WHAT MAKES YOU DEFICIENT?

An increase in skin pigmentation, aging, and the topical application of a sunscreen diminishes the cutaneous production of cholecalciferol. Latitude, season, and time of day as well as ozone pollution in the atmosphere influence the number of solar ultraviolet B photons that reach the earth's surface, and thereby, alter the cutaneous production of cholecalciferol. In Boston, exposure to sunlight during the months of November through February will not produce any significant amounts of cholecalciferol in the skin. Because windowpane glass absorbs ultraviolet B radiation, exposure of sunlight through glass windows will not result in any production of cholecalciferol. It is now recognized that vitamin D insufficiency and vitamin D deficiency are common in elderly people, especially in those who are infirm and not exposed to sunlight or who live at latitudes that do not provide them with sunlight-mediated cholecalciferol during the winter months."

- Aging
- Changes in latitude
- Cold weather
- Glass windowpanes
- Increased skin pigmentation
- Indoor lifestyle
- Ozone pollution
- Sunscreen use
- Time of day

HOW DO WE ABSORB <u>INGESTED</u> VITAMIN D, WHAT MAY AFFECT THIS ABSORPTION?

When vitamin D is ingested, it is absorbed with fats through the intestinal walls, with the aid of *bile*. Once it has reached the blood stream, *calciferol* is taken mainly to the liver, where it is either utilized or stored. Vitamin D is also stored in other tissues: skin, brain, spleen, and bones. Vitamin D intake must be more finely tuned in regard to the right therapeutic level than most other vitamins, and it is considered by many authorities to be the most potentially toxic vitamin. Symptoms of vitamin D toxicity can easily occur when vitamin D is taken in large amounts or with excessive sun exposure. (It is possible that part of sun poisoning symptoms are due to vitamin D toxicity.)

D, in the provitamin form, is found mainly in foods of animal origin. *D3*, or "natural" vitamin D, is found in

fish liver (cod liver) oil	butter
oily fish (mackerel salmon sardines herring)	liver
egg yolks	

Homogenized milk and some breakfast cereals are "fortified" (or poisoned) with synthetic vitamin D. Foods of plant origin are fairly low in D; mushrooms and dark leafy greens contain some. Strict vegetarians who do not get adequate exposure to sunlight need to take positive steps to get their 400 IUs of vitamin D daily.

FUNCTIONS

Vitamin D helps to regulate calcium metabolism and normal calcification of the bones in the body, influences our utilization of the mineral phosphorus, is closely tied to the work of the parathyroid glands. Vitamin D3 main functions:

- Decreases excretion from the kidneys
- Helps to maintain normal blood levels of calcium and phosphorus
- Helps put calcium and phosphorus into teeth
- Helps increase the absorption of calcium from the gut
- Stimulates resorption of calcium and phosphorus from bone

Straight calcium intake, without vitamin D is not likely to do much good unless the patients are sunbathing.

Because of its regulation of calcium and phosphorus metabolism, vitamin D is very important to balanced growth in children, especially to healthy bones and teeth. It is also indirectly helpful in maintaining the nervous system, heart function, and for normal blood clotting–all of which are affected by calcium levels.

The connections which exist between vitamin D and certain hormones may surprise the reader.

■ Vitamin D works together with *parathyroid hormone* in the regulation of calcium metabolism.

■ Vitamin D itself is actually a hormone as well as a vitamin; as all hormones are, it is produced in one part of the body (the skin) and released into the blood to affect other tissues (the bones). There is a feedback system with the parathyroid to produce active vitamin D3 when the body needs it, and this "vitamin" is closely related structurally to the body hormones estrogen and cortisone.

If vitamin D is low, mineral absorption lessens, blood levels of calcium and phosphorus decrease, and the body, in the fundamental effort to keep the blood levels normal, pulls these minerals from the bones. This results in demineralized, weak bones, a condition called osteomalacia (loss of bone mineral), or adult rickets. The decreased level of calcium in the blood also affects the heart and nervous system.

Uses of vitamin D or vitamin A and vitamin D (some not very well known):

■ Aiding the healing of fractures, osteoporosis, and other bone problems
■ Maintaining healthy bones and dentition
■ Prevention or cure rickets, the vitamin D deficiency disease
■ Reducing the incidence of colds
■ Treatment of allergies
■ Treatment of arthritis
■ Treatment of asthma

- Treatment of cataracts, visual problems
- Treatment of diabetes
- Treatment of hypocalcemia (low blood calcium) secondary to such problems as hypoparathyroidism, which may occur after thyroid surgery.
- Treatment of menopausal symptoms such as hot flashes and depression (*vasomotor symptoms*)
- Treatment of muscle spasms, especially when related to anxiety states
- *Myopia* (nearsightedness) and *conjunctivitis* (pink eye)
- Treatment of sciatica pain
- Treatment of skin problems

DEFICIENCY AND TOXICITY

There are some toxicity problems related to hypervitaminosis D: it is wise to be careful with supplemental vitamin D (with high doses of more than 1,000—1,500 IUs daily for a month or longer in adults, more than 400 IUs in infants, or more than 600 IUs daily in children) Some people have poor fat digestion and assimilation, they may handle higher amounts of oral vitamin D.

Symptoms of excess include:
- Abnormal calcification of soft tissues may occur
- Diarrhea, nausea
- Excessive thirst
- Headaches
- Increased levels of calcium and phosphorus in the blood and urine
- Speeds the atherosclerosis process
- Weakness

Fortified vitamin D (synthetic, irradiated ergocalciferol-D2) milk, raises concerns with toxicity. It may be contributing to calcification of the arteries, or atherosclerosis, from infancy through old age. "The added 400 IUs per quart of milk is about 15 times the amount normally found in milk and may increase the amount of calcium in the circulation, which could be a problem."

Older people are more prone to vitamin D deficiency since their skin production is lower, their digestion and absorption may be diminished, and their liver function may be reduced. Vitamin D may be deficient in people with gastrointestinal disease, such as ulcerative colitis. The sun's action on the skin to produce vitamin D is inhibited by pollution, clouds, clothing, window glass, skin pigmentation, and sunscreens. The occurrence of several of these factors together may make the development of the symptoms of rickets more likely.

- *General bone loss* and osteoporosis in the elderly
- Multiple sclerosis may be influenced by low vitamin D levels in puberty
- Nearsightedness and loss of hearing may also develop from vitamin D deficiency because of the vitamin's influence on the eye muscles and from loss of calcium in the ear bones
- *Osteomalacia* poor mineralization of bone and the inability of the bones to handle stress
- *Rickets* in children
  - Bowing of the legs
  - Fragility of bones
  - Increase in the size of the joints, such as the wrists, ankles, and knees
  - Muscle spasms (tetany) which also causes tingling and weakness
  - Muscular development diminished
  - Soft skull bones
  - Spinal curvature
  - Teeth may have poor structure

REQUIREMENTS

Vitamin D is best utilized if accompanied by vitamin A. Most of our calciferol needs are met with some vitamin D in foods and regular sunlight exposure. If we live in smoggy cities or where tall buildings block the sunlight, we may need more vitamin D. Those who have darkly pigmented skin, work nights, or cover their bodies with lots of clothes, as do members of some religious orders, probably need more vitamin D than the avid sunbather. In winter, we usually require more D from supplements or from our foods.

VITAMIN D SUPPLEMENTATION

It is generally recommended for individuals with indoor life styles, especially home-bound patients, but it also should be considered for all older individuals. The recommended daily allowance is 400-800 IU daily. The most convenient sources of vitamin D are as additions to calcium supplements or multivitamins. Daily doses of vitamin D over 800 IU daily are usually not needed or recommended. On the rare occasions where *Rocaltrol*® is indicated, serum and urine calcium levels should be appropriately monitored.

The RDA for vitamin D is 400 IUs, or roughly 10 mcg. per day. Infants and growing children probably need more vitamin D relative to body size than do adults. During pregnancy and lactation, more D is needed than the 400 IUs. Therapeutic doses for problems treated with vitamin D are about 1,000—1,500 IUs maximum per day, though some doctors may prescribe even more, mainly of the natural vitamin D3. In general, however, it is wise for adults to limit any supplemented vitamin D to the 400 IUs per day commonly found in multivitamins and to limit use of vitamin-D-fortified milk for a variety of reasons (it is synthetic and toxicities may result).[H009]

In a study intended to determine whether vitamin D supplementation reduces the incidence of hip and peripheral bone fractures among elderly people, researchers in Amsterdam[L120] randomly assigned 2578 people aged 70 years or older to receive vitamin D3 (400 IU/d) or a *placebo* (sugar pills) for a maximum of 3.5 years. Participants were advised to eat at least three servings of dairy products per day; the mean dietary calcium intake achieved was 868 mgr./d. The treatment group was found to have adequate serum 25-hydroxyvitamin D concentrations in the third year of the study, whereas the placebo group was deficient in vitamin D. However, vitamin D supplementation was not found to reduce the risk of hip or peripheral bone fractures. These results were unaffected by the participants' age, sex, residence, level of compliance or outdoor activity, exposure to sunshine and mobility scores.

A personally tailored program of weight bearing and strength training exercise is necessary to prevent the bone mass from declining.

CALCIMAR® INJECTION (SYNTHETIC), MIACALCIN® INJECTION, MIACLCIN® NASAL SPRAY

According to "Stedman's Medical Dictionary", calcitonin (kal-si-to'nin). A peptide hormone, of which eight forms in five species are known; composed of 32 amino acids and produced by the parathyroid, thyroid, and thymus glands; its action is opposite to that of parathyroid hormone in that c. increases deposition of calcium and phosphate in bone and lowers the level of calcium in the blood; its level in the blood is increased by glucagon and by Ca2+, and thus opposes postprandial hypercalcemia. thyrocalcitonin; [calci- + G. tonos, stretching, + -in]

It is a synthetic hormone very similar to that found in *calcitonin* of salmon origin, which is a hormone secreted by the thyroid gland in mammals and by the *ultimobranchial* gland of birds and fish. *Calcitonin-salmon* appears to have actions essentially identical to calcitonins of mammals, its potency per mgr. is greater and it has a longer duration of action.

Calcitonin acts on bone in ways not fully understood, also on kidneys and the gastrointestinal tract. It produces a marked transient inhibition of the ongoing bone resorptive process. With prolonged use, there is a persistent, smaller decrease in the rate of bone resorption. Calcitonin and *parathyroid hormone* share in the regulation of blood calcium: high blood calcium levels cause increased secretion of calcitonin which, in turn, inhibits bone resorption.

It is used in the treatment of post-menopausal osteoporosis, provided there is adequate calcium and vitamin D intake, to prevent the progressive loss of bone mass. The PDR states that no evidence currently exists to indicate whether or not CALCIMAR® decreases the risk of vertebral crush fractures or spinal deformity. The manufacturers tell us that:

> "a recent controlled study, which was discontinued prior to completion because of questions regarding its design and implementation, failed to demonstrate any benefit of CALCIMAR® on fracture rate. No adequate controlled trials have examined the effect of calcitonin-salmon injection on vertebral bone mineral density beyond one year of treatment. Two controlled studies with CALCIMAR have shown an increase in total body calcium at one year, followed by a trend to decreasing total body calcium (still above baseline) at two years. It has been suggested that those post-menopausal patients having increased rates of bone turnover may be more likely to respond to antiresorptive agents such as CALCIMAR."

SIDE EFFECTS AND RISKS

Because calcitonin is protein in nature, the possibility of a generalized allergic reaction exists; in a few cases the reactions are very serious (E.G. bronchial spasms, swelling of the tongue or throat, and anaphylactic shock), in one case, even fatal. Generalized flushing and blood pressure drops may occur, but these are not necessarily due to allergy.

Patients receiving this drug may experience very low serum calcium leading to severe Charley horses and cramps. There may be kidney damage. Pituitary tumors were increased in rats getting this drug, rabbits had a lower birth rate, and it inhibits lactation in animals.

- Blood pressure drops
- Generalized allergic reaction
    anaphylactic shock
    bronchial spasms
    swelling of the tongue or throat
- Generalized flushing
- Inhibition of lactation in animals
- Kidney damage
- Lower birth rate in rabbits
- Pituitary tumors increase in rats
- Very low serum calcium
    severe Charley horses
    cramps

MIACALCIN® (CALCITONIN-SALMON) NASAL SPRAY

Only injectable forms of calcitonin-salmon have been available in the United States until recently. Calcitonins are antiresorptive agents which allow bone formation to catch up with bone breakdown in the bone remodeling process. Calcitonin-salmon is a synthetic product with the chemical structure of natural calcitonin found in salmon. It is the only calcitonin approved by the FDA for the treatment of osteoporosis.

Manufactured by Sandoz Pharmaceuticals Corporation, available since 1995. Mostly used in a dosage of 200 IU (International Units) per day (gently in alternate nostrils) in conjunction with adequate calcium and vitamin D supplementation. Miacalcin® Nasal Spray is usually used for individuals who resist using the injectable form of calcitonin because of inconvenience, nausea, flushing, or other side effects. It has been recommended for women who refuse or cannot tolerate estrogens, or in whom estrogens should not be used, it is however more effective with estrogen, than either it or estrogen alone.

The reader needs to be appraised that in normal tissue there are small networks of minute canals that pick up contaminants and clean the areas, the **lymphatics**. But there are no lymphatics in the triangular area which goes from the corners of the mouth to the bridge of the nose. Also, the olfactory nerves (smelling nerves) open a direct pathway to the brain, without the benefit of the protection offered by the blood-brain barrier. *Inhaled* substances can go *directly* to the brain.

Accordign to current knowledge, nasal administration of **calcitonin** has been shown to result in a 2-3% increase of vertebral bone density with a possible a reduction in fracture rate as well, (30%-40%). However, these data are not conclusive. An added benefit of calcitonin-salmon is that it controls pain. Side effects are said to be few, just some nasal irritation.

BONE PASTE, NORIAN SRS® (SKELETAL REPAIR SYSTEM)

"And all the king's horses
And all he king's men,
Could not put Humpty Dumpty together again."

Norian SRS® (Skeletal Repair System), a really bionic medicine, is a new substance for mending bone made of calcium and phosphoric acid. Prior to use a sodium phosphate solution is added to make a compound that has the consistency of a thick paste. The physician, using x-ray guidance, injects the paste into the fracture site. It begins hardening in about 10 minutes, drying to a strength equal to that of natural bone within 12 hours. Over time the person's own bone cells grow into the hardened paste and replace it with new bone. It is said to be accepted by the body without rejection or adverse side effects.

THE PHARMACEUTICAL TREATMENT OF PAIN

Pain can be demeaning, exhausting, depressing. As previously stated, it is the most serious threat to quality of life. Pain is, too often, under-treated or improperly treated, due to the ignorance of the public and the professionals. Inflammatory pains yield fairly well to aspirin and many over the counter analgesics. Neurologic pain, including disc and spinal problems, neuralgias, etc., require opiates, from the lighter Darvon® and codeine preparations, to stronger, more powerful and feared drugs such as Demerol® and others. Misinformation and prejudice has deprived many from proper treatments, as the professionals exhibit irrational fears that the patients will become victims of drug addictions, and as they themselves have to fear reprisals by ignorant medical examiner boards.

ANALGESICS (PAIN RELIEVERS)

How is the pain associated with osteoporosis treated? Variably, and often not very well. A Scottish[P070] study on drugs employed in treating osteoporosis, listed the drugs mostly used (this listing being alphabetical in this book, and not by frequency) as:

- *Anti-epileptic* agents (drugs for the control of seizures)
- *Anxiolytics* (tranquilizers)
- *Chymopapain* (an enzyme derived from the papaya fruit, which can be injected in the spine)
- *Colchicine* (a drug for gout)
- Corticosteroids
- NSAIDS (non-steroidal anti-inflammatory drugs)
- *Opiods* (similar to morphine)
- *Tricyclic antidepressants* (a family of antidepressants)

In the Scottish protocol,[P070] Paracetamol (Tylenol®, acetaminophen) was recommended as the standard treatment for transient back pain. More severe pain was said to require the addition of an *opioid*, such as *codeine* or *dextropropoxyphene* (*Darvon®*). *Morphine* and *pethidine—meperidine* or *Demerol®*, they said, might be necessary in patients with back pain due to malignancy or osteoporotic fracture. However, they stated, opioid analgesics are associated with dependence, tolerance and adverse effects. As far as nonsteroidal anti-inflammatory drugs (NSAIDs), they felt they had analgesic efficacy comparable with paracetamol or Tylenol. They confirmed that individual patients responded differently to different NSAIDs, and several agents might have to be tried. Therapy was necessary for a long term in diseases with inflammation.

Peculiarly, the use of the very wonderful drug aspirin was not addressed, showing that the usual prevalent issues of money and patents prevail over medical reasoning.

A PRIMER ON SOME PAIN MEDICATIONS

I list aspirin first, not only because of its alphabetical location, but because of its many advantages. What is the story behind this best known of analgesics?[P030]

It used to be that aspirin and other *salicylates* (the aspirin family of drugs) were the only medications available for nonprescription relief of minor ailments, from headaches and fever to muscle strain and minor arthritis. Today, consumers looking for temporary relief have their pick of what can be a bewildering array of "regular," "extra-strength," and "maximum pain relief" tablets, caplets and gel caps on the drugstore shelf.[P030] Though this cornucopia can seem confusing, the products' pain-relieving ingredients fall into just four categories:

- Acetaminophen (Tylenol® and others)
- Aspirin (and other salicylates)
- *Ibuprofen* (a *non-steroidal analgesic* or *NSAID*)
- *Naproxen sodium* (a *non-steroidal analgesic* or *NSAID*)

As of today we can also find *Orudis*, another member of the NSAIDS.

For the most part, these over-the-counter (OTC) analgesic ingredients are equally effective. However, some may be more effective for certain types of ailments, and some people may prefer one type to another because of their varying side effects. William T. Beaver, M.D., professor of pharmacology and anesthesia at Georgetown University School of Medicine in Washington, D.C. is quoted stating that "Knowing the pros and cons of each type of pain reliever will allow you to choose among them"

ASPIRIN

Ken Flieger[F050] tells us that in purses and backpacks, in briefcases and medicine chests the world over, millions of people keep close at hand a drug that has both a long past and a fascinating future. Its past reaches at least to the fifth century B.C., when Hippocrates used a bitter powder obtained from willow bark to ease aches and pains and reduce fever. Its future is being shaped today in laboratories and clinics where scientists are exploring some intriguing new uses for an interesting old drug. The substance in willow bark that made ancient Greeks feel better, *salicin*, is the pharmacological ancestor of a family of drugs called *salicylates*, the best known of which is the world's most widely used drug—aspirin. Americans consume an estimated 80 billion aspirin tablets a year. The Physicians' Desk Reference lists more than 50 over-the-counter drugs in which aspirin is the principal active ingredient.

"...aspirin's beginnings were rather unspectacular. Nearly 100 years ago, a German industrial chemist, Felix Hoffmann, set about to find a drug to ease his father's arthritis without causing the severe stomach irritation associated with *sodium salicylate*, the standard anti-arthritis drug of the time. In the forms then available, the large doses of salicylates used to treat arthritis—6 to 8 grams a day—commonly irritated the stomach lining, and many patients, like Hoffmann's father, simply could not tolerate them. Figuring that acidity made salicylates hard on the stomach, Hoffmann started looking for a less acidic formulation. His search led him to synthesize *acetylsalicylic acid* (*ASA*), a compound that appeared to share the therapeutic properties of other salicylates and might cause less stomach irritation....Hoffmann was confidant [sic] that ASA would prove more effective than salicylates then in use. His superiors, however, did not share his enthusiasm. They doubted that ASA would ever become a valuable, commercially successful drug because at large doses salicylates commonly produced shortness of breath and an alarmingly rapid heart rate....Hoffmann's employer, Friedrich Bayer & Company, gave ASA the now-familiar name aspirin, but in 1897 Bayer didn't think aspirin had much of a future." [emphasis added]

HOW DOES IT WORK?

This drug that, at small doses, interferes with blood clotting, at somewhat higher doses reduces fever and eases minor aches and pains, and at comparatively large doses combats pain and inflammation in rheumatoid arthritis and several other related diseases. Most authorities agree that aspirin achieves some of its effects by inhibiting the production of inflammatory chemicals called *prostaglandins*.   What are prostaglandins? "Prostaglandins are hormone-like substances that have the following properties:

- Cause redness and fever
- Control uterine contractions
- Direct the functioning of blood platelets that help stop bleeding
- Influence the elasticity of blood vessels
- Regulate numerous other activities in the body

In the 1970s, a British pharmacologist, John Vane, Ph.D., noted that many forms of tissue injury were followed by the release of *prostaglandins*. In laboratory studies, he found that two groups of prostaglandins caused redness and fever, common signs of inflammation. Vane and his co-workers also showed that, by blocking the synthesis of prostaglandins, aspirin prevented blood platelets from aggregating, one of the initial steps in the formation of blood clots." [emphasis added]

Ruth Papazian, author of an article about over-the-counter pain relievers, calls aspirin "Old Faithful", and tells us that "Americans have been reaching for aspirin for almost 100 years as an all-purpose pain reliever.[F030]

> **"AMERICANS HAVE BEEN REACHING FOR ASPIRIN FOR ALMOST 100 YEARS AS AN ALL-PURPOSE PAIN RELIEVER.[F030]**

It is available in both prescription and over the counter (OTC) products, in various strengths.

- Regular strength aspirin contains 325 milligrams (mgr.) per tablet;
- Extra or maximum strength contains 500 mgr. per tablet.

"Some manufacturers add *caffeine* to aspirin. 'There is no evidence that caffeine relieves pain, but it can enhance the effects of aspirin, possibly by lifting a person's mood,' says Michael Weintraub, M.D., director of FDA's Office of OTC Drug Evaluation. Since a two-tablet dose provides roughly the same amount of caffeine as a cup of coffee, you can get the same effect by taking two plain aspirin with coffee."[F030] [emphasis added] Incidentally, in the "land down under", caffeine combinations are unknown, but they sell codeine in small doses over the counter.

Some aspirin products are specially formulated in an attempt to decrease stomach irritation. The various processes may be:

- *Buffered* (balanced as far as their acidity goes, with calcium carbonate, magnesium oxide, and other antacids)
- *Enteric coated* so that they don't dissolve until they reach the small intestine, but they may take up to twice as long to provide pain relief as plain aspirin

However, aspirin also causes gastrointestinal upset indirectly by inhibiting mucus production, and buffering does nothing to offset this effect.

Aspirin should not be taken by people who have/are:

- Asthma (it can trigger an attack in some asthmatics)
- Bleeding disorders (it may cause bleeding)
- Liver or kidney disease
- Taking anticoagulant medication (it may cause bleeding)
- Ulcers
- Uncontrolled high blood pressure

Continual high dosages of aspirin can cause hearing loss or *tinnitus* —a persistent ringing in the ears.

BUFFERIN® IS A "BUFFERED" ASPIRIN PREPARATION

Buffered aspirin compounds contain alkaline ingredients to diminish the acid potential of acetyl-salicylic-acid or aspirin.

ACTIVE INGREDIENTS

Aspirin 325 mgr	Aspirin 325 mgr
Magnesium Oxide	Magnesium Carbonate

OTHER INGREDIENTS

Benzoic Acid	Hydroxypropyl Methylcellulose
Simethicone Emulsion	Carnauba Wax
Magnesium Stearate	Sorbitan Monolaurate
Citric Acid	Polysorbate 20
Titanium Dioxide	Corn Starch
Povidone	Zinc Stearate
FD&C Blue No 1	Propylene Glycol

The manufacturer recommends this product for the temporary relief of:

arthritis pain (minor)	menstrual pain
toothaches	headaches
muscle pains	inflammation
pain and fever of colds	

WARNINGS supplied by the manufacturer address mostly children, teenagers and pregnant women, but for those who would be in the osteoporotic category, we still have:

"...DO NOT TAKE THIS PRODUCT IF YOU ARE ALLERGIC TO ASPIRIN, HAVE ASTHMA, HAVE STOMACH PROBLEMS (SUCH AS HEARTBURN, UPSET STOMACH OR STOMACH PAIN) THAT PERSIST OR RECUR, OR IF YOU HAVE ULCERS OR BLEEDING PROBLEMS UNLESS DIRECTED BY A DOCTOR. IF RINGING IN THE EARS OR LOSS OF HEARING OCCURS, CONSULT A DOCTOR BEFORE TAKING OR GIVING ANY MORE OF THIS PRODUCT."

PRECAUTIONS

Advice for patients presenting with signs and symptoms of *transient ischemic attacks* (*TIA's*) or small strokes:
- Small increases in blood pressure
- Small increases in blood urea nitrogen (*BUN*), an indication of waning kidney function
- Small increases in serum *uric acid* levels, usually associated with gout

The simultaneous use of antacids and aspirin can:
- Decrease the absorption of aspirin (nonabsorbable antacids)
- Increase the elimination of aspirin (absorbable antacids)

ACETAMINOPHEN

Twenty years ago, FDA approved *acetaminophen* (*Tylenol®*), and other brands and generics, in dosages of 325 mgr. and 500 mgr. for OTC use. "Nobody knows exactly how acetaminophen works, but one theory is that it acts on nerve endings to suppress pain," says Weintraub. Acetaminophen, he adds, is as effective as aspirin in relieving mild-to-moderate pain and in reducing fever, but less so when it comes to soft tissue injuries, such as muscle strains and sprains. The usual adult dosage is two 325-mgr. tablets every four hours.

Though acetaminophen is no better or faster at pain relief than aspirin, the drug is touted to be gentler on the stomach and reduce fever without the risk of *Reyes syndrome* in children. However, even at moderate doses, acetaminophen can cause liver damage in heavy drinkers, and abnormal lab values in the liver functions of many users. At press time of the

Papazian article, FDA was planning to require a warning about this on the labels of OTC products containing the drug.

Reyes syndrome is a rare bleeding disorder that occurs when aspirin is used in some immunosuppressed children suffering from chickenpox. It has never ceased to amaze me that the drug industry takes great pains in expounding about Reyes Syndrome and its connection to aspirin (actually, acetaminophen may also be risky), a problem of extremely rare occurrence, maybe one in a million, but does not inform the public about the danger for kidney failure in individuals who are afflicted with a genetic disturbance called *6-Glucose-monophosphte-dehydrogenase* or *6-GMPD*, a problem that affects one out of four blacks, who are unable to properly handle this substance, and have constant low grade urinary bleeding. In an article in the Los Angeles Times, a few years ago, it has been publicized that blacks who take acetaminophen with regularity have a higher level of kidney failure, but when I phoned the journalist who wrote one of these articles, he refused to do a follow-up story to explain the reasons behind it.

**EVEN AT MODERATE DOSES ACETAMINOPHEN CAN CAUSE
LIVER DAMAGE IN HEAVY DRINKERS**

MAY ALSO CONTAIN:

"This product should not be taken by any adult or child who is taking a prescription drug for anticoagulation (thinning of blood) diabetes, gout or arthritis unless directed by a doctor"

An example of an acetominophen preparation is *Arthritis Foundation*™ *Aspirin Free Caplet*

Each *Arthritis Foundation*™ *Aspirin Free Caplet* contains

ACTIVE INGREDIENT
Acetaminophen 500 mg

INACTIVE INGREDIENTS:

Cellulose	Magnesium Stearate
Red No 40	Cornstarch

Polyethylene Glycol   Hydroxypropyl Methylcellulose
Sodium Starch Glycolate

The PDR tells us that:
"Acetaminophen is a clinically proven analgesic and antipyretic. Acetaminophen produces analgesia by elevation of the pain threshold and *antipyresis* (fever control) through action on the *hypothalamic* (mid-brain) heat-regulating center. Acetaminophen may be used safely by most persons with peptic ulcers, when taken as directed for recommended conditions. Since Arthritis Foundation® Aspirin Free Pain Reliever contains no aspirin, it is not likely to cause a reaction in those who are allergic to aspirin."[P051]

It is recommended for the temporary relief of :
aches   fever pains
arthritis (minor pain)   headaches

There is only a veiled reference to the fact that acetaminophen is toxic to the liver, especially if alcohol is consumed in more than small amounts. A little more obvious is the warning of liver damage with overdose, for which the antidote is the amino acid *acetylcysteine* (available at health food stores as *NAC*. It probably would be a good move for people who take a lot of Tylenol® to supplement this amino acid.

NSAIDS

Ibuprofen and *naproxen sodium* have a pharmacological function similar to aspirin: their effects are due to inhibiting the production of inflammatory substances (*prostaglandins*). They are more potent pain relievers, especially for menstrual cramps, toothaches, minor arthritis, and injuries accompanied by inflammation, such as *tendinitis* (inflammation of the leaders). Taken at the recommended adult dosage, OTC ibuprofen (*Advil*® and others) and naproxen sodium (*Aleve*®) are touted to be somewhat gentler on the stomach than aspirin. However, people who have ulcers or who get GI upset when taking aspirin are told by manufacturers they should avoid both. In addition, asthmatics and people who are allergic to aspirin are strongly warned to avoid ibuprofen and naproxen sodium. These products often cause rashes when people are exposed to sunlight (*photosensitivity*).

> **ASTHMATICS AND PEOPLE WHO ARE ALLERGIC TO ASPIRIN ARE STRONGLY WARNED TO AVOID IBUPROFEN AND NAPROXEN SODIUM**

"An FDA advisory panel has recommended labeling on ibuprofen products like that recommended for aspirin, warning heavy drinkers about increased risk of gastric bleeding and impaired liver function (products with naproxen sodium labels already include this information)."

IBUPROFEN TABLETS, IBUPROFEN CAPLETS

ACTIVE INGREDIENT
Ibuprofen 200 mg.

INACTIVE INGREDIENTS:

Acetylated Monoglyceride	Microcrystalline Cellulose
Sodium Lauryl Sulfate	Beeswax and/or Carnauba Wax
Pharmaceutical Glaze Povidone	Starch
Croscarmellose Sodium	Propylparaben
Stearic Acid	Iron Oxides
Silicon Dioxide	Sucrose
Lecithin	Simethicone
Titanium Dioxide	Methylparaben
Sodium Benzoate	

Used for the temporary relief of:
common cold (minor aches/ pains)

muscular aches	menstrual cramps
headache	backache
reduction of fever	toothache
minor pain of arthritis	

ORUDIS®, ORUVAIL® (KETOPROFEN)

Ketoprofen is defined as a "nonsteroidal anti-inflammatory drug" (NSAID). The chemical name for ketoprofen is 2-(3-benzoylphenyl)-propionic acid."

Orudis capsules contain the "*inactive* ingredients":

D&C Yellow 10*	FD&C Blue 1*
Lactose	D&C Red 28 (25 mg)*
FD&C Yellow 6*	Magnesium stearate
FD&C Red 40 (25 mg)*	Gelatin
Titanium dioxide	
* Industrial colors	

Each ***Oruvail*®** [long acting, prescription strength of Orudis®] capsule (100 mg, 150 mg, or 200 mg) contains the *inactive* ingredients:

D&C Red 22	FD&C Blue 1
Sodium lauryl sulfate	D&C Red 28
Gelatin	Starch
D&C Yellow 10 (100 & 150 mg caps.) other proprietary ingredients.	
Sucrose	Ethyl cellulose
Shellac	Talc
FD&C Green 3 (100 & 150 mg caps.)	Silicon dioxide
Titanium dioxide	

In the PDR we find:
"WARNINGS: ASPIRIN SENSITIVE PATIENTS. DO NOT TAKE THIS PRODUCT IF YOU HAVE HAD A SEVERE ALLERGIC REACTION TO ASPIRIN, E.G.—ASTHMA, SWELLING, SHOCK OR HIVES, BECAUSE EVEN THOUGH THIS PRODUCT CONTAINS NO ASPIRIN OR SALICYLATES, CROSS-REACTIONS MAY OCCUR IN PATIENT'S ALLERGIC TO ASPIRIN" The PDR further advises that ketoprofen should not be taken with aspirin and acetominophen unless it is by a doctor's direction, and not to combine this product with ibuprofen-containing products.

"CONTRAINDICATIONS: "Ketoprofen should not be given to patients in whom aspirin or other nonsteroidal anti-inflammatory drugs induce asthma, urticaria, or other allergic-type reactions, because severe, rarely fatal, anaphylactic reactions to ketoprofen have been reported in such patients."[P051]

"NSAIDs are often essential agents in the management of arthritis and have a major role in the treatment of pain, but they also may be commonly employed for conditions which are less serious. Physicians may wish to discuss with their patients the potential risks (see "WARNINGS," "GENERAL PRECAUTIONS," and "ADVERSE REACTIONS" sections) and likely benefits of NSAID treatment, particularly when the drugs are used for less serious conditions where treatment without NSAIDs may represent an acceptable alternative to both the patient and physician."

> "...WARNINGS — RISK OF GI [GASTROINTESTINAL] ULCERATION, BLEEDING, AND PERFORATION WITH NSAID THERAPY". [EMPHASIS SUPPLIED]

Abnormal production of sperm (*spermatogenesis*) or inhibition of spermatogenesis developed in rats and dogs given NSAIDS at high doses, and a decrease in the weight of the testes occurred in dogs and baboons at high doses.

DRUG INTERACTIONS:

- *Aspirin:* Concurrent use is not recommended.
- *Diuretics*: greater risk of developing renal failure.
- *Lithium* levels may increase, should be monitored
- *Methotrexate*: may cause changes in the elimination leading to elevated serum levels and increased toxicity.
- *Probenecid*: the combination is not recommended.
- *Warfarin* (*coumadin*): requires close monitoring of patients on both drugs.

ADVERSE EVENTS OCCURRING IN MORE THAN 10% OF PATIENTS
Dyspepsia (11%)

Adverse events occurring in 3% to 9% of patients

abdominal pain	Flatulence
Nausea	Constipation
Headache	Nervousness
Diarrhea	Increased BUN
Swelling fluid retention	Dreams
Insomnia	

ADVERSE EVENTS OCCURRING IN 1% OF PATIENTS

Anorexia	Rash
Urinary- tract irritation	Depression
Somnolence	Vomiting
Dizziness	Stomatitis
Malaise	Tinnitus visual disturbance

ADVERSE EVENTS OCCURRING IN LESS THAN 1% OF PATIENTS

Agranulocytosis	Impotence
Peripheral vascular disease	Allergic reaction
Gastrointestinal perforation	Pharyngitis
Alopecia	Hearing impairment
Photosensitivity	Amnesia
Hematemesis	Prolonged menstrual bleeding
Anaphylaxis	Hematuria
Pruritus	Anemia
Hemolysis	Purpura
Appetite increased	Hemoptysis
Purpuric rash	Blood
Hepatic dysfunction	Rectal hemorrhage
Bronchospasm	Hypertension
Renal failure	Bullous rash
Hypocoagulability	Retinal hemorrhage
Chills	Hyponatremia
Retinal pigmentation	Confusion
Infection	Rhinitis
Congestive heart failure	Interstitial nephritis
Salivation	Conjunctivitis conjunctivitis sicca
Intestinal ulceration	Skin discoloration
Dry mouth	Laryngeal edema
Sweating	Eructation (burping)
Melena	Tachycardia
Dyspnea	Migraine
Taste perversion	Myalgia

Thirst	Epistaxis
Nephrotic syndrome	Thrombocytopenia
Exfoliative dermatitis	Onycholysis
Urticaria	Eye pain
Pain	Uterine hemorrhages
Facial edema	Palpitation
Vasodilation	Fecal occult
Paresthesia	Vertigo
Gastritis	Peptic ulcer
Weight gain/loss	

OF RARE OCCURRENCE, NOT CONCLUSIVELY RELATED TO THE DRUG:

Acute tubulopathy	Gynecomastia
Nightmares	Aggravation of Diabetes mellitus
Hallucination	Pancreatitis
Arrhythmias	Jaundice
Personality disorder	Aseptic meningitis
Libido disturbance	Septicemia
Buccal necrosis	Microvesicular steatosis
Shock	Dysphoria
Myocardial infarction	Ulcerative colitis

Increased interactions may occur when Orudis® doses greater than 50 mg as a single dose or 200 mg per day are used in conjunction with other drugs that bind heavily to proteins.

"...borderline elevations of one or more liver function tests may occur in up to 15% of patients. These abnormalities may progress, may remain essentially unchanged, or may disappear with continued therapy. The *ALT* (*SGPT*) [a common liver function test]... is probably the most sensitive indicator of liver dysfunction. Meaningful (3 times the upper limit of normal) elevations of ALT or AST (SGOT) occurred in controlled clinical trials in less than 1% of patients. A patient with symptoms and/or signs suggesting liver dysfunction, or in whom an abnormal liver test has occurred, should be evaluated for evidence of the development of a more severe hepatic reaction while on therapy with ketoprofen. Serious hepatic reactions, including jaundice, have been reported from post- marketing experience with ketoprofen [Orudis®] as well as with other nonsteroidal antiinflammatory drugs."[P051]

ANTIDEPRESSANTS

Antidepressant medications are commonly prescribed for patients with chronic low back pain, but also cause significant sedation and drops in blood pressure.

CLONIDINE

One less classic approach to low back pain is the use of *clonidine* [antidepressant].[C020] It usually gives very good analgesia but causes a high incidence of adverse effects, including significant sedation and decreases in arterial pressure and heart rate.[T090]

CHAPTER V

OSTEOPOROSIS: ALTERNATIVES

THE ALTERNATIVES

What are the alternative treatments? We could define them many ways, but all of these definitions would be missing this or that detail. For our purpose, we could refer to alternatives as those treatments that look at the patient as a *whole* (*wholistic or holistic*). Alternatives go beyond the scope of what *Establishment* medicine studies, including all collateral observations, the co-factors of a problem, the nutritional approaches to removing a deficiency, chiropractics, acupuncture, homeopathy, chelation, all the modalities that are not patentable or capable of being financially monopolized. They emphasize the importance of the environment, the toxic exposures, the mind and the spirit. They retain the trust of their users and increase their user base hour by hour because they *work*.

Many times alternative practitioners have been suppressed and ridiculed. Patients even express fear that they might be punished for not doing what the doctors from the "Church" (of Medicine, a name coined by Dr. Robert Mendelsohn) tell them to do. But the law is on the *Establishment's* side, as expressed in the Position Paper from ACAM (American Council for Alternative Medicine):

> "Under the common law, the State may not deny an individual the right to exercise a reasonable choice in medical care, nor the correlative right of licensed practitioners to provide such care, and the United States Constitution precludes unfair burdening of choice in treatment decisions. Under both the Doctrine of the Right of Privacy and the Commercial Speech Doctrine, substantial deference is given to the individual to make important decisions regarding his own body. As recently reiterated by the Supreme Court, 'At the heart of [protected] liberty is the right to define one's own concept of existence, of meaning, of the universe, and of the mystery of human life.' Planned Parenthood v. Casey, supra, 112 S.Ct. at 2807.''

"Complementary physicians take a broader view with regard to osteoporosis. In addition to confronting the many risk factors long before menopause occurs, they supplement with the full range of nutrients necessary for building bone. For example, complementary physicians believe that it is a mistake to give calcium without balancing it with magnesium, since the imbalance created may lead to soft tissue calcification of blood vessels and other tissues, resulting in disease. At least 22 nutrients have been shown to contribute to building bone and a preventive program should include all of them."[S040]

In order to understand alternative approaches to osteoporosis, we must learn what feeds our bodies and what poisons and damages them. Ultimately, we must learn how to deal with the problems.
■ What poisons or damages us?
■ What feeds us?
■ How do we deal with the problem of osteoporosis?

We must know who and what our enemies are. One set of enemies are the poisons from our food and our environment.

POISONS IN OUR FOOD AND DRINK

TABLE SALT

Salts are combination molecules. There are many salts made from innumerable compositions of atoms. Table salt, one of these salts, is a compound that is made of the elements sodium and chlorine. Sodium is a soft metal which reacts violently with water. To form salt, the sodium has given up an electron to form positively charged sodium ions. Chlorine alone is a yellow gas. To form salt, the chlorine atom accepts an electron and becomes a negatively charged chloride ion. Since we have all seen table salt, we know that the sodium and chloride ions which form salt have completely different physical and chemical properties from the metal and gas from which they were formed.

The confusion that reigns over the role of salt in our lives is enormous. This is not so difficult to explain since it has been subject to the multiple manipulations of politics and industry.

Salt is a necessary part of life, not only because it flavors and protects foods, but because we need sodium to:
■ Maintain blood volume
■ Perform other vital functions
■ Regulate water balance
■ Transmit nerve impulses

The element **sodium** is naturally present in most foods. It is added to canned, packaged, and frozen foods in order to flavor and preserve them. We add it during cooking. We sprinkle it on our food at the table because it makes food taste good. And,in limited amounts, it is good for us. But many people consume far too much sodium in the form of table salt. Salt consists of 40 percent sodium and 60 percent chloride. One teaspoon has 2 grams of sodium. Without intending to say that the following statement should be endorsed as the gold standard, the Food and Nutrition Board of the National Academy of Sciences believes that an adequate and safe level of sodium (the main element in table salt) each day is 1.1 to 3.3 grams. Americans now consume between 2.3 and 6.9 grams daily.

From my point of view, the main problem with table salt is not the content of sodium, but the dangerous addition of all, or some, of the following damaging substances:

- **Aluminum hydrochloride**, to prevent it from caking (some salt companies, like Morton, use calcium silicate, dextrose and KI—potassium iodide—in the iodized version of its salt: "when it rains, it pours"*)

- **Potassium iodide** (**KI**), allegedly to protect Chinese and other children from retardation

- **Potassium nitroprusside**, a precursor of **cyanide**.

*Morton International, Inc., Morton Salt

DOES SALT INTAKE IMPACT ON THE DEVELOPMENT OF OSTEOPOROSIS?

Maybe a little—especially in males—so we are told.[G090] Since the studies are made with these contaminated mixtures of salt (not with pure sodium chloride) it is impossible to tell, but since we know that the additives are harmful, we must presume that commercial salt does impact on the development of osteoporosis.

Studying daily intake of any substance in humans is extremely difficult, due to the many individual diets. When an attempt was made to evaluate the effects of dietary sodium intake on osteoporosis, A small, statistically significant protective effect of sodium was found at the wrist end of the larger of the arm bones (the radius) and in men only. At other body sites in both women and men, no effect of sodium on BMD was apparent.[G090]

There was no detrimental effect of dietary sodium on bone mineral density, and, in the range measured, sodium was not a major osteoporosis risk factor.

Since blood pressure medicines and diuretics increase the risk for osteoporosis, we need to avoid developing high blood pressure and, subsequently, the medications used for its treatment. We need to pay attention to problems with the use of table salt.

"SALT-SENSITIVE" PEOPLE AT GREATER RISK FOR HYPERTENSION

09/23/1996

BY DENISE MANN

DR. DONALD BRIAN THOMAS, M.D., PhD.

"1996 Medical Tribune News Service reported at the annual meeting of the American Heart Association's Council for High Blood Pressure Research in Chicago, that some people are more likely to develop high blood pressure when they eat salt, because they retain high amounts of it, have difficulty excreting the excess in their urine. It remains in their blood, drawing water to it. This increases the volume of the blood, and creates greater pressure as the blood is pumped through the arteries. The condition is known as *salt sensitivity*. They state that "Salt sensitivity is marked by a rise in blood pressure after salt consumption is increased, or a fall in high blood pressure after consumption is cut."

"If you are sensitive to salt, you will develop hypertension if you don't cut down your salt intake, was the summarized conclusion of Dr. Robert Phillips, director of the hypertension section at the cardiovascular institute at Mount Sinai Hospital in New York. African-Americans, Latinos and elderly whites are at increased risk for hypertension and may be salt-sensitive. A diet higher in potassium, (beans, chick peas, potatoes, broccoli and fresh fruits) is better for them. But unfortunately, the average American diet contains about 4 grams of salt per day. This is double a more acceptable amount of 2 grams.

"The Salt Institute, an organization based in Alexandria, Va., that represents North American salt producers, would prefer that any links between salt and high blood pressure be omitted on product labels."

Because most commercially available salt is *contaminated* with **iodine** (under the guise that this is to protect our poor little children from mental retardation), and because iodine taken inappropriately may harm the thyroid glands it alleges to support, it may affect bones and hormones very adversely. Therefore, iodized salt is covered a little more in depth than other subjects.

STABILITY OF IODINE IN SALT

Iodization of salt with potassium iodide will, unfortunately, ensure reasonable retention of iodine in the salt for some months. To add insult to injury, salt iodization levels were recently increased from 7-15 ppm (parts per million—1 ppm is usually equivalent to 1 mg per quart) to 20-25 ppm.

EFFECT OF IODIZED SALT ON THE COLOR AND TASTE OF FOOD

Reports of studies on a variety of foods such as meats, cheese, pickled olives, canned vegetables, white bread, etc. suggest that salt iodized with iodide has no influence on the palatableness of these foods. Experiments conducted on the appearance and taste of boiled potatoes and rice with high levels of iodine (400 mgr. I/kg) did not show any effect of iodine. However, "off" flavors were produced in the presence of *cresol*, a constituent of lemon flavoring.

How can table salt impact on high Blood Pressure? Older people in particular should be cautious about using too much salt (restrictions are far less for sea or rock salt). The main reason for caution adduced by the *Establishment* is that overuse of sodium is one factor that is associated with high blood pressure (HBP). They fail to mention that the *aluminum* in it is probably the real problem. Having a family history of HBP and being overweight are major factors too. HBP in turn can lead to heart disease, stroke, and kidney failure. Blood pressure rises with age, and all of these disorders are much more common among older people.

THE ALUMINUM IN **TABLE SALT** IS PROBABLY THE REAL PROBLEM

Restricting the amount of packaged, commercially polluted table salt (which is not necessarily identical with the commonly used word *sodium)*, in the diet, can control HBP in many people who already have the disease. Patients are often told it also can increase the effectiveness of drug treatment, making a lower dose possible. Unfortunately many do not know that the very popular diuretic *furosemide* (*Lasix*) depends on sodium to do its job.

How to ease cutting back? As people grow older, their sensitivity to flavors and smells often decreases. Because of this, there may be a desire for more salt to combat the flat taste of foods. If they have been told to cut back on salt, there are several steps they can take.

It is easy to change a few dietary habits that will reduce the levels of contaminated commercial table salt, without greatly changing the diet. First, one must learn which foods are lower in table salt (and sodium). Fresh foods usually have less sodium than processed ones. Fresh meat is lower in sodium than lunch meat, bacon, hot dogs, sausage, and ham—all of which have iodized, chemicalized salt added to flavor and preserve them.

Among vegetables, some are higher, others lower in sodium. On a *decreasing* scale:

1. canned vegetables	* * * * * *	(highest)
2. vegetable juice	* * * * *	
3. frozen vegetables without sauces	* * * *	
4. frozen and canned fruit and fruit juices	* * *	
5. fresh fruit and fruit juices	* *	
6. fresh vegetables	*	(lowest)

Commercially prepared foods, canned soups, frozen dinners, and other "fast food" items usually have unwholesome commercial salt added in their preparation. Snacks foods, such as potato chips, pretzels, corn chips, popcorn, crackers, and nuts—normally have a great deal of bad salt added. Ketchup, mustard, relish, salad dressings, sauces, brines, and dips contain sodium. Pickles and olives are also prepared with a good amount of table salt.

Many food manufacturers list the sodium content of their products on the labels. (Foods labeled "salt-free," "sodium-free," "low-salt," or "low-sodium" must have this information.) If sodium is one of the first three ingredients listed, the product is high in sodium.[N071] The sodium is often probably not the problem, but the junk added to table salt is.

COLAS AND SODAS

Drinking sodas is notoriously bad on teeth (a form of bone), probably because of the sodas' content of phosphoric acid. In a study performed to evaluate the effects that Coca Cola had on rat teeth when the animals drank it, the conclusion was that it did erode teeth, but that if calcium lactate —a common calcium supplement—was added to Coca Cola, this mixture resulted in significantly reduced tooth erosion in rats. We may assume that the phosphoric acid may affect skeletal bone in a similar fashion.[B070]

THE CHEMICAL TOXINS IN THE ENVIRONMENT (INCLUDING OUR WATER)

There are many substances in our immediate environment which are harmful to the body, and which cause illness, even death. Some are mined, others derive from the petroleum industry, some are found in air and water, others are organic compounds often added to foods. They act individually and potentiate each other in forms unpredictable because of the multitude of variables that exist. Frequently, these substances are totally ignored by the *Establishment* which does not like to offend industrialists and large corporations of which the medical people may own profitable shares. All of them impact on health, affecting from blood circulation to protein metabolism, and hence, on osteoporosis, but for the scope of this book we will only highlight the most directly related to this problem.

THE TOXIC METALS

These are substances which either don't belong in the human body, or belong only in limited amounts. The substances that don't belong are in this section, the others are dealt with as "toxic effects" of nutritional minerals.

Toxic metals can affect bone metabolism and osteoporosis directly—by action on the bone—and indirectly—by action on steps of protein formation or nutrient absorption. For instance, the collagen molecules of the bone are usually broken down into smaller portions by actions of enzymes, to then self-assemble into collagen fibrils. In an American study, several *toxic* metal salts, cadmium, copper, zinc, nickel, cobalt and mercury chlorides, inhibited this important step, but the results were of variable intensity, depending on the source of the collagen.[H111]

Toxic metals and their combination harm bones, and also other organs and tissues. "Cadmium, lead, mercury, and aluminum are toxic metals that may interact metabolically with nutritionally essential metals. Iron deficiency increases absorption of cadmium, lead, and aluminum. Lead interacts with calcium in the nervous system to impair cognitive development. Cadmium and aluminum interact with calcium in the skeletal system to produce *osteodystrophies* [mal-development of the bone]. Lead replaces zinc on *heme* [blood pigment] enzymes and cadmium replaces zinc on *metallothionein* [a zinc containing amino acid]. Selenium protects from mercury and methyl-mercury toxicity. Aluminum interacts with calcium in bone and kidneys, resulting in aluminum osteodystrophy. Calcium deficiency along with low dietary magnesium may contribute to aluminum-induced degenerative nervous disease."[G082]

THE TOXIC METAL ALUMINUM

Aluminum is everywhere, we are exposed to it daily, in cooking pots, soft drink cans, antacids, tea, etc. Aluminum induces osteoporosis and neurologic disorders.

Hundreds of recent reports from research initially focused on cancer, show as an additional finding "that positively charged, trivalent aluminum ions AL (III) are one important, previously unrecognized cause of bone resorption and osteomalacia (bone softening, crushing, and breaking) not associated with Vitamin D deficiency, in all mature vertebrates and, in particular, the loss of surface bone. AL (III) in bone causes bone pain and proximal *myopathy* (disorders of adjoining muscles and tissues) in all vertebrate species tested."[A030]

"In test animals, phosphate intestinal absorption was strongly suppressed by aluminum. Although calcium absorption did not appear to be affected by aluminum, a negative calcium balance occurred due to increased urinary excretion of calcium. Presumably, calcium was excreted in urine, as it could not be used in the formation of bone crystals because of the lack of phosphate. Plasma calcium was always elevated and plasma phosphorus was always depressed when test animals (ponies) were fed a 4500 ppm aluminum diet. Plasma hydroxyproline [a substance which results from bone metabolism] concentration was increased with high aluminum intake, showing bone turnover was increased due to aluminum effects on phosphorus and calcium metabolism. Magnesium, zinc, iron and copper metabolism were not affected by aluminum intake."[S080]

We must wonder why aluminum, being as old as the planet, is becoming a problem <u>now</u>? "Aluminum is the third most abundant element on the surface of the Earth. It has been held captive in rock biologically unavailable for 3 billion years. Now, industrialization has resulted in acid rains that have decreased the pH of lake waters to the point where AL (III) ion is readily leached out of rocks and soil." AL (III) ion is so toxic that fish that can survive in acidic water, can not live in equally acidic water containing even a very small amount of aluminum ion.[B210]

All vertebrate species, including man, pick up biologically available AL (III) ion from plants contaminated with aluminum leached from rock by acid rain. Tea from plants grown in acidic soil, especially if acidic lemon juice is added, is believed to be a significant source of biologically available aluminum, which over many years of ingestion, may be the primary cause not only of osteoporosis, but of dementias associated with aging. Adding milk to tea (a custom strongly adhered to in England and South America, is believed to detoxify aluminum by strongly binding it with phosphate.[B210]

"Aluminum (III) ion has no positive biological role in most animals, being toxic to cells at large (*cytotoxin*) and the nervous system in particular (*neurotoxin*). Typical clinical signs of AL (III) ion toxicity in humans are [B210] :

- Dialysis dementia
- Iron adequate microcytic anemia
- Vitamin D-resistant osteomalacia

ALUMINUM ANTIDOTES?

As you may remember, molecules have numerous concentric circles of electrons. Aluminum's outer layer of electrons, is similar in number to the outer electron layer of **boron**. In some complex boron-containing biomolecules, boron prevents bone resorption in laboratory animals, which is exactly the reverse of aluminum; however, it is implicated as causal for some neurologic disorders. It has been used as a nutritional supplement.

GALLIUM

We can antidote aluminum in many ways: one way is to learn how to use the mineral Gallium. We can, of course, also *chelate* aluminum out. You will read more about these processes in the section on alternative treatments.

THE TOXIC METAL ARSENIC

Bone is often destroyed by arsenic. In a study about combating the toxic effects of arsenic with natural means, "crude aqueous extract of garlic bulbs (*Allium sativum L. single clove variety*) was administered to [poor little] mice of both sexes daily for up to 30 and 60 days, in doses corresponding to 6 g [1/5 oz.] for a 60 kg [132 lbs] human body. *Sodium arsenite* [an arsenic salt]... was injected subcutaneously to mice on every 7th day of the experiment. The damaging "...affects [sic] of prolonged exposure to sodium arsenite...was reduced by a highly significant amount when crude garlic extract, in the dose used, was given daily to the mice...for the same period." [C081]

Osteoporotic individuals on hormonal replacement therapy are usually concerned about two subjects: bones and cancer. So, they need to watch out for arsenic, because "There exists a strong relation between exposure to arsenic in air and deaths from respiratory [and other] cancer[s]. The increase in deaths is not always linear, that is, the increase in dosage causes increases in death not according to how it doubles or triples, but whether this doubling or tripling happens at light or higher dosages."[E041] Arsenic poisoning "...also shows significant increases in cancer of the large intestine and bone, buccal cavity and pharynx, rectal cancer, and kidney cancer. There was a positive relation between exposure to arsenic in air and kidney and bone cancer, but none for the other cancers, except respiratory." [E041]

Is there a medical test to show whether I am toxic? *Establishment* will tell you there is no routine medical test to show whether you have been contaminated, however, a test on human hair (*hair analysis*) is a simple and inexpensive way to tell if a person has been exposed.

The treatment of most effectiveness is chelation therapy, discussed later on in the "alternatives" section.

THE TOXIC METAL BARIUM

What is *barium*? (Pronounced bar'e-um). Barium is a silvery-white metal found in nature. It occurs combined with other chemicals such as sulfur or carbon and oxygen. These combinations are called compounds. Barium compounds can also be produced by industry. Industrial exposure to barium occurs mostly in the work place or from drinking contaminated water. Ingesting high levels of barium can cause problems with the heart, stomach, liver, kidneys, and other organs. Barium gets into the air during the mining, refining, and production of barium compounds, and from the burning of coal and oil. Some barium compounds dissolve easily in water and are found in lakes, rivers, and streams. Barium is found, at low levels, in most soils and foods. Fish and aquatic organisms accumulate barium.

Barium has no needed biological role. The British Pharmaceutical Codex from 1907 indicates that *barium chloride* [*"barii chloridum"*, $BaCl2.2H2O$] has a stimulant action on the heart and other muscles, and that it "raises blood pressure by constricting the vessels and tends to empty the intestines, bladder, and gall bladder". Its poisonous nature was also pointed out. *Barium sulphide* (*BaS*) was used as a depilatory agent (removes hair). *Barium sulphate* (*BaSO4*) is insoluble and used for body imaging (barium meal).

Barium compounds are used to make:
- Bricks
- Drilling muds made by the oil and gas industries: it is easier to drill through rock by keeping the drill bit lubricated
- Cosmetics
- Glass
- Paint
- Rubber
- Tiles
- X-ray contrast materials (barium sulfate)

Barium compounds that dissolve well in water may cause harmful health effects in people. Ingesting high levels of barium compounds that dissolve well in water has, over the short term, resulted in:
- Brain swelling
- Changes in heart rhythm

- Damage to the liver, kidney, heart, and spleen (It can affect protein formation and cause osteoporosis)
- Difficulties in breathing
- Increased blood pressure
- Muscle weakness
- Stomach irritation

We don't know the effects, in people, of ingesting low levels of barium over the long term. Animal studies have found increased blood pressure and changes in the heart from ingesting barium over a long period of time. We do not yet know the effects of barium from breathing it or from touching it.

The Department of Health and Human Services, the International Agency for Research on Cancer, and the Environmental Protection Agency (EPA) have not classified barium in regards to its human carcinogenicity. Barium has not been classified because there are no studies on people and the two available animal studies were inadequate to determine whether or not barium causes cancer.

Is there a medical test to show whether I've been exposed to barium?

Establishment will tell you there is no routine medical test to show whether you have been exposed to barium. A test on human hair (*hair analysis*) is a simple and inexpensive way to tell if a person has been exposed. *Establishment* doctors can measure barium in the blood, bones, urine, and feces, using very complex instruments. Due to the complexity of the tests, they are usually done only for cases of severe barium poisoning and for medical research.[U009]

Patients who are tube fed often "develop metabolic bone diseases. Because of the chemical relationship between barium and calcium, and the barium bone affinity, a possible responsibility of this element in...bone pathology has been [re]searched."[B200] A French study on tube feeding showed that significant concentrations of barium have been found in the nutrition components.

The most effective treatment is chelation therapy.

THE TOXIC METAL BISMUTH

BISMUTH SUBSALICYLATE

Bismuth Subsalicylate is usually ingested in the pharmaceutical suspension Pepto-Bismol.

Is there a medical test to show whether I am toxic? *Establishment* will tell you there is no routine medical test to show whether you have been contaminated, however, a test on human hair (*hair analysis*) is a simple and inexpensive way to tell if a person has been exposed.

THE TOXIC METAL CADMIUM

Cadmium is a malleable, ductile, toxic, bluish-white metallic element that occurs in association with zinc ores. Cadmium is an environmental poison, is toxic to humans, and has no known useful biological function.

Sources of cadmium are:

- Car exhaust: the wind blows traces of the cadmium in battery and engine parts
- Car tires: cadmium enters the atmosphere as the tires wear down.
- *Catalyzing* reactions (chemically speeding up the process)
- Cigarette smoke (it comes from the cigarette paper and is especially bad in second hand smoke.)
- Electroplating other metals
- Metal alloys
- Nickel-cadmium electrical storage batteries
- Nuclear reactor rods (as a neutron-absorber in the control of nuclear fission)
- Old galvanized pipes
- Paint
- Photoelectric cells
- Pigments
- Process engraving
- Solder
- Stabilizers for plastics

"Cadmium enters the environment primarily through industrial effluents and landfill leaching.... "Cadmium is slightly soluble in water. Concentrations of less than 1 milligram will mix with a liter [quart] of water. Cadmium is highly persistent in water, with a *half-life* of greater than 200 days. The half-life of a pollutant is the amount of time it takes for one-half of the chemical to be degraded."[A022]

*"**Cadmium** (**Cd**)* exposure induces bone resorption *in vitro* and *in vivo* that can lead to low bone mass and increased incidence of fracture."[W068] "... Cd accelerates the differentiation of new *osteoclasts* [bone destroying cells] from their *progenitor* [parent] cells[,] and activates or increases the activity of mature osteoclasts."[W069]

Severe cadmium poisoning from industrial sources in Japan, resulted in a bone disease known as *Itai-Itai* disease, literally "it hurts, it hurts". Bone in severe cadmium poisoning shows areas of abnormal configuration and appearance of bone loss and fractures, known as *looser zones* and *healing bands*, especially of the ribs. These bones are abnormal, full of woven, thickened areas and areas of over-hardened bone.[Y009] We may see low grades of this and confuse it with other conditions.

Scientists in Israel studied the effect of cadmium on the healing of bones of young rats subjected to the form of animal abuse euphemistically called medical research. "The effect of cadmium (Cd) in drinking water [supplied to rats], on repair of bone at a site of hole injury to the tibia [leg bone]..., was followed...A slight reduction (about 10%) in body weight and water and food consumption was observed in cadmium-exposed rats as compared to control rats."[G140] The lab tests done on them, at this stage, "... did not indicate changes related to Cd toxicity,..."[G140] but there were changes in the bone enzymes. "Calcium accumulation in the newly formed repair tissue at the site of injury was also significantly reduced to one half. Cadmium, a toxin so common that almost everybody is contaminated with it, to various levels [just see what your hair analysis shows] "... probably exhibits an effect on the bone repair process as reflected by reduction in [the]... activity [of]...osteoblastic cells...and mineralization at the site of injury in the tibia of young rats."[G140]

FROM PERFECTION AND SYMMETRY, TO DISORDER.
HOW DOES CADMIUM DAMAGE THE BONES?

To understand how cadmium (Cd) is so ubiquitously (widespread) harmful to bone, researchers in New York studied the formation of the crystalline, calcium containing, bone mineral *hydroxiapatite* (*HA*) under normal conditions, and then, with the addition of cadmium. Under normal conditions, HA has a very typical crystalline lattice structure. Cadmium incorporation in HA introduced little strain in the lattice itself, but resulted in a decreasing crystal size. A crystal usually has a typical symmetry that manifests as an image created by the beams of various types of light going through it—the *spectrum*. Light beam studies, "(*Infrared spectroscopy*) of Cd-HA showed a complex series of small changes in the spectra as a function of Cd concentration, resulting from some distortion in the crystal perfection and symmetry.[B172]

Is there a medical test to show whether I am toxic? *Establishment* will tell you there is no routine medical test to show whether you have been contaminated, however, a test on human hair (*hair analysis*) is a simple and inexpensive way to tell if a person has been exposed.

The treatment of cadmium poisoning which is most effective is, of course, chelation therapy.

THE (TOXIC) MINERAL FLUORIDE

WOULD YOU CARE FOR RAT POISON IN YOUR WATER?
THE SAGA OF SODIUM FLUORIDE

Do you want to take rat poison in order to get hard but brittle bones? The *Establishment* purports that sodium fluoride, an abominable industrial residue scraped from chimneys after the processing of aluminum ore and also frequently a contaminant of drinking water, otherwise sold as rat poison, may have a useful role to play in patients afflicted with severe osteoporosis. In osteoporosis, the main metabolic problem is increased bone resorption, rather than a decrease in bone formation. Fluoride *enhances* bone formation, it *does not reduce* bone resorption. The bone formed when fluoride is part of the process, is very hard and prone to splintering as it has substituted some of the bone's elasticity by increased hardness. People living in areas in which the water has a high-fluoride content have, for instance, higher dental density than people living in a low fluoride area (of course, those areas also usually have higher contents of other minerals such as *calcium, boron, strontium*, etc.). These higher density teeth are rather brittle.

The use of artificial fluoride supplements is a love affair of many grant-hungry, politically correct professionals and academicians. When used in post-menopausal women fluoride causes unequal results in different types of bones. A study done by the Mayo Clinic found that fluoride therapy increases bone density in trabecular bone, yet decreases cortical bone density, which may increase osseous fragility, and increase the risk of hip fractures. The Mayo Clinic abandoned the use of fluoride therapy, as a wise consequence of this study. Fluoride's side effects are many, I recommend the reading of FLUORIDE, THE AGING FACTOR, by John Yamouyannis.

FLUORIDE THERAPY DECREASES CORTICAL BONE DENSITY

Fluoride becomes part of the bone elements, therefore, it can impact on bone development. The higher the dose, the more serious the consequences. In a study supplying rats with a very high intake of fluoride, growth rate was depressed in all groups receiving fluoride, but most severely in those receiving a diet with 50% fat; that group had an increased amount of absorption, probably because of a delaying effect of fat and fluoride on the emptying of the stomach.[M011]

Is there a medical test to show whether I am toxic? Fluorine can be tested in the urine.

Fluoride does not chelate out.

THE TOXIC METAL LEAD

What is *lead* and where is it found? Lead is a mineral found in the environment all around us, generally occurs in nature in the form of ores and as a by-product in the smelting of silver. Its versatility, its physical and chemical properties, account for its extensive use. Lead can be rolled into sheets and made into rods and pipes. It can also be molded into containers and mixed with other metallic elements. Lead has been mined, smelted and compounded for thousands of years. Once mined, processed and introduced into man's environment, it becomes a potential problem forever. It has even been found in the Egyptian tombs. We find it in gasoline residues, lead paint, lead water pipes, lead joints in copper pipes, newsprint, mini blinds and *Grecian Formula*® products.

Poisoning can occur either due to inhalation or swallowing of lead paint chips[B130] and/or due to dust, (Most houses built before 1978 used lead paint both on the inside and outside), street dust containing exhaust residue, or contaminated water sources. Once in the body, it goes from blood to tissue, and remains there for a lifetime.

It also affects the formation of cartilage. In an animal study where rats and guinea pigs were given **lead acetate** for 3-6 months, the formation of proper cartilage protein..."[Z010] measured in the cartilage forming cells (**chondrocytes**) decreased, and abnormalities occurred in the growth and in development of cartilage and of the structural elements of bone.[Z010]

WHO GETS LEAD POISONING?

Children, especially those below six, are the most vulnerable to lead poisoning. However, it is equally widespread in other segments of the population, more pronounced in printers, welders, plumbers, mechanics, etc.

HOW DOES ONE GET LEAD POISONING?

- Contaminated drinking water
- Eating paint chips
- Inhaling paint dust
- Playing in contaminated dirt and putting their fingers in their mouth

WHAT ARE THE SYMPTOMS OF LEAD POISONING?

- Colicky pains
- Dark line along the gums
- Dementia
- Hypertension
- Local muscular paralysis
- Personality changes
- Tooth decay

Is there a medical test to show whether I am toxic? *Establishment* will tell you there is no routine medical test to show whether you have been contaminated, however, a test on human hair (**hair analysis**) is a simple and inexpensive way to tell if a person has been exposed.

A LINK TO TOOTH DECAY?

In a 1997 edition of New Scientist magazine, dental researchers from the University of Grenada reported that children with 10 or more sites of decay in their mouths also had about triple the amount of lead in their bodies compared to children with no decay. Lead may replace natural protective traces of metals in tooth enamel which then renders teeth more prone to attack by cavity-causing bacteria. This may explain why older people, who have had additional years to accumulate lead in their bodies from traffic fumes, tap water, etc., suffer from tooth decay. A similar harmful effect may be expected in skeletal bone.[B120] Additional references can be found in the appendix after the regular references.

LEAD IN COSMETICS

To make things really bad, lead acetate is frequently introduced into the organism in the form of hair cosmetics. "Lead acetate is used as a color additive in "progressive" hair dye products. These products are applied over a period of time to achieve a gradual coloring effect. In order to be approved for this use, a color additive petition was required to establish safety.

"The safety data submitted in support of this petition included results from trials on humans using the products. In the trials, people using the product under controlled conditions of use were monitored for the amount of lead in their bloodstream. No significant increase in blood levels of lead was seen in the trial subjects and the lead was not shown to be absorbed into the body through such use. [The article does not state what criteria were used, who sponsored the study, and for how long the individuals were evaluated. My personal experience is different].

"This data allowed FDA to determine that safe conditions of use could be established and a color additive regulation allowing the use of lead acetate in hair dyes was established. The regulation requires that specific labeling instructions appear on the product labels. These include cautions to use the product externally, not to use on cut or abraded skin, and to wash hands thoroughly after use. Consumers are advised to carefully follow all label directions."[U010]

A new study published in the Journal of the American Pharmaceutical Association raises the possibility of danger to children. The agency has not yet evaluated the new study, but will review it carefully to determine if the information warrants further attention or action. The data in hand, however, indicates that lead acetate containing hair dye products can be used safely. It is important, however, that consumers carefully follow the directions on the package and keep the products out of the hands and away from children.

Consumers can determine if lead acetate is used in a particular hair dye product by reviewing the product ingredient declaration appearing on the label of the cosmetic in package form.

LEAD IN THE SKELETON

Is there any connection between blood lead levels, urinary lead level (after *chelation* or chemical extraction) and lead in bones? In a Swedish study, a close correlation was found between the blood lead level of 20 lead workers and their urinary excretion of lead for 24 hours after intravenous infusion with 1 gram of the chelating agent *EDTA* or *calcium di-sodium edetate*. There was a significant correlation between chelated lead and bone lead in currently exposed workers. It was concluded that chelatable lead mainly reflects the blood and soft-tissue lead pool, which is only partly dependent upon the skeletal lead content that comprises the biggest share of the total body burden.[T040] The skeleton harbors more than 90% of the body burden of inorganic lead.[B140]

The most effective treatment is chelation therapy.

THE TOXIC METAL MERCURY

Mercury is a substance which is highly toxic to animals and humans. Even very low levels may suppress necessary selenium function. Mercury can be responsible for arthritic and neurologic symptoms, which may add to, or mimic, osteoporotic pains and disabilities.

Elemental mercury is a heavy and relatively inert liquid which is oxidized to inorganic mercury under natural conditions. Mercury may combine with an organic fraction to from methyl-mercury. Both mercury and methyl-mercury are of environmental concern. Mercury may enter the environment in industrial or municipal waste treatment discharges, from previously contaminated sediments, and from the weathering of natural rocks. Bacteria may then convert it into methyl-mercury. The concentration of mercury in bodies of water may be elevated with acid rain due to the scouring of mercury from the air and increased partitioning from the sediment into the water.[U122]

Chronic toxic effects may include:
- Arthritic symptoms
- Changes in appearance or behavior
- Lower fertility
- Mimicking osteoporotic pains and disabilities
- Neurologic symptoms
- Reproductive problems
- Shortened life span

"Chronic effects can be seen long after first exposure(s) to a toxic chemical."[U122]

Dental amalgam fillings are the most important source of mercury exposure in the general population, a few decades ago mercury was also used medically as *Mercurochrome*, *Merthiolate*, *diuretics*, *laxatives*, etc.[H150] Other sources are:
- Hemorrhoidal preparations
- Seafoods
- Skin lightening agents
- Water supplies

In studies using the involuntary cooperation of mice, it was clearly demonstrated that "Not only mercury but also silver accumulated in the spleen and kidneys after amalgam implantation. Dental amalgam implantation in a physiological body...[environment]...causes chronic stimulation of the immune system. Implantation of *silver alloy* [similar to the silver fillings in teeth] not containing mercury also induced autoimmunity, suggesting that other elements, especially silver, have the potential to induce autoimmunity in genetically susceptible vertebrates....[Mixed] heavy metals, from dental amalgam and other sources, may lower the threshold of an individual metal to [develop]...immunological [anomalies]...[and] lead to overt autoimmunity."[B020]

What are other, lesser known but no less important problems with mercury? There exists a possible inhibitory effect of mercury for the conversion of the inactive thyroid hormone T4 to the active hormone T3. This may affect protein synthesis, indirectly aggravating osteoporosis.

There is a remarkable correlation between illness and mercury contamination (measured by hair levels) in certain individuals. In a Japanese study Dr. R. Nakagawa, an environmental scientist, evaluated the connection between the levels of the toxic metal mercury in human hair, and the prevalences of diseases such as atopic dermatitis [rashes of undetermined origin], asthma, dementia, cerebral infarct [stroke], osteoporosis, hypertension and diabetes in 133 volunteers from Tokyo an surrounding areas from Oct. 1992 to June 1993. "The total mercury concentrations in the hair of...diseased people were from 2.08 ppm to 36.5 ppm. Those values were considerably higher than that of healthy people of the same age groups."[N010]

There are numerous forms of hyperactivity, mental and emotional changes, neuromuscular disorders and loss of appetite linked to mercury toxicity. Close associations between multiple sclerosis and dental amalgam fillings are also encountered. The expression "mad as a hatter" derives from the fact that hatters had frequent exposure to felts treated with mercury salts, and hatters had notoriously bad tempers.

Is there a medical test to show toxic levels? *Establishment* will tell you there is no routine medical test to show whether you have been contaminated, however, a test on human hair (*hair analysis*) is a simple and inexpensive way to tell if a person has been exposed. There are special *chewing gums* that can be used for the evaluation of leaching amalgams.

The most effective treatment is chelation therapy.

THE TOXIC METAL TIN

Would you put a lethal poison in things which go in your mouth. Would you *tin*ker with your health (pardon the pun). Tin is present in cans, containers, make up, and, unfortunately, tooth paste. The word *stannuous*, which you can see as *stannuous fluoride*, means: containing tin.

In rats deliberately poisoned with tin, concentrations of other minerals in

various tissues were quite frighteningly disturbed. The mineral disturbances would be the equivalent in humans to decreasing plasma and tissue
concentrations of iron, copper and zinc, by up to 15%.[P052]

Is there a medical test to show whether I am toxic? *Establishment* will tell
you there is no routine medical test to show whether you have been contaminated, however, a test on human hair (*hair analysis*) is a simple and
inexpensive way to tell if a person has been exposed.

The most effective treatment is chelation therapy.

HAIR MINERAL ANALYSIS (HAIR ANALYSIS)
What is hair mineral analysis?

Hair tissue mineral analysis (HTMA) is an analytical test which measures
the mineral content of the hair. The sample of hair is prepared in a licensed
clinical laboratory through a series of chemical and high temperature
digestive procedures. Testing is then performed using highly sophisticated
detection equipment and methods to achieve the most accurate and precise
results.

Why use hair instead of blood? Because hair is ideal. It can be cut easily
and painlessly, and it can be sent to the lab without special handling
requirements. Also, clinical results have shown that a properly obtained
sample of hair can give an indication of mineral status and toxic metal
accumulation following long-term or even acute exposure. The body
removes toxins from the serum as a protective measure, depositing them
into tissues, including hair. Hair is used as one of the tissues of choice by
the Environmental Protection Agency in determining toxic metal exposure. A 1980 report from the E.P.A. stated that human hair can be effectively used for biological monitoring of the highest priority toxic metals.
This report confirmed the findings of other studies in the U.S. and abroad,
which concluded that human hair may be a more appropriate tissue than
blood or urine for studying community exposure to some trace elements.

Why test for minerals? Trace minerals are essential in countless metabolic functions in all phases of the life process. In the words of the late author
and noted researcher, Dr. Henry Schroeder, trace elements (minerals) are
"...more important factors in human nutrition than vitamins. The body can

manufacture many vitamins, but it cannot produce necessary trace minerals or get rid of many possible excesses."

Is Hair Analysis supported by research? Hair analysis is supported by extensive literature in a variety of respected national and international scientific publications. Each year in the United States alone, federally licensed clinical laboratories perform over 150,000 hair mineral assays for health care professionals interested in an additional screening aid for a comprehensive patient evaluation. This does not take into consideration the thousands of subjects used in numerous continuing research studies conducted by private and government research agencies.

In osteoporosis, calcium loss from the body can become so advanced that severe bone disease can develop without any appreciable changes noted in the calcium levels in a blood test. Among the trace elements in bone and hair, significant differences were found in the contents of zinc, copper and manganese between normal subjects and osteoporotic patients. However, exact involvements of the trace elements in osteoporosis have not yet been clarified.[0139]

THE IMPORTANCE OF GOOD NUTRITION

NUTRIENTS
Individual nutrients fulfill many varied functions in human metabolism. Some are directly related to the treatment and prevention of osteoporosis, others only relate to general health. Because of the scope of this book, I will concentrate mainly on specific functions, without completely disregarding the generalities as they impact on general health. If particular features about a specific nutrient, you may find particularly enlightening appear to be missing, it is only because of space constraints, and future books on other health issues will treat those items in depth.

NUTRITIONAL DEFICIENCIES
Much of the research has been done with laboratory species on very exacting diets, yet total deficiency states are almost impossible to induce in humans, which self select foods. Findings in the various species do not automatically extend to findings in humans. Various harmful effects may occur in the fetus/neonate, the actively growing young animal, and in the adult.

CARBOHYDRATES IN THE DIET

Carbohydrates are made from various numbers of molecules responding to the same basic structural formula containing variable number of atoms of *C* (*carbon*), *O* (*oxygen*) and *H* (*hydrogen*), arranged in different structural patterns.

They are classified as:
- **Simple:** glucose, sucrose, fructose
- **Complex:** starches, dextrines and maltoses

SIMPLE CARBOHYDRATES

Fructose, fruit sugar, touted to be a simple sugar of a much "higher" nutritional quality than glucose, can actually represent a slight health hazard. It is oversupplied in our diet, for it does not just appear as a component of table sugar and a natural ingredient in fruits and vegetables, but high fructose corn syrup, and other corn syrup ingredients are part of most sodas, juice drinks, etc. It has been found that white blood cells do not grow well in a solution that has a high *fructose* concentration, and that high *fructose* may interfere or deplete the energy substance *adenosine triphosphate* (*ATP*), because *fructose* may bind to the energizing phosphate groups. Actually, we have reports that any deficiency of *kinase enzymes*, a widespread problem since all immunosuppressive viruses deplete *tyrosine-phospho-kinase*, may cause a *fructose intolerance* even at low levels of this sugar, that can further weaken *virus* victims and victims of *hypoglycemia*. Victims of osteoporosis certainly do not need any depletion of their energy.

COMPLEX CARBOHYDRATES

Starches are the complex carbohydrates so highly touted by vegetarians and lovers of so called *whole* or *health foods*. Without denying the nutritional value of these foods, it is worth mentioning that the grains and legumes which contain them, are often depleted of trace elements, and have absorbed massive amounts of environmental toxins. Starches promote more drops in body blood sugar levels than do meats, cheeses, and eggs, but less than simple sugars such as sucrose, glucose, and fructose.

Vegetarianism, inspired by certain philosophical ideas, and the need to find diets tolerable to those suffering from chronic, degenerative diseases, have popularized fruits, vegetables and complex carbohydrates. However well these diets may fit patients suffering from cancer and other serious illnesses, they are not really suited to the majority of us, living in an environment full of pollutants and under heavy stress. As early as the 1930s, high carbohydrate diets became linked with chronic infection, rheumatic fever, even colds. Abuse of table sugar (*sucrose*) appears to be the main offender—at least in those metabolically intolerant to it.

Despite the ingrained belief among vegetarians, (today's nutritional correctness)—that high carbohydrate diets are the best for good health and wholesome bones, temporary increases in the elimination of calcium in urine have been noted after high carbohydrate meals, independent of dietary calcium: this is probably due to impaired renal calcium reabsorption mediated by an increase in plasma insulin levels. Based on these observations, some investigators believe that long term intake of high carbohydrate diets may increase the risk of *nephrolithiasis* (kidney stones), and possibly osteoporosis. As science usually does, contradictions are often found. In a different study, despite higher all day levels of plasma insulin on the high carbohydrate diets compared to the high fat diet in both normal and non-insulin-dependent diabetic subjects, no changes in daily urinary excretion of calcium or other constituents associated with renal stone risk, were observed. Furthermore, there was no change in fractional intestinal *47Ca* absorption. Although hypercalciuria may ensue transiently after high carbohydrate meals, the authors of that particular study concluded that substitution of simple or complex carbohydrates for fats, calorie by calorie, for a longer duration, does not result in significant urinary calcium loss. They believe that high intakes of digestible carbohydrates may not increase the risk of nephrolithiasis or osteoporosis via this mechanism.[G020]

PROTEINS AND AMINO ACIDS

There is much debate whether protein intake is beneficial or harmful to bone structure, but as most things are with nutrition, the effect is quantity and balance-related. Excessive protein intake, whether animal or vegetable, unopposed by the buffering effect of fruits and vegetables, may cause some calcium loss. Protein malnutrition is also definitely associated with poor bone protein metabolism. In an Italian study about the beneficial effects of several proteins and amino acids, it was determined that a preparation of *arginine-lysine-lactose* improved BMD.[A010]

The comparison between the two groups studied showed that those with the Italian supplementation experienced the following favorable outcomes:

- Evident and significant reduction of parathormone (parathyroid hormone, which breaks down bone) levels
- Evident and significant reduction of hydroxyprolinuria (amino acids found in urine, which indicate bone loss levels)
- Greater reduction in painful symptoms
- Marked increment in BMD in subjects treated with arginine-lysine-lactose

These effects appear to be due to a distinct improvement in intestinal calcium absorption mediated by lysine and lactose, and probably to a positive action played by the amino acid at the level of support structures.

PROTEINS

Proteins are primary components of muscle (meat), milk, cheese, eggs, etc., and are also represented in lesser amounts in beans and some grains.

Proteins are not directly absorbed, they have to be broken down into smaller components, the amino acids. These are the building blocks of the human body proteins: muscles, skin, immunoglobulins, etc. In the nervous system, they act as neurotransmitters (facilitating interaction between nerve connections).

Amino Acids, according to whether they are manufactured in the body, or have to be provided from the food we eat, can be classified into essential and non-essential (which does not mean they are more or less necessary, but simply refer to their sources):

Essential: (They are *not* manufactured by the human body, and must be provided by food intake). There are eight in the adult; in children as many as ten of the amino acids may qualify as *essential.*
Nonessential: manufactured in the human body.

Although there are many different amino acids, the total number represented in the human protein makeup is nineteen.

Proteins can be classified according to whether their composition includes *all* of the essential amino acids, or not, into:

- **Complete** (all essential amino acids are present)
- **Incomplete** (not all essential amino acids are present)

What determines the body's capacity to utilize dietary protein to its best efficiency? The capacity of the body to use dietary proteins for the building of proper protein is dependent on the levels in which *all* essential amino acids are present in the digestive tract *at the same TIME and in the PROPER PROPORTIONS*. This is known as the *NPU* (*net protein utilization*) of that food. If a person eats an apparently *high protein diet*, with much meat, but overcooks it, at temperature levels that may destroy or denature essential amino acids, that person will actually become protein deficient.

To be properly digested, proteins need *hydrochloric acid* in the stomach; people who do not produce sufficient hydrochloric acid to appropriately break food down into usable amino acids also develop protein deficiencies despite apparently adequate supply.

**THE NUTRITIONAL VALUE OF PROTEINS IS QUITE VARIABLE:
ONLY "COMPLETE PROTEINS"
CAN BUILD ADEQUATE HUMAN PROTEIN**

Most animal proteins are **complete** (They contain *all* essential amino acids). But turkey meat is not complete. *Vegetable proteins*, with the exception of *soy bean* protein, are mostly *incomplete*. Foods of non-animal origin, if properly combined, supply amino acid pools that permit complete proteins to be synthesized. Proper combining of foods requires knowledge and foresight to prepare nourishing meals. The best source of information I have ever found about this subject, is "Diet for a Small Planet", by Frances Moore Lappe.

The beneficial effects of a high protein diet on the maintenance of health and prevention of disease were studied with great interest from the 1920s to the 1940s. In those days, the treatment of patients suffering from syphilis was carried out with *arsenic* derived compounds. These caused severe side-effects, even shock, liver damage, etc. A high protein diet was remarkably protective for the experimental subjects. Similar beneficial effects were noticed in studies utilizing **cadmium** as the toxic test agent. Not only were the amounts of protein found to be of importance, but also the type of protein used. The most protective seemed to be egg-white.

Certain proteins active in the immune process (**immunoglobulins or Ig**) can be supplied through mother's milk, from the mother to the infant, or through a *bovine* **colostrum** (the first secretion of the cow's udders after giving birth) preparation that is commercially available (**Immugen**).

AMINO ACIDS
Amino acids are the building blocks of all protein, protein that forms skin and hair, muscles and bones. The health effects of taking *individual* amino acids are still being explored, and more and more interesting effects are found. Amino acid deficiencies often *must* be identified and singled out in order to institute proper therapy. Although amino acid studies of the patient's blood or urine are not an everyday test, they are available at many labs. It is important to learn as much as possible about them, their function, and their balance.

Commercially, they exist in two series (**D** and **L**). The letters indicate a difference in the way a light beam acts when passing through a transparent container of an amino acid solution. The light may turn to the right (**D/Dextro**), or the left (**L/Levo**). The L series is the most compatible with the way they exist in the human body.

L-ALANINE
L-Alanine is a co-factor in metabolizing the sugar glucose, and creating energy for the body.

L-ARGININE
L-Arginine is strongly recommended because of its stimulating effect on the production of Human Growth Hormone (HGH). It acts directly on pituitary cells, especially those connected with tyrotropin-releasing hormone, a hormone related to thyroid metabolism, and it needs the presence of calcium to impact on this process.[V041] It is a part of certain nutritional mixes and powders to replenish osteoporotic bones. It is included in drops and pills touted to induce the let-down of growth hormone.

A note of caution: arginine, when unopposed by lysine, *activates* herpes virus growth in experimental studies. It may do so with other viruses.

L-ASPARAGINE

L-Asparagine is needed to balance the nervous system.

L-ASPARTIC ACID

It combats fatigue, activates energy production in the cell

L-CARNITINE

L-Carnitine is a normal component of animal protein, and has documented activity as:

- Aid in the transport of certain fatty acids
- Controlling and strengthening the heart muscle
- Helping many antioxidants to protect the cardiovascular system
- Preventing buildup of fat

It is closely related to the metabolism of the amino acid lysine (very important to bone metabolism), and may well be one of the therapeutic miracles of the future. In my practice, I have frequently had the opportunity of treating people who had *cardiovascular failure* or weak heart (characterized by leg swelling towards the evening, shortness of breath upon walking and lying flat, and other symptoms) with *carnitine,* and have accomplished the reversal of the problem. Some patients who were already on the medication *digitalis*, used therapeutically in treating this problem, were able to discontinue their medication when supplementing their diet with *carnitine*.

L-CITRULLINE

L-Citrulline has important energy functions, and can be converted into L-Arginine, so important to the metabolism of Human Growth Hormone (HGH).

L-CYSTINE

L-Cysteine is a *sulphur containing amino acid*, well known to reduce testicular damage by *cadmium* in rodents used for experiments. The protective effects against this toxic heavy metal, are highly interesting in a society where everyone is exposed to cadmium-toxicity due to industrial pollution. However, *cysteine* seems to have such a strong effect on the elimination of cadmium through the kidneys that the intake of this toxic mineral with *cysteine* accelerates kidney damage. The toxicity of cobalt, copper, and nickel is also reduced. *N-acetyl-cysteine (NAC)*, a commercial *cysteine*, has gained much favor as a nutritional, therapeutic, and antitoxic factor. Edward J. Calabrese, from the Environmental Health Program, Division of Public Health, of the University of Massachusetts, author of "NUTRITION AND ENVIRONMENTAL HEALTH", tells us that "It has been shown that the administration of a variety of sulphur-containing amino acids including *methionine*, *cystine* and *cysteine* may affect the toxicity and/or carcinogenicity of over 40 compounds....In the overwhelming number of cases, these amino acids clearly reduce both the incidence and severity of the particular adverse condition."

L-CYSTEINE

L-Cysteine is also a *sulphur containing amino acid*, with properties similar to L-cystine, being instrumental in post-surgical healing and skin maintenance.

L-GLUTAMIC ACID

L-Glutamic acid is a unique amino acid, insofar that it can be brain fuel, just like glucose, and stimulate brain cell activity.

L-GLUTAMINE

Glutamine may lower calcium levels. By my own observation, individual supplementation with this amino acid may unleash a herpes outbreak. Strangely enough, Ross Laboratories is selling a commercial form of *glutamine,* adducing that it "increases CD4/CD8 ratio (one aspect of the immune system)," and that it is good for the "metabolically stressed patient."[R091] It certainly does not explain how this CD4/CD8 ratio comes into being, or how it works on the *metabolically stressed patient.*

L-GLUTATHIONE

L-Glutathione is a powerful antioxidant. it protects the body from the free radicals created by cigarettes and radiation, chemotherapy, X-rays and alcohol poisoning.

L-GLYCINE

L-Glycine is unique insofar that it does not split into D and L series, being very important to a healthy prostate and stable nervous system. It can enhance energy, but, if taken to excess, damage the energy level.

L-HISTIDINE

L-Histidine can act as a virus growth promoter, yet it is instrumental in unleashing allergic reactions.

L-LEUCINE

L-Leucine is a **branched** (an allusion to chemical structure) amino acid, which is suppressive to immunity under experimental settings, but only if general nutrition is poor.

L-LYSINE

L-Lysine has been shown to protect experimental animals against the depressant and hypnotic effects of alcohol; it is also protective against herpes and other viruses. Over the years of my practice, innumerable patients added lysine to their program and remained free from uncomfortable herpes outbreaks. Lysine has also been used in the form of creams.

CHOLINE AND METHIONINE

Choline and *methionine*: are necessary for the full development of the *thymus* (the gland of immunity). If young rats are deficiently nourished in these amino acids while *intra utero* (in the womb), or while nursing, they will have a poorly functioning immune system throughout life.

METHIONINE

Methionine is a sulfur containing amino acid. and a powerful antidote against many toxins. One of the mechanisms by which methionine may protect from many and varied chemicals is that it can give certain chemicals, *methyl* groups, (*methyl donor*) to other substances. As early as 1942, it was already known that this amino acid could prevent *Chloroform*-induced liver damage (chloroform was a frequently used anesthetic), as well as jaundice from the many arsenic containing drugs used in those days. Patients who were severely ill for undetermined reasons improved with the addition of choline and methionine to their diets. It is also effective against *cobalt* and *copper* toxicity, and, as a very important quality, it is protective against *lead, **thallium, selenium, silver**,* and ***mercury*** intoxication.

Maintaining mice on a ***choline*** deficient diet results in mice afflicted with hepatic methyl donor deficiency (HMDD), which can not detoxify many harmful substances or drugs.[T051]

PATIENTS WHO WERE SEVERELY ILL FOR UNDETERMINED REASONS IMPROVED WITH THE ADDITION OF CHOLORINE AND METHIONINE TO THEIR DIETS

In 1945 it was clearly demonstrated that the jaundice and hepatitis that ensued from exposure to ***carbon tetrachloride*** (cleaning fluid), could be markedly *lessened* by the increased intake of ***methionine*** and protein.

Methionine defeats marijuana and tobacco smoke: In our marijuana-happy society, it may be a bit of good news that the conjoint use of ***methionine*** and vitamin C markedly *reduced* the cancer-causing capacity that marijuana and tobacco smoke exercised on the lungs of animals used in experiments.

Mothballs may kill more than just moths. In 1919 it had already been established that the deficiency of certain nutrients, especially ***methionine*** and other sulphur-containing amino acids increased the toxicity of ***naphthalene*** (the chemical in mothballs). It was not long until other interactions between methionine and other members of this family of compounds (***azo-dyes***, such as create the purplish-red or maroon color in bladder pills) were found. These dyes are used as food colorings, fabric dyes, and medicine coloring material. This is important to know because of naphthalene's widespread industrial use, and its presence in the form of moth repellents and moth balls in most households. It is unconscionable that with this very pedestrian substance in such widespread use, which residually contaminates clothes worn close to the skin—the largest absorptive surface of the body, that the public is not informed that individuals who suffer from ***G-6-PD deficiency*** (an enzymatic disorder afflicting as many as 1 in 4 blacks, and also present in whites who have leukemia.), should never be exposed to this very toxic substance; it can cause skin rashes, ***intravascular hemolysis*** (disintegration of red blood cells inside blood vessels), ***renal tubular blockade*** (impaired kidney function), ***ocular neuritis*** (nerve damage of the eyes), digestive problems, vomiting, sweating, etc.

Because methionine is necessary to detoxify medicines and substances that osteoporotics may be exposed to, it is important that they are aware of the importance of this amino acid.

To those using *laetrile* (a derivative of bitter almonds and the pits of several fruits, used in cancer therapies, also known as *vitamin B_{17}*), *methionine* and the other sulphur containing amino acids represent an extra insurance against potential *cyanide* poisoning from the metabolism of *laetrile*.

To those exposed to *nitrites* and *nitrates* in unwholesome diets (in preserved meats of all kinds), or drugs, or by handling explosives, *methionine*, particularly in association with vitamin C, offers a strong defense mechanism against damage to the blood pigment, which in the presence of nitrates or nitrites may convert into useless and harmful *methemoglobin*. Good blood pigment is necessary for the appropriate metabolism of bone.

Since the maintenance of unadulterated DNA is so very important, understanding that *methionine* and other sulphur containing amino acids block DNA damage by substances known as *N-nitroso compounds*, is of paramount importance.

Pyridines, commonly used chemicals, are also less toxic to subjects well supplied with *methionine*.

Another remarkable property of *methionine* is its protective effect against *acetaldehyde* toxicity (a toxin resulting from the metabolism of alcohol drinkers and cigarette smokers, who are especially highly at risk for osteoporosis).

L-ORNITHINE

L-Ornithine has numerous important functions in healing, detoxification, and helping the release of human growth hormone (HGH), when accompanied by L-arginine and L-carnitine.

L-PHENYLALANINE

L-Phenyalanine is effective in mood elevation, aids in the control of memory, and obesity. It is good to assist in the control of pain.

DL-PHENYLALANINE (DLPA)

DL-Phenyalanine is quite effective in many cases of pain or addictions. It is used in the DL forms, what is called a *racemic mixture*.

L-PROLINE

L-Proline is fundamental to healthy tissues, being part of the production of collagen, which strengthens ligaments, needed in bone building, etc. One form, *Alpha-methyl-proline*, is necessary for the synthesis of *collagen type I*, the major protein of bone matrix, which is significantly reduced in osteoporosis. In tests performed on unfairly exploited rats, *alpha-methyl-proline* treatment significantly increased collagen formation, as compared to untreated rats who had had their ovaries removed, even those who were given estrogen.[L130]

L-TAURINE

L-Taurine has numerous metabolic functions aiding in fat digestion, bile production, helping with cardiovascular disorders and hypoglycemia.

L-THREONINE

L-Threonine has been found to be protective against alcohol-induced personality changes in the behavioral performance of rats used in experiments, and is necessary to maintain good protein balance.

L-TRYPTOPHAN

L-Tryptophan is necessary to maintain calmness, synthesize niacin, B3. It has enjoyed enormous popularity for its sleep inducing effect, has been persecuted and maligned after a mysterious outbreak of eosinophilia-myalgia-syndrome, which has increased white blood cells and muscle pain, and was tracked down to a contaminated product.[153]

L-TYROSINE

L-Tyrosine is a basic building block of the all-important *thyroid hormones*, and of skin pigments. It is necessary to other glandular function. Deficiencies may lead to depression and mood disorders.

L-VALINE

L-Valine contributes to tissue repair and has a stimulant effect.

ENZYMES

Enzymes are defined as *activators of chemical processes, without being part of the chemical process themselves.* Some work inside the cells, bio-logic-process enzymes, others are part of the digestive process in the stomach and other sections of the digestive tract.

Digestive enzyme supplements, and certain biologic enzymes such as *co-enzyme Q*, etc., are commercially available. Some enzyme supplements are based on an enzyme of vegetable source (*papaya* enzyme), and have received much notoriety. However, digestion is a complex process, and complete enzyme supplements, containing those which digest protein, starch and fats, as well as hydrochloric acid and bile salts, are probably the best to buy. Proper digestion enhances proper assimilation, and improves health.

> **PROPER DIGESTION IS NECESSARY FOR GOOD ASSIMILATION WHICH IS INDISPENSABLE TO HEALTH**

To me, it is always surprising and at the same time disappointing, that despite the prevalence of digestive disturbances in our culture, those unnecessarily suffering are not taking digestive enzymes.

METABOLIC MODIFIERS

DMAE

Dimethyl Amino Ethanol (*DMAE*) is a nutritional supplement, mainly found in fish, that supports the old wives' tale that fish is a great brain food. DMAE is normally present in small amounts in our brains, and is known for its mental stimulation and enhancement.

Because fish is naturally abundant in DMAE, a diet high in sardines and anchovies will provide higher than average levels of DMAE and choline to the brain, to serve as raw materials for the production of the *neuro-transmitter acetylcholine*. Acetylcholine is responsible for conducting nerve impulses within the brain, and by accelerating the brain's synthesis of this important neurotransmitter, DMAE may aid in improving memory and learning, as well as preventing loss of memory in adults.

DMAE helps elevate mood, improve memory and learning, increase intelligence and physical energy, and extends the life span of laboratory animals. It is used by many people for its mild, safe stimulant effect, yet DMAE also makes it easier for most people to get to sleep. Many people report less fatigue in the day and sounder sleep at night, as well as needing less sleep when taking DMAE.

The stimulant effect of DMAE is significantly different from the stimulation produced by coffee, amphetamines, or other stimulant drugs. DMAE does not have a drug-like quick up and down. People who take DMAE have reported that they feel a mild stimulation continually, without side effects. Many athletes using DMAE report an improved energy output in addition to better concentration on form and technique. Also, when DMAE use is discontinued, no depression or let-down occurs. This is of great importance to osteoporotic individuals who have lost their zest for life and are not getting the necessary exercise.

GINSENG

Panax Ginseng is the *stress herb*. It is reported to be mildly estrogenic (having functions similar to estrogen), and anabolic (protein building), and is commonly found in many of the traditional formulas which are used for fatigue, insomnia, poor stamina, or any stress symptoms, world wide. Since it helps the mood and the adaptation to stress, it has been classified as an *adaptogen*.

There are *true* and *false* ginsengs. *True* ginsengs are of the **genus Panax**. This is a word always included in their scientific name. There are only two commonly used varieties of true Ginseng. The most widely known is **Panax Ginseng**, also called **Asian**, **Chinese**, or **Korean Ginseng**. The second is **Panax Quinquefolius** or **American Ginseng**. Both Asian and American Ginseng are **adaptogens** (substances that help adapt to stress). "Ginseng contains several **saponin glycosides**. Saponins are **4-ring steroid-like chemicals** with attached sugar molecules that make a foam when shaken in water. In the early '60's, Russian and Japanese scientists identified specific saponins unique to ginseng, called '**ginsenosides**' or '**panaxosides**'."

"There have actually been many scientific experiments on the effects of Ginseng, and it's interesting to note that most of them have confirmed

Chinese claims. There have also been many scientific experiments which showed no effect from taking Ginseng which may also correspond to what the Chinese have been telling us for generations. That sounds confusing and obviously requires an explanation.

"...The Chinese believe that Panax Ginseng is effective when used by the elderly while American Ginseng is better used by active, fit persons. Many of the studies that show that Ginseng had no effect were conducted on the wrong group, according to traditional Chinese medicine.

"The Chinese believe that Panax Ginseng, which is the *Yang* or hot, energizing Ginseng, is more effective when used to bolster health and prevent disease in autumn and winter, not summer. The reason is that Panax Ginseng, being hot, will tend to work better against cold weather diseases. Panax Ginseng helps prevent "cool" diseases, such as poor circulation, digestion, slow metabolism and decreased sexual activity. Panax Ginseng, being stimulating, should be used by those who need stimulation, such as the old and infirm and persons who are inactive and out of shape.

"Panax Quinquefolius (American Ginseng), on the other hand, is considered *Yin*, cool and rejuvenating rather than stimulating and therefore should be used more in spring and summer and in hotter weather, where it will tend to be more effective. Panax Quinquefolius should be used 'as a sedative rather than a stimulating tonic, and used by people who need vitality but are already constitutionally yang, that is, active, agitated, nervous, or hot. For such people, the Asian root might create excessive stimulation while the American root could help build their strength and allow proper rest' (Stephen Fulder—The Ginseng Book, 1996). American Ginseng should be used more often by young, fit and active persons."[G091]

In comparison with the effects of usual stimulants, the anti-fatigue action of ginseng shows an essential difference. The stimulants give effects under most situations, whereas ginseng reveals its action only under the challenge of stress.

DMSO

DMSO—dimethyl sulfoxide—is a chemical product that has been around a long time, but is totally strange to the orthodox medical community. It has been used for years by athletes to help them with painful muscles and joints.

It is not a drug which treats disease symptoms. "DMSO treats altered cellular function or damaged cells. The cells become healed and restored by changing and stabilizing the *water structure* within the cell. It exerts its effects on biological systems by changing the liquid structure of water. Therefore, changes occur in protein and other molecules."

DMSO has certain unique physiological characteristics which stem from its molecular makeup: It is a simple small molecule with unusual properties. It is largely not harmful or toxic. When DMSO is diluted with water, the solution warms up.

WHAT ARE ITS MAJOR THERAPEUTIC PROPERTIES?

- It blocks pain by interrupting conduction in the small *c-fibers*, the *non-myelinating* 9not covered by the myelin sheath) nerve fibers.
- It affects cardiac contractility by inhibiting calcium, to reduce the workload of the heart.
- It increases *interferon* (an anti-viral substance) formation.
- It is a potent diuretic.
- It is a scavenger of the hydroxyl free radical.
- It is a vasodilator, probably related to histamine release in the cells and to prostaglandin inhibition.
- It is anti-inflammatory.
- It is anti-bacterial, anti-fungal and anti-viral.
- It reduces the incidence of platelet *thrombi* (clots in vessels).
- It softens collagen (gristle).
- It stimulates the immune system.
- It stimulates wound healing.
- It transports all molecules (drugs, etc.) across cell membranes.[E011]

"It can be effective in multiple sclerosis, systemic lupus erythematosus, rheumatoid arthritis, thyroiditis, ulcerative colitis, cancer, etc."[E011]

Osteoarthritic patients, sometimes also suffering from osteoporosis, have often had a remarkable relief from pain and increase in mobility from the use of DMSO.[M012]

FATS OR LIPIDS*

This classification covers many and very diverse substances, and is, probably, the most unfortunate generalization in nutritional sciences. Although all the substances classified under its umbrella feel **unctuous** (greasy) to touch and share a few other characteristics, they are the most misunderstood, wrongly classified and maligned of all macro-nutrients.

FATTY ACIDS

- Major building blocks of **fats** in foods and the body
- Structural parts of membranes surrounding cells and, within the cell, of the organelles (subcellular structures), principally as **phosphatides**

Because knowledge of the chemical structure of a substance is very important, since it permits us to predict and understand certain properties of that substance, we may say that:

....
* This section adapted from SAY NO! TO HERPES, AIDS AND CHRONIC FATIGUE, by Eva Lee Snead, M.D., AUM publications, 1997

Structurally, **fatty acids** are:
- A chain of **C** (**carbon**) and **H** (**hydrogen**) atoms, *insoluble* in water, arranged like beads in a necklace. (The Cs make the main string of the necklace, the Hs dangle from the Cs).
- A weak **organic** acid group called a **carboxyl** (**-COOH**) on one end, located where a latch would be.

The chain part of the fatty acid ends in a **methyl** group (1 **C**, 3 **H**). The ends have been assigned Greek symbols (**omega**, and **delta**) to identify which one we are talking about. The length of the C chain is variable, the most common lengths varying between 4 and 24 carbons. The shorter lengths are soluble in water, and usually *not* considered to be *fatty* acids. They are **formic** acid (bee sting and ant bite), with only 1 carbon and **acetic** acid (vinegar), with 2.

Chemists assign numbers to the carbons in a chain, to be able properly to describe the structure of a fatty acid. The numbering begins at the omega (ω) end, with numeral *1*, and is therefore called the omega (ω) system.

Chemically speaking, we accept that the **molecules** that make up substances are arrangements of diverse atoms. Organic molecules are defined as made from chains of **carbon** (**C**) atoms. **C** atoms are built in such a fashion that they have the power to attach to 4 other atoms. These potential linking sites are called **valences**.

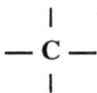

$$-\overset{|}{\underset{|}{C}}-$$

To these, atoms such as **oxygen** (**O**), or others are attached. These chains are electrically held together by what we call **bonds**. Bonds can be **single** or **multiple**.

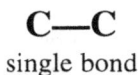

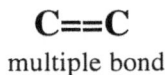

C—C	**C==C**
single bond	multiple bond

Since **C** has 4 valences, 3 linking sites are left over in single bonds and 2, or 1 in multiple bonds, which are attached to other substances. Each carbon can attach up to 4 other atoms, usually other carbons and/or hydrogens.

According to how many atoms other than carbons are attached to the carbon (C) atoms in the fat, they will have room for 1 or more bonds in chaining together. On that basis they are classified as **saturated** (all one bond) and **unsaturated** (more than one bond). Humans, animals and plants differ in their ability to insert double bonds at various locations of the chain, and these structural differences determine properties and biologic functions of **fatty acids**: energy production, shock absorbers, etc.

ESSENTIAL FATTY ACIDS
(LINOLEIC, LINOLENIC, ARACHIDONIC, GABA)

These **must** be provided in a diet, as the body can not synthesize them. The two most important unsaturated fatty acids in the human diet both have 18 C atoms: they are **linoleic** (**LN**) and **linolenic** (**LNA**) acids. Deficiencies of these are frequently widespread. Their prevalent symptoms are:

Linoleic acid deficiency creates eczema-like conditions, hair loss, degeneration of the liver and kidney, drying up of glands with excessive water loss through the skin, thirst, poor healing of wounds, sterility in males, miscarriages in females, problems of the circulatory system and heart, retardation of growth, behavioral problems and susceptibility to infections.

Linolenic acid deficiency may cause growth retardation, visual problems, learning disabilities, motor incoordination, tingling feelings in extremities, changes in personality and behavior.

Essential fatty acids absorb *oxygen* and *sunlight*, being in some fashion related to the *breathing* processes. Fats provide caloric energy. Unsaturated fatty acids *accelerate* the metabolism.

Because their molecules repel each other, fatty acids can spread into a very thin layer. You can observe this when pouring oil on water. This property is called *surface activity*. This permits them to carry toxins to the surface of cells for discarding. It also is the basis of *electrical properties* which are essential to the functioning of nerves and muscles. They can bond to the *sulphydril groups* in proteins, an activity essential to the processes of life. They are precursors of *prostaglandins,* hormone-like substances which regulate many body processes. They assist in the growth process and weight loss. In the *genetic apparatus* they *stabilize* the chromosomes and appear to be connected to stopping and starting gene expression.

Daily need of essential fatty acids is variable from person to person, but higher in males. Although minimum requirements have been set at 3-6 grams a day, many believe 9-30 grams to be necessary, and higher in obese people and those on a high intake of olive oil. Diets high in *essential fatty acids* must also be high in vitamins A, E, C, B_3, B_6, and the mineral zinc.

The natural sources of fatty acids are vegetable fats. The very best source is *flax seed oil*. Safflower oil has *LA*, but not *LNA*.

Because in some studies an apparent link appears to exist between the intake of foods which may, among other variables, have a high saturated fat content (but not just fats by themselves) and cardiovascular diseases, researchers have often discouraged the intake of foods from animal sources, such as red meat. The recommendation is based in at least as much faith and preconception as in scientific accuracy. We must consider that these investigative diets are prepared from food that has proteins, carbohydrates, nutrients and contaminants, and that fat is certainly *not* the only variable.

On the other hand, the *unsaturated fatty acids*, touted as safe, really are only wholesome if eaten as complete unrefined oils, where natural antioxidants accompany the *unsaturated fatty acids*. Actually, commercial oils, clear and colorless, margarine and shortening, are extremely harmful substances: the originally *unsaturated fatty acids* have been artificially saturated by the addition of hydrogen that, to become chemically active, was passed over a *nickel catalyst*. Trace amounts of this metal are carried in the hydrogen gas. The *unsaturated fatty acids* that are left require certain nutrients (vitamins E, C and the trace element *selenium*) to be properly metabolized and prevent certain chemical damage to tissue. These nutrients are naturally contained in unadulterated oil, but are vastly lost due to heating and processing. These heat-modified oils may cause more harm than good when ingested, by promoting the formation of the dangerous free radicals, damaging cells and the system. This does not intend to mean that we should not ingest the unsaturated fatty acids, just do so with a complete supply of defensive *co-factors*. The most important dietary *unsaturated fatty acids* are: *Linoleic, Linolenic and Arachnidonic*: they are essential to health and are often referred to as *Vitamin F.*

Vitamin E is the major fat-soluble antioxidant in human subjects and is crucial in protecting the unsaturated fats normally contained in vegetable oils (PUFAs) against lipid peroxidation (fat-rusting). Dietary PUFAs have been accused of making it hard for the body to absorb vitamin E, and experimentation seemed to substantiate this. In a Dutch study on rats, the concentration of vitamin E in liver and plasma was significantly lower in animals fed a high concentration of linoleic acid compared with those fed on the lowest level.[T060]

Does vitamin E decrease the harmful biologic "rusting" of nutrients and fat (lipid peroxidation)? In a study comprising twenty heart failure patients and ten matched healthy controls, it was noticed that oxidized or damaged chemicals, such as *malonyldialdehyde* and *superoxide anion,* were present in amounts larger than in healthy individuals, and that the more severe the heart failure, the higher the damaged chemicals tested. The beneficial antioxidants, or protectors, *catalase, glutathione reductase* and *superoxide dismutase* were decreased. The addition of vitamin E in doses of 400 mgr. once a day orally for 4 weeks significantly reduced the levels of damaged chemicals, and produced an elevation of the antioxidant enzymes. There was an apparent normalization of the lab values for oxidative stress following treatment of heart failure, and a markedly improved response to vitamin E supplementation.[G050]

GABA (*GAMMA-aminoButiriC acid*) and *GLA* (*Gamma-linoleic acid*)*:*
These are transformation products of dietary fatty acids. They can be naturally found in:
■ Evening primrose oil
■ Flax-seed oil
■ Kelp
■ Lard

Some people are unable to synthesize these transformation products, which are enormously important to the brain and immune factors. *Penicillin* is not only a well known antibiotic, but one of the substances that facilitates conversion of the basic fatty acids to GABA. Maybe that is why it helps patients with viral sore throat, even if it does not destroy the virus.

TRIGLYCERIDES
They are the largest component of storage and food fats, by volume and weight. They are composed of:
■ One (1) molecule of *glycerol* (a three carbon structure)
■ Three (3) fatty acid chains

Some have more saturated, others more unsaturated fatty acids. They are a source of energy storage and shock absorption.

What is the danger in having high levels of triglycerides? The word triglyceride often is accompanied by a negative connotation, because the presence of high levels of this fat metabolite in the blood is associated with:
■ Clumping of blood cells
■ Decrease in oxygen carrying capacity
■ Degenerative disease

Much confusion exists in terminology and information: the public is lead to believe that high intake equals high levels. This is an erroneous conclusion, and good nutrition will result in proper blood concentration.

Phosphatides are similar to triglycerides, in their structure
■ One (1) molecule of *glycerol* (a three carbon structure)
■ Three (2) fatty acid chains
■ One (1) *phosphate*

These substances are soluble in water, and capable of forming thin layers. They form the skins of the cells, and also of the organelles inside them. They hold proteins *inside* the cell and keep toxins *out*. Unfortunately some pharmaceuticals and carcinogens are able to pass through membranes despite the phosphatides' defensive role.

Lecithin is the best known member of the phosphatides. It supplies *choline*, a substance that is needed for numerous liver and brain functions. It is a detoxifier and a component of bile.

FATS ARE ABSOLUTELY ESSENTIAL IN HUMAN NUTRITION

The media bombard us day and night with warnings about the supposed dangers of fats. They try, at the same time, to sell us oils and margarines contaminated with nickel, imitation eggs, and convince us not to eat good quality protein, but they are simply engaged in a brainless overkill. Are *fat-free diets* healthy? FAT FREE DIETS CAN actually BE DANGEROUS! Consider that fat soluble substances depend for their absorption on the presence of concentrated bile from the *gall-bladder*. The gall-bladder only opens in the presence of certain fats. Fat-free diets can, therefore, be very dangerous. But bile and bile salts are very important in the prevention and treatment of osteoporosis, because they help the absorption of fat soluble substances, including vitamin D.

CHOLESTEROL IS UNFAIRLY MALIGNED

Is cholesterol really a villain? Nothing more inaccurate! This is just a media hype to play into the hands of unscrupulous drug manufacturers and suppliers of certain dietary foods. Cholesterol, chemically speaking, is not really a fat, yet it is often classified with these substances because of its waxy, greasy-to-touch texture. Cholesterol is essential to life and health. It is constantly produced in the body itself, from 2 *C acetate* groups. Because of its capacity to protect the organism against the very dangerous lipid peroxidation (biologic rusting) reactions, it is classified as an *antioxidant*. If it is not supplied in the diet, the body will rapidly form some. It is the basic molecule from which bile salts, sex hormones and *corticosteroids* (hormones produced in the adrenal glands), are formed. Although accumulations of cholesterol are found in damaged arteries, lesions colloquially known as *arteriosclerotic*, this in no way suggests or supports that cholesterol is the cause of such hardening. Accumulations seem to be due to a generally faulty diet, to toxins or to genetic disorders, not to superabundance of this substance in the food. Studies are usually inappropriately designed to arrive at any such conclusion because the variables are infinite in the composite diets that are used.

CHOLESTEROL IS THE SCAPEGOAT, AN UNSUNG HERO IN HUMAN NUTRITION

It may be the vitamin E deficiency (often due to the intake of commercially adulterated unsaturated fatty acid products), and not the cholesterol by itself, that causes all the problems. Cholesterol is probably only the scapegoat.

Accumulating body fat in the form of obesity (a problem which may occur without ever eating fats) appears to be associated with health problems. In most studies of overweight subjects, the very dietary habits that promoted overweight also appear to promote deficiency of that body's defenses against illness. It is unclear, however, whether obesity is purely diet-related, or whether it is primarily a genetic predisposition activated by dietary habits and imbalances in nutrients. At any rate, it still is a highly misunderstood condition.

The concept of a *high fat diet* or a *diet high in animal fats* is a very unclearly formulated idea because the foods classified as such contain many other variables, both in the natural composition of the products, and in adventitious pollutants. Therefore, conclusions that may be drawn of such studies are certainly not always correct. Shifting to a so called *low fat diet*, which most construe to be one very low in foods derived from the animal kingdom, inappropriately supplied with necessary fats and essential fatty acids may actually be a much worse choice, diminishing absorption of minerals and causing poor development of organs. For instance, one of its undesirable consequences is that it reduces the growth rate of the thymus gland, essential to many facets of immunity.

Olive oil, when used in experimental studies, activates the clearing of foreign matter from the human system. It is not considered essential: life may go on without ingesting it, since it is manufactured by the body. However, addition of this to white blood cells, makes them more active.

DEFICIENCY OF FATTY ACIDS

When you are sick and osteoporotic, when you could develop fractures that need surgery, you certainly can not afford wound infections. Chronic undersupply of fatty acids renders all tissues vulnerable to infection, especially the nervous tissue. In a study using rats as test subjects, Drs. Clausen and Molnar demonstrated this important relationship, increasing the rodents' sensitivity to a certain form of encephalitis, through deprivation of these nutrients.

Is artificial as good as natural? Not where it comes to fatty acids! It is dangerous to tamper with Mother Nature: the effect fatty acids on the body is highly dependent on their **chemical structure**. Clausner tells us that naturally occurring fatty acids have a completely different effect on the immune system than those synthetically manufactured.

VITAMINS

By definition, they
- Are *essential* (indispensable to life)
- *Can not* be synthesized in the human body
- *Must* come from food, or living things

(Vitamin D can be metabolized on the skin, by the action of the ultraviolet rays on body lipids, some of the of the B vitamins, also vitamin K are manufactured by the friendly bacteria living in the digestive tract, but *not* by human tissue itself).

All natural vitamins are organic food substances found only in living things, that is, plants and animals. With few exceptions the body cannot manufacture or synthesize vitamins. They must be supplied in the diet or in dietary supplements. Vitamins are essential to the normal functioning of our bodies. They are necessary for our growth, vitality, and general well-being.

People often think that vitamins can replace food. They cannot. In fact, vitamins cannot be assimilated properly without ingesting food. That is why many authors suggest taking them with a meal. Vitamins help regulate metabolism, help convert fat and carbohydrates into energy, and assist in forming bone and tissue.

One of the systems of classification of vitamins, which is based on their solubility in diverse media, is as follows:

- Soluble in fat, or *fat soluble*: may be stored in tissue: **A, D, E, K**.
- Soluble in water, or *water soluble*: need to be replenished daily: C and **B** group

The fat soluble vitamins *A* and *D* are fashioned of a structure chemically classified as **steroids**. They serve an important stabilizing function at genetic level, interacting with receptors and being direct modifiers (*modulators*) of genetic processes.

As to the daily need of nutrients, the government has set a value, **RDA** or *recommended daily allowance*, that in their opinion, should be appropriate for daily intake or supplements. This value is way below anything a reasonable nutritionist would usually prescribe, at least in the vitamin department. These RDAs, according to the researchers of the time they were established, are the amounts of a nutrient which would preserve health in an already perfectly healthy 20 year old. Obviously, such a creature barely exists, the environmental and dietary conditions of people are vary varied, and this RDA has very little meaning and is usually insufficient for most individuals.

VITAMIN A

VITAMIN A is classified as a fat soluble vitamin, of the family of the **carotenoids**. It must always be borne in mind that vitamin A *must* coexist in the body with *vitamin E* to be effective. Absence of E causes very rapid destruction of A.

It actually forms part of the cell wall; it is essential to the formation of the *first barrier* against infection, the skin and mucous membranes, which line the oral cavity, vagina, rectum, etc. Vitamin A is rapidly used up under the stress of an infection. The liver normally stores reserve volumes of this vitamin. In people who die of an overwhelming infection, when the liver tissue is examined at an autopsy, the stores of A have disappeared.

Vitamin A is not to be confused with **beta-carotene**, a **pro-vitamin A** that must be converted in real vitamin A by the liver, a process which is often not functioning properly, especially in individuals with liver damage or diabetes.

The average American diet is often marginally or heavily deficient in vitamin A; this is worsened by the fact that it is rapidly destroyed (oxidized) if vitamin E supply is insufficient, since A and E work on a buddy-system. Many commercial fats and environmental toxins destroy vitamin A, so its deficiency is really a widespread problem, even if the intake of vitamin A rich foods occurs. Contrary to what would be expected, in a politically incorrect move of nature, vitamin A deficiency runs rampant in the US, but is not very prevalent in poor countries. Poor children in South Carolina, studied by High in the late 60s, had up to a 50% prevalence of low or marginally low vitamin A nutrition.

In laboratory studies where conditions can be controlled, it is possible to sort out which problems are caused by *general malnutrition* and which by the specific lack (*hypovitaminosis*) of vitamin A. It is quite apparent that the deficiency must be coupled with a severe level of infection to really create a problem, because vitamin A deficient animals live an almost normal life in a *totally* germ free environment. Addition of vitamin A to the diet of normal animals increases their resistance against infectious agents. In the late eighties, the medical establishment in the United States invited a study among physicians, where these were voluntarily adding (*beta*) β-*carotene* (a form of this vitamin) to their diet, and long before the protocol was completed, the doctors reported marked improvement to their health. (As usual, the results of the study were misreported, implying that beta-carotene was harmful). Similar effects are seen in protection against pesticides, chlorinated hydrocarbons, heavy metals, etc. Not only chemicals are counteracted, but even harmful effects of noise, X-ray radiation, AND SENSITIVITY TO COLD TEMPERATURES, are mitigated by vitamin A intake.

"Vitamin A levels drop rapidly in people who are *malnourished* and live mostly under artificial light."[S160]

HOW DOES VITAMIN A IMPACT ON OSTEOPOROSIS?

Not only because of its more general health impact, but since bone development at an early age is an important precedent for healthy bones later in life, we must pay attention to obtaining a good supply of vitamin A, and to the role played by *breast feeding* in vitamin A nutrition. Breast milk is virtually the only source of vitamin A the first few months for many infants and often continues to be one of the most important sources through age 2. Without breast milk, newborns cannot maintain optimal vitamin A nutrition for more than a few weeks. Although vitamin A concentrations in human milk are dependent on the mother's vitamin A status, vitamin A deficiency is rare among breast-fed infants, even in parts of the world where vitamin A deficiency is prevalent most of the time (**endemic**). Promotion of breast feeding for 4-6 months as the only nutrition, and continued breast feeding with complementary foods thereafter should form part of any dietary intervention to improve vitamin A status.

A form of vitamin A commonly used today is β *carotene*, the yellow pigment found in carrots and other vegetable sources, which is actually only a *provitamin* (a precursor). Each molecule can yield two vitamin A molecules, when converted. It has a distinctive antioxidant potential. The purported advantage of using beta-carotene is, that in healthy individuals it can be converted to real vitamin A upon demand, preventing overdosing. Its great disadvantage is that certain liver disorders, diabetes and other conditions, may render the patient unable to convert the provitamin into the vitamin. Certain carnivores such as cats are unable to convert beta-carotene into vitamin A.

> **IN CERTAIN LIVER DISORDERS, DIABETES AND OTHER CONDITIONS, THE PATIENT IS UNABLE TO CONVERT BETA-CAROTENE INTO VITAMIN A**

MAIN FUNCTIONS
- Aids in bone and teeth formation.
- Counteracts night-blindness and weak eyesight
- Growth and repair of body tissues
- Maintain skin that is smooth, soft, disease-free
- Protect the mucous membranes of the throat and lungs
- Protect the mucous membranes of the mouth
- Protect the mucous membranes of the nose
- Protects against air pollutants

DEFICIENCY SYMPTOMS
- Defective teeth and gums
- Frequent fatigue
- Increased susceptibility to infections

- Loss of smell and appetite
- Night blindness
- Retarded growth
- Rough, dry, scaly skin
- Slow healing

Toxic symptoms are usually not noticed in humans, only a few instances are reported. But in animal studies, such symptoms have been found, and since they apply to bone growth, they should be of interest in a book on osteoporosis:

DISEASE STATES IN ANIMALS WITH AN EXCESS OF VITAMIN A

What happens in growing and adult animals?

- Bone overgrowth around vertebrae
- Decreased length of long bones
- Decreased bone production
- *Exostoses* and *osteophytes* in joints
- Loss of *proteoglycans* from the matrix
- Osseous metaplasia in the insertions of muscles and tendons
- Osteogenic activity in connective tissue around joints
- Osteoporosis—thin cortices, reduced diameter, metaphyseal flaring in long bones
- Reduced numbers of *chondrocytes* (cells which build cartilage)
- Suppression of osteoblasts in long bones
- Suppression of chondrocytes in growth plates
- Unbalanced bone growth in the axial skeleton

Vitamin A is important in prevention and supplementation for osteoporotic patients because of its effect on bone (see above), and its general protective effects which ease the repair and growth processes of body cells, glandular integrity and hormonal function.

How does vitamin A impact on treatment and prevention of cancer? Hormone receptors are sites in the chromosomes which attach to certain hormones. Tumors with high levels of hormone receptors usually respond better to certain cancer therapies. Since osteoporotic patients frequently have to take estrogens, and there is always a concern about an increase in breast cancer due to this therapy, it may be some comfort to know that in a study performed in 1996, it was concluded that the *carotenoid* (precursors of vitamin A) substances were protective and made the outlook for therapy in case of a cancer much brighter, because of higher frequency of hormone receptors in the tissue of people who took in more carotenoids. However, this was a statistical study, not a clinical experiment.[R080]

The protean (varied) effects of Vitamin A in normal metabolism, are reflected in the diversity of the consequences which can result from its deficiency. Vitamin A deficiency can impact upon the fetus, the young and growing and the adult, and can perturb a wide range of tissues and organ systems. Some of the effects on the fetus and young growing animals are the same. We may surmise that similar effects occur in humans. What happens in the fetus with vitamin A deficiencies?

- Basic cellular disturbance
- Impaired *differentiation* (transformation into specific adult cells, such as kidney, liver, etc.) of fetal cells in many developing organ systems
- Impaired growth of fetal cells in many developing organ systems

What are the pathologic consequences of vitamin A deficiencies?

Malformations (*teratogenesis*), occur in various animals studied. For the purpose of its relationship to osteoporosis, we may notice that in the calf, bone disorders, such as thickening of the basal bones of the skull with narrowing of the occipital foramina, may occur.

What happens in the growing animal with vitamin A deficiencies? This is even more closely connected to our interest in bone formation:

- Basic cellular disturbance
- Defective remodeling in membranous bone (most significant in the bones of the skull)
- Hormonal changes
- Inadequate activity by osteoclasts

Hormonal changes leading to suppression of ovulation compound the metabolic problems. Similar hormonal changes may affect bone structure.

EXCESSIVE INTAKE—TOXICITY SYMPTOMS OF BETA-CAROTENE

- Hair loss
- Headaches
- Yellow/orange skin color, especially on the palms of the hands and the soles of the feet

RDA AND COMMON DOSAGE

"Vitamin A is measured in Retinol Equivalents (RE's). Retinol Equivalents measure the vitamin A activity of a food."[E001] RDA for adults is 800-1000 RE's.

DIETARY SOURCES OF VITAMIN A AND BETA-CAROTENE

The best dietary sources of vitamin A and beta-carotene are:

"FOOD	AMOUNT	RETINOL QUIVALENTS
Liver, beef	3 ounces	9,124
Cod liver oil	1 tablespoon	4,080
Sweet potato	1 medium	2,487
Carrot, whole	1 medium	2,025
Pumpkin, fresh, boiled	1/2 cup	1,325
Egg yolk	one large	97
Cheese, cheddar	1 ounce	86
Milk, fortified, whole	1 cup	76
Cream, heavy, whipping	1 tablespoon	63" [E001]

VITAMIN B1 (THIAMINE)

"Thiamine is a water soluble vitamin. Major dietary sources of thiamine include pork, legumes (dried beans), peanuts, sunflower seeds, whole grains and enriched breads and cereals. Like most water soluble vitamins, excess intake of thiamine is excreted and not stored in the body. Thiamine is sensitive to heat and, like other water soluble vitamins, leaches into cooking water."[E001]

MAIN FUNCTIONS

- Aids in the digestion of carbohydrates
- Functioning of the nervous system, muscles and heart
- Metabolic cycle for generating energy
- Promotes growth and good muscle tone
- Stabilizes the appetite

DEFICIENCY SYMPTOMS

- Amnesia
- Beriberi
- Heart and gastrointestinal problems
- Insomnia
- Loss of appetite
- Mental depression and constipation
- Mental confusion
- Muscle wasting
- Muscular incoordination
- Neurologic symptoms
- Paralysis and nervous irritability
- Vague aches and pains
- Weakness and feeling tired
- Weight loss
- Wernicke-Korsakoff syndrome

EXCESSIVE INTAKE AND TOXICITY SYMPTOMS

Thiamine is easily cleared by the kidneys, and no thiamine toxicity has been caused by oral intake.

RDA AND COMMON DOSAGE

RDA for adults is 1.1-1.5 mg.

DIETARY SOURCES OF THIAMINE - B1

THE BEST DIETARY SOURCES OF THIAMINE - B1, ARE:

"FOODS	AMOUNTS	MILLIGRAMS
Brewer's yeast	1 tablespoon	1.3
Pork center loin chop	3.5 ounces	1.2

Sunflower seeds. dry	1/4 cup	0.8
Ham steak, cured	2 ounces	0.5
Wheat germ, raw	1/4 cup	0.5
Green peas,cooked	1 cup	0.4
Black beans, cooked	1 cup	0.4
Watermelon	1 slice, 1 x 10 inch	0.4
Canadian bacon, cooked	2 pieces	0.4
Oatmeal, cooked	1 cup	0.3
Black-eyed peas, cooked	1 cup	0.2
Oysters, raw	1 cup	0.2"[C160]

VITAMIN B2 (RIBOFLAVIN)

It is a water soluble B vitamin, which confers the yellow color to many B complex preparations.

"Riboflavin is a water soluble vitamin. Major dietary sources of riboflavin include milk, yogurt, cheese, organ meats, meat, poultry, dark green leafy vegetables, whole grain and enriched breads and cereals. Like most water soluble vitamins, excess intake of riboflavin is excreted and not stored in the body. Riboflavin is sensitive to ultraviolet light and, like other water soluble vitamins, leaches into cooking water."[E001] Its main functions are:

MAIN FUNCTIONS
- Alleviates eye fatigue
- Carbohydrate, fat and protein metabolism
- Formation of antibodies and red blood cells
- Maintains cell respiration
- Necessary for the maintenance of good vision
- Necessary for the maintenance of skin, nails and hair
- Promotes general health

DEFICIENCY SYMPTOMS
- *Blepharitis* (cracking and crusting of eyelids)
- Bloodshot eyes
- Cracks and sores in the mouth and lips
- Dermatitis

- Digestive disturbances
- Itching and burning eyes
- Oily skin
- Purplish tongue
- Retarded growth
- Scaly eye lids
- Sluggishness
- Trembling

EXCESSIVE INTAKE—TOXICITY SYMPTOMS
May interfere with chemotherapeutic agents.

RDA AND COMMON DOSAGE — DIETARY SOURCES
RDA for adults is 1.2-1.7 mg.
THE BEST DIETARY SOURCES OF RIBOFLAVIN—B2 ARE:

"FOOD	AMOUNTS	MILLIGRAMS
Kidney, beef	3 ounces	4.1
Liver, beef	3 ounces	3.6
Liver,chicken	3 ounces	1.5
Yogurt, nonfat, plain	8 ounces	0.6
Milk	1 cup	0.4
Brewer's yeast	1 tablespoon	0.3
Soybeans, dried	1/4 cup	0.2
Swiss cheese	2 ounces	0.2
Black-eyed peas, cooked	1 cup	0.2
Green peas, cooked	1 cup	0.2
Chicken, white meat	3 ounces	0.1
Chick peas, dried	cup	0.1
Kidney beans, dried	1/4 cup	0.1
Egg, hard-cooked	1	0.1
Peanuts,chopped	1/4 cup	0.1
Broccoli, cooked	1 cup	0.1
Kale, cooked	1 cup	0.1
Spinach,cooked	1 cup	0.1 "[C160]

NIACINAMIDE (NIACIN- VITAMIN B-3)

Niacin is a water soluble vitamin, which can also be synthetized in the body, deriving from the amino acid triptofan. Major dietary sources of niacin include meat, poultry, fish, organ meats, milk, eggs, whole grain and enriched breads and cereals. Excess intake of niacin is excreted and not stored in the body. Niacin leaches into cooking water.

MAIN FUNCTIONS

- Helps metabolize protein, sugar and fat
- Helps maintain a healthy skin, tongue and digestive system
- Improves circulation
- Increases energy through proper utilization of food
- Maintains the nervous system
- Prevents *pellagra* (a deficiency disease that has a typical group of three symptoms, or *triad* of the three Ds: diarrhea, dementia and dermatitis (red, rough skin disease)
- Reduces high blood pressure
- Reduces the cholesterol level in the blood

DEFICIENCY SYMPTOMS

- Bad breath
- Canker sores
- Fatigue
- Gastrointestinal disturbance
- Headaches
- Indigestion
- Insomnia
- Irritability
- Loss of appetite
- Mental depression
- Muscular weakness
- Nervousness
- Pellagra
- Skin disorders
- Vague aches and pains

EXCESS INTAKE—TOXICITY

- Liver damage
- Rash
- Ulcers
- Vascular dilation, resulting in flushing

RDA AND COMMON DOSAGE

The RDA for adults is 13-19 mg.
THE BEST DIETARY SOURCES OF NIACIN-B3 are:

"FOOD	AMOUNTS	MILLIGRAMS
Liver, beef	3 ounces	14
Tuna, light, packed in water	3 ounces	11
Chicken, white meat	3 ounces	10.6
Kidney, beef	3 ounces	9.1
Salmon steak	3 ounces	8.4
Peanuts, chopped	1/4 cup	6.2
Halibut, steamed	3 ounces	6
Beef, lean	3 ounces	3.9
Rice, brown, cooked	1 cup	3
Sunflower seeds, dried	1/4 cup	2
Soybeans, dried	1/4 cup	1.2
Navy beans, dried	1/4 cup	1.2
Kidney beans, dried	1/4 cup	1.1
Chick peas, dried	1/4 cup	1
Pacific oysters, raw	1 each	1 "C160

PANTOTHENIC ACID (VITAMIN B-5)

Pantothenic acid, also known as vitamin B5, is named after the Greek word pantos (pantos), meaning "everywhere", because it is found in both plant and animal food sources. Pantothenic acid is a water-soluble B vitamin: it cannot be stored in the body but must be replaced daily, either from diet or from supplements. Excess intake of pantothenic acid is excreted, and not stored in the body. Pantothenic acid is sensitive to heat.

It is also referred to as "antistress vitamin" due to its fundamental role in:

- Contributing to the production of important brain neuro-transmitters such as *acetylcholine*
- The formation of various *adrenal hormones*, *steroids*, and *cortisone*

In addition to helping to fight depression, pantothenic acid also supports the normal functioning of the gastrointestinal tract and is required for the production of cholesterol, bile, vitamin D, red blood cells, and antibodies.

Under severe dietary conditions a lack of vitamin B5 can lead to a variety of symptoms including hypoglycemia, skin disorders, fatigue, depression, digestive problems, lack of coordination and muscle cramps. The current RDA for pantothenic acid is 10 mgr.

MAIN FUNCTIONS
- Cell building
- Development of the central nervous system
- Fights infections by building antibodies
- Helps the adrenal glands
- Improves resistance to stress
- Production of acetylcholine
- Production of steroids, cholesterol, bile
- Production of vitamin D
- Red blood cell formation
- Release of energy from carbohydrates, fats, and protein
- Utilization of vitamins

DEFICIENCY SYMPTOMS:
- Burning soles of feet
- Constipation
- Depression
- Digestive disturbances
- Dizzy spells
- Fatigue
- Muscle cramps
- Painful and burning feet
- Restlessness
- Retarded growth

- Skin abnormalities
- Stomach stress
- Vomiting

EXCESSIVE INTAKE — TOXICITY SYMPTOMS

"Doses of 10 to 20 grams may result in diarrhea and water retention."[E001]

■ FOOD SOURCES

avocados	dates	potatoes
beans	eggs	salt-waterfish
beef	green	whole grain breads
cauliflower	liver	whole grain cereals
chicken	nuts	
cheese	peas	

RDA AND COMMON DOSAGE

Most common B-complex formulas contain from 10 to 100 mgr. of B5, though therapeutic dosages daily doses up to 1000 mgr. are not uncommon, especially for treatment of arthritis and allergies. The dose estimated safe for adults is 4-7 mg.

DIETARY SOURCES OF PANTOTHENIC ACID

THE BEST DIETARY SOURCES OF PANTOTHENIC ACID ARE:

"FOOD	AMOUNT	MILLIGRAMS
Liver, beef, cooked	3 ounces	6.04
Egg, whole	1 medium	1.1
Avocado	1/2 medium	1.1
Mushrooms, canned	1/2 cup	1
Milk, skim	1 cup	1
Soybeans, cooked	1/2 cup	0.5
Banana	1 medium	0.5
Orange, raw	1 medium	0.5
Collard greens, cooked	1/2 cup	0.4

Potato, baked	1 medium	0.4
Broccoli	1/2 cup	0.3
Cantaloupe	1/4 melon	0.3
Peanut butter	1 tablespoon	0.2
Apple	1medium	0.2
Wheat germ	1 tablespoon	0.1 [C160]

VITAMIN B6 (PYRIDOXINE)

Vitamin B6, also called *Pyridoxine*, is a water soluble nutrient that cannot be stored in the body, but must be obtained daily from either dietary sources or supplements. excess intake of pyridoxine is excreted and not stored in the body. Pyridoxine is sensitive to heat and ultraviolet light. It is not just one, but a family of substances, including *pyridoxine, pyridoxal, and pyridoxamine*, closely related in form and function. It supports more vital bodily functions than any other vitamin. Why is its scope of functions so widespread? Because it is a *co-enzyme* (assists enzymatic function).

> WE WANT TO WATCH B6 VERY CLOSELY,
> BECAUSE OF ITS CLOSE ASSOCIATION WITH THE METABOLISM OF PROTEIN
> AND ITS INCREASED REQUIREMENT WHEN HORMONES ARE TAKEN.

Among its many benefits, vitamin B6 is recognized for:

- Co-enzyme involved in the metabolism of carbohydrates, fats, and proteins
- Helping to maintain healthy immune system functions
- Manufacturing of enzymes
- Manufacturing of hormones
- Manufacturing of neurotransmitters (*serotonin*, a brain neurotransmitter that controls our moods, appetite, sleep patterns, and sensitivity to pain)
- Manufacturing of prostaglandins
- Manufacturing of red blood cells
- Protecting the heart from cholesterol deposits
- Preventing kidney stone formation

- Treatment of allergies
- Treatment of arthritis
- Treatment of asthma and arthritis
- Treatment of carpal tunnel syndrome
- Treatment of night leg cramps
- Treatment of premenstrual syndrome

MAIN FUNCTIONS

- Aids in fat and carbohydrate metabolism
- Aids in the removal of excess fluid of premenstrual women
- Aids in the formation of antibodies
- Helps maintain a proper balance of sodium and phosphorous in the body
- Maintains the central nervous system
- Promotes healthy skin
- Reduces muscle spasms
- Reduces leg cramps
- Reduces nausea
- Reduces hand numbness
- Reduces stiffness of hands
- Synthesis and breakdown of amino acids, the building blocks of protein

DEFICIENCY SYMPTOMS

- Anemia
- Anxiety (especially in infants)
- Arm and leg cramps
- Convulsions (especially in infants)
- Depression
- Dermatitis
- Increased susceptibility to diseases due to a weakened immune system
- Insomnia
- Irritability (especially in infants)
- Kidney stones
- Lethargy

- Loss of muscular control
- Loss of hair
- Mouth disorders
- Muscular weakness
- Nervousness
- Profound malfunctioning of the central nervous system
- Skin eruptions
- Slow learning
- Vomiting
- Water retention

SUPPLEMENTATION
B6 is commonly used as a supplement when people are suffering from:
- Depression
- Morning sickness and
- Nausea
- Patients suffering from heart disease
- Patients undergoing radiation treatment
- Persons taking amphetamines
- Persons on high protein diets require extra vitamin B6
- Persons taking oral contraceptives
- Persons taking antidepressants
- Persons taking estrogen
- Pregnant women have an increased need for supplemental vitamin B6

EXCESSIVE INTAKE—TOXICITY SYMPTOMS
- Neuropathy (Numbness and damage to the nervous system)

RDA AND COMMON DOSAGE — DIETARY SOURCES
The RDA for vitamin B6 is 1.6 to 2 mgr. per day. Most strong B-complex formulas contain between 10 to 75 mgr. of vitamin B6.
THE BEST DIETARY SOURCES OF PYRIDOXINE— B6 ARE:

"FOOD	AMOUNT	MILLIGRAMS
Banana	1 medium	0.7
Watermelon	1 slice (1 x10 inches)	0.7

Salmon	3 ounces	0.6
Chicken, white meat	3 ounces	0.5
Pork, center loin chop	3.5 ounces 0.5	0.5
Potato, baked, with skin	1 medium	0.4
Soybeans	1/4 cup	0.4
Brewer's yeast	1 tablespoon	0.4
Sunflower seeds, dry	1/4 cup	0.3
Tuna, light, packed in water	3 ounces	0.3
Pacific Halibut	3 ounces	0.3
Brown rice, long grain	1 cup	0.3
Wheat germ, raw	1/4 cup	0.3
Navy beans, cooked	1 cup	0.3
Green peas, cooked	1 cup	0.3
Spinach, cooked	1 cup	0.1"C160

Doses up to 500 mgr. per day are uncommon but safe, but doses above 2 grams per day can lead to irreversible neurological damage if not balanced out properly by other vitamins.

VITAMIN B-12 (COBALAMIN)

It is a water soluble B vitamin, it has a typical red color. Its main functions are:
- Carbohydrate, fat and protein metabolism
- Formation and regeneration of red blood cells
- Increases energy
- Maintains a healthy nervous system
- Needed for calcium absorption.
- Promotes growth in children

DEFICIENCY SYMPTOMS
- Brain damage
- Degeneration of spinal cord
- Depression
- Growth failure in children
- Lack of balance
- Nervousness

- Neuritis
- Pernicious anemia
- Poor appetite
- Tiredness

DIETARY SOURCES OF VITAMIN B12

The RDA for adults is 2 mcg.
THE BEST DIETARY SOURCES OF VITAMIN B12 are:

"FOOD	AMOUNT	MILLIGRAMS
Liver, beef	1 ounce	20
Kidney, beef	3 ounces	19
Liver, chicken	3 ounces	16.5
Salmon, steak	3 ounces	3
Tuna, light, packed in water	3 ounces	2.5
Yogurt, nonfat, plain	8 ounces	1.4
Beef, lean	3 ounces	1.4
Pacific Halibut	3 ounces	1.2
Milk, whole	1 cup	0.9
Pork, center loin chop	3.5 ounces	0.6
Swiss cheese	1 ounce	0,5
Egg, whole, raw	1 medium	0.4
Chicken, white meat	3 ounces	0.3
Cheese, American, processed	1 ounce	0.2" [C160]

BIOTIN AND PTEROYLGLUTAMIC ACID

These members of the water-soluble B vitamin family are not as well known and studied as their other B group cousins.

Specific roles of both vitamins in relationship to the immune system have been demonstrated. In study after study it has been shown that both synthesis and function of immune antibodies *decreases* if **biotin** and **pteroylglutamic acid** are undersupplied. Lymphocytes cultured in a **biotin** deficient environment grow poorly.

BIOTIN

Biotin is a water-soluble vitamin and member of the B-complex family. Originally isolated in 1901, over the years numerous researchers attached different names to this nutrient, referring to it alternately as *bios*, *vitamin H*, *protective factor X*, *and coenzyme R*. Today the scientific name for this sulfur-bound vitamin is biotin, though occasionally it may be incorrectly referred to as vitamin B6. "Major dietary sources of biotin include yeast, organ meats, milk, egg yolks, nuts, legumes (dried beans), and whole grains. Like most water soluble vitamins, excess intake of biotin is excreted and not stored in the body."[E001]

Biotin is an essential nutrient that is required for:
- Carbohydrate and protein metabolism
- Cell growth
- For the production of fatty acids
- Healthy skin and hair
- May play a role in preventing hair loss
- Metabolize the amino acid *leucine*
- Produce glucose from protein
- Proper utilization of the other B-complex vitamins

Biotin has achieved some notoriety as a hair growth stimulator.

BIOTIN-DEFICIENCY

A biotin deficiency of is rare, as biotin is easily synthesized in the intestines by bacteria, usually in amounts far greater than are normally required for good health. Some symptoms of biotin deficiency are:
- Anorexia
- Decreased red blood cells and anemia
- Depression
- Dermatitis
- Eczema
- Inflammation of the tongue
- Lethargy
- Muscle pain
- Nausea
- Poor appetite and nausea
- Red, scaly patches of the skin

- Retardation
- Tiredness and grouchiness
- Vomiting

Those at highest risk to develop biotin deficiency are:
- Alcoholics
- Pregnant women or nursing mothers
- Those taking antiepileptic drugs
- Those who are taking too many antacids or ulcer therapies
- Those who have low hydrochloric acid
- Those who have poor digestion and absorption
- Those who have stomach surgery
- Those eating too many raw egg whites over a prolonged period can contribute to biotin deficiency, as eggs whites contain a protein called avidin, that binds to biotin and interfere with its absorption. This is not a problem when consuming cooked eggs, which are a good dietary source of biotin
- Those subsisting on I.V.s that have too little biotin
- Those having low counts of the friendly bacteria in the colon (acidophilus) due to antibiotic therapies
- Those who are elderly
- Those taking a lot of antibiotics or sulfa drugs, which can inhibit the growth of the intestinal bacteria that produce biotin

Infants with *seborrheic dermatitis*, evidenced by dry and scaly face and scalp may also be suffering from a biotin deficiency.

EXCESSIVE INTAKE—TOXICITY SYMPTOMS:
- No evidence of biotin toxicity has been seen from oral intake

DIETARY SOURCES OF BIOTIN
The adult RDA for biotin is 300 micrograms.
THE BEST DIETARY SOURCES OF BIOTIN are:

FOOD	AMOUNT	MICROGRAMS
Yeast	3.5 ounces	85

Liver, beef	3 ounces	82
Oatmeal, cooked	1 cup	58
Soybeans, cooked	1/2 cup	22
Egg, whole, cooked	1 medium	13
Salmon	3 ounces	10
Milk, whole	1 cup	10
Mushrooms, canned	1/2 cup	7
Halibut	3 ounces	7
Banana	1 medium	6
Peanut butter	1 tablespoon	6
Cantaloupe	1/4 melon	3
Cottage cheese	1/2 cup	2
Wheat germ	1 tablespoon	1.3
Cheese, cheddar	1 ounce	1

Other good sources are:

brewer's yeast	milk
egg yolks	rice
grains and legumes	salt-water fish
intestinal bacteria	royal jelly
liver	soybeans

Biotin is found in virtually all B-complex supplements in doses ranging from 25 micrograms to 300 micrograms. There are no known toxic levels or symptoms for biotin.

Acidophilus (the friendly intestinal bacteria) supplementation will protect the *intestinal flora* of those who take antibiotics.

PTEROYLGLUTAMIC ACID

Main functions
- Promotes healthy hair
- Protein metabolism
- Utilization of folic acid
- Utilization of Pantothenic acid
- Utilization of Vitamin B-12

DEFICIENCY SYMPTOMS

- Depression
- Drowsiness,
- Extreme exhaustion
- Grayish skin color
- Loss of appetite
- Muscle pain

FOLIC ACID

FOLIC ACID: Folic acid is another one of the B vitamin group which is essential to the production of circulating antibodies and the vitality of the white blood cells. "Folate (folic acid or folacin) is a water soluble B vitamin. Major dietary sources of folate include green leafy vegetables, organ meats, meat, poultry, seafood, legumes (dried beans), seeds, and whole grain breads and cereals. Folate requirements are increased during pregnancy. Like most water soluble vitamins, excess intake of folate is excreted and not stored in the body. Folate is sensitive to heat, oxygen and ultraviolet light. Like other water soluble vitamins, folate leaches into cooking water."[E001]

Folic acid has an important role in detoxifying *XO* (*xanthine oxidase*), an aggressive enzyme normally present in milk, that interacts with substances in the *caffeine* family. When *raw milk* D is drank, fat globules of normal size envelop the XO, so it does not filter into the blood stream through the mucous membranes of the colon. *Homogenizing* the milk (processing THE LIQUID to minimize the size of the fat globules), disables this protective mechanism, the XO is no longer coated to form a larger particle, and passes into general circulation where it exerts its harmful effects, and forms the dangerous *free radicals*.

Some studies that brought out the effectiveness of folic acid on the optimizing of the immune functions, were done on guinea pigs. These animals are some of the better suited for comparison studies with humans, because they share with us a genetic inability to synthesize *vitamin C*. When these animals were made deficient in *folic acid*, their *thymus* development was slowed down.

MAIN FUNCTIONS

- Amino acid synthesis
- DNA and RNA synthesis
- Formation of red blood cells by its action on the bone marrow
- Growth and reproduction of all body cells
- Metabolism

DEFICIENCY SYMPTOMS

- Anemia
- Gastrointestinal disorders
- Premature gray hair*
- Vitamin B-12 deficiency

* May we remember that premature graying hair is listed among the characteristics for increased osteoporosis risk.

EXCESSIVE INTAKE—TOXICITY SYMPTOMS

- It may mask symptoms of vitamin B12 deficiency

DIETARY SOURCES OF FOLATE

The RDA for adults is 180-200 mcg.
THE BEST DIETARY SOURCES OF FOLATE, from high to low, are:

FOOD	AMOUNT	MICROGRAMS
Kidney beans, cooked	1 cup	735
Liver, chicken	3 ounces	654
Brewer's yeast	1 tbsp.	313
Pinto beans, cooked	1 cup	294
Black beans, cooked	1 cup	256
Navy beans, cooked	1 cup	255
Black-eyed peas, cooked	1 cup	210
Liver, beef	3 ounces	187
Asparagus, cooked	1 cup	172
Turnip greens, cooked	1 cup	170
Split peas, cooked	1 cup	127
Spinach, cooked	1 cup	109

Green peas, cooked	1 cup	101
Soybeans, dried	1/4 cup	90
Sunflower seeds	1/4 cup	82
Broccoli, cooked	1 cup	62
Lima beans, cooked	1 cup	40

INOSITOL

It is a water soluble B vitamin. Its main functions are:

MAIN FUNCTIONS

- Breakdown of fats
- Formation of lecithin
- Prevents thinning of hair
- Reduces blood cholesterol

DEFICIENCY SYMPTOMS

- Constipation
- Fat metabolism disorders
- Hair loss
- High blood cholesterol

It has been reported that the use of inositol decreases the experimental development of cancer by the powerful cancer promoter DMBA. Cancer prevention information appeals to menopausal women who worry about real or imaginary side effects of supplemental hormones.[V050]

Inositol hexaphosphate (InsP6) reproducibly inhibits experimental mammary carcinoma, therefore having great potential as a chemo-preventive and adjuvant therapeutic agent for this disease as well. One more plus for the osteoporotics on ERT.

CHOLINE

While closely related to the B complex family of vitamins, *choline* is not truly considered a vitamin, because it does not satisfy the vitamin criteria (being essential to health). Researchers cannot agree on any common deficiency symptoms of choline. Choline is found in all living cells, and is known to play a vital role in maintaining the central nervous system and in numerous metabolic functions:

■ Activity in the brain and central nervous system
■ Component of *lecithin*
■ Helps to protect the liver from the accumulation of fatty deposits
■ Is a precursor of the important neurotransmitter *acetylcholine*, a chemical used in the transmission of brain impulses between nerves, muscles and organs. In this role it is involved directly with cognition, long and short term memory, stimulus response, and mental energy. Since acetylcholine levels increase rapidly after consuming choline, researchers have employed choline supplements in the treatment of various disorders marked by lowered levels of acetylcholine in the brain, including Huntington's disease, Parkinson's disease, Alzheimer's disease, and *tardive dyskin esia* (a neurologic condition characterized by awkward twisting movements which are not voluntarily controllable).
■ Required for the production and metabolization of fats and cholesterol
■ Used in the manufacture of cell membranes

There is at present, no FDA recommended daily intake for choline.
A deficiency of choline can result in:
■ Increased fatty deposits in the liver
■ Memory loss
■ Poor muscle coordination

Excess consumption of choline can lead to over-stimulation of muscles, leading to tightening of the shoulders and neck, resulting in a tension headache.

Foods highest in choline include:

brewers yeast	liver
whole grain cereals	egg yolks
meats	legumes
milk	

Choline can be manufactured in the human body, but usually not to optimum levels, with the help of vitamin B12, folic acid, and the amino acid methionine. Choline is also available as a dietary supplement, in several compounds:
- Choline *bitartrate*
- Choline *chloride*
- *Phosphatydil* choline

Choline supplements should be avoided by persons who suffer from manic depression, as they may deepen the depressive phase of this disorder.

MAIN FUNCTIONS
- Controlling fat and cholesterol buildup in the body
- Facilitates the movement of fats in the cells
- Helps regulate the kidneys, liver, and gallbladder
- Helps improve memory
- Important for nerve transmission
- Prevents fat from accumulating in the liver

DEFICIENCY SYMPTOMS
- Cirrhosis and fatty degeneration of the liver
- Hardening of the arteries
- Heart problems
- Hemorrhaging kidneys
- High blood pressure

PABA (PARA AMINO BENZOIC ACID)

> **PABA SUNSCREENS SHOULD BE USED FOR PROTECTION BY SENSITIVE INDIVIDUALS**

Among its many and varied functions in the organism, *PABA* (*para-amino-benzoic acid*) has two very important roles in the fight against harmful peroxidation (the damage caused by oxygen and *free radicals*).

- In the gut, PABA stimulates the friendly acidophilus bacteria to produce folic acid, a strong detoxifier of xanthine oxidase.

■ PABA is a *selective* protector of the skin against the damaging frequencies of the ultraviolet rays of the sun, and of fluorescent lights. If PABA is undersupplied in the outer layers of the skin, a genetically determined condition in certain persons of Scottish-Welsh-Irish descent, there is little protection against these rays, and **keratoses** (areas of hardened, darkened, abnormal skin, also known as age spots) and **skin cancers** occur.

MAIN FUNCTIONS
■ Aids healthy bacteria in producing folic acid
■ Aids in the formation of red blood cells
■ Aids in the assimilation of pantothenic acid
■ Contains sun screening properties
■ Returns hair to its natural color

DEFICIENCY SYMPTOMS
■ Constipation
■ Depression
■ Digestive disorders
■ Eczema
■ Extreme fatigue
■ Hair turning prematurely gray
■ Headaches
■ Irritability
■ Nervousness

BIOFLAVONOIDS

Bioflavonoids are also referred to as **vitamin P**, yet, often not considered true vitamins, and are *companion substances* to vitamin C. Two of the most active forms are **hesperetin, hesperidin, quercetin, rutin**, etc., (very high in the white membranous fibers of citrus and in blue-green algae.). They are well known for preventing small blood vessel breakage, being quite effective in pain control of sport injuries, simulating the production of bile, cholesterol metabolism, etc.

VITAMIN C (ASCORBIC ACID)

Vitamin C, also known as ascorbic acid, is a water-soluble, antioxidant vitamin, essential to the body's health. It is located in the **extracellular** (outside the cells) areas of the body. It easily dissolves in water. This is advantageous because ascorbic acid will be converted from the body more readily. Vitamin C is able to react with aqueous free radicals and reactive oxygen. Vitamin C is the first antioxidant that is used up when the body engages in defending against damaging free radicals. Are there any beneficial interactions between vitamin C and other antioxidants? Vitamin C and Vitamin E complement each other because they are found in different areas of cells and tissues. Vitamin E localizes to fatty substances and vitamin C localizes in the watery areas of tissues. Vitamin C prevents the conversion of **nitrates** (a common contaminant of tobacco smoke, smog, bacon, lunch meats, and some vegetables) into cancer-causing substances.[S160]

Most animals can manufacture ascorbic acid in large amounts. Primates, humans, and the fruit eating bat, cannot make their own vitamin C. With vitamin C being part of more than 300 bodily functions, life itself depends on its daily replenishment. Its primary function in protein metabolism, is to maintain collagen, a protein necessary for the formation and support of skin, ligaments, bones and teeth, and for the strength of blood vessel walls. In addition, PUFAs play an important part in the absorption of iron necessary for the formation of red blood cells. They also play a role in the utilization of **folic acid**, one of the B-complex vitamins.

Natural vitamin C is destroyed by food preparation (heating) more than any other nutrient. Synthetic vitamin C is destroyed by stomach acid, but not by normal heating. The body does not store vitamin C. "Like most water soluble vitamins, excess intake of vitamin C is excreted and not stored in the body. Vitamin C is sensitive to heat and oxygen. Like other water soluble vitamins, vitamin C leaches into cooking water."[C160]

MAIN FUNCTIONS

- Aids in the prevention and treatment of the common cold
- Aids in the absorption of iron
- Builds resistance to infection
- Essential for healthy teeth, gums, and bones
- Extends life span
- Gives strength to blood vessels
- Glutathione (an antioxidant peptide) levels vary with vitamin C intake

- Helps heal wounds, scar tissue, and fractures
- One of the major antioxidant nutrients
- Prevents the conversion of nitrates (from tobacco smoke, smog, bacon, lunch meats, and some vegetables) into *carcinogens* (cancer-causing substances)
- Prevents *scurvy*
- Reduces gum disease
- Reduces cataracts
- Reduces cancers
- Reduces heart disease
- Required for the synthesis of *collagen*, the intercellular "cement" which holds tissues together

Vitamin C can induce production of collagen bone protein, bone formation and markers of bone formation, and protect bone from the effects of blockers of bone formation.[F081]

Vitamin C aids in bone formation and upkeep, impacting on the *deoxypyridinoline: pyridinoline cross-links ratio*, especially in bone (femur). *Scurvy*, an advanced form of vitamin C deficiency is known o be associated with improper bone formation.[M010] It manifests with bone-specific anomalies, such as:

- Decrease in *mRNA* (*messenger RNA*, a measure of genetic function) for osteocalcin, a bone-specific marker
- Decreased *alkaline phosphatase* (an enzyme involved in bone mineralization) in bone
- Decreased *alkaline phosphatase* in serum
- Inhibition of collagen synthesis
- *Osteopontin* (referring to a location in the nervous system) mRNA concentrations increased

Vitamin C is important to the person's ability to cope with stress: from a British study on guinea-pigs we learn that ascorbic acid intake significantly affected the level of vitamin C in the adrenal glands which produce anti-stress hormones.[T080]

VITAMIN C PROTECTS YOU FROM RADIATION AND POISONS!

Vitamin C even protects from the deleterious effects of radiation. Egyptian "albino rats were treated with aqueous vitamin C solution and vitamin E solution dissolved in olive oil at two concentrations...for 6 months. Some of the animals were ...subjected to whole-body irradiation."[E021] Both vitamin C and olive oil protected the animals from the radiation. Other similar studies using gamma rays, also brought out this fact, and that vitamin E was also effective in this case.[S021]

In studies done in India, it was also proven that vitamin C protects the body from certain toxins: "Vitamin C, when administered concurrently with a pesticide (*endosulfan, phosphamidon or mancozeb*), could significantly decrease the frequency of pesticide-induced clastogenic [breakdown] and mitosis-disruptive [cell division damaging] changes in the bone marrow cells of young Swiss albino mice."[K081]

CANCER PREVENTING ABILITY OF VITAMIN C

Of great importance to those who may need to use hormones and worry about cancer, is that, according to Nobel laureate Dr. Linus Pauling, the foremost authority on Vitamin C, Vitamin C will decrease the risk of getting certain cancers by 75%. He has been ridiculed, his theories poohpooed, but for us who want to lead a healthy, cancer free life, it is interesting to learn that in a study done in Japan, not only was vitamin C an effective destroyer of leukemia cells, but this effect improved in the presence of a variety of *tannin* and *lignin*-related compounds (green tea, black tea, pine cone (*Pinus parviflora Sieb. et Zucc.*), and various wines.[S030]

An antiepilepsy drug (*Clofazimine-CLF*) used in India is known to cause cell abnormalities, but the concurrent use of vitamins A and C, or C alone—but not A alone—prevents these problems. "A scavenging effect of the vitamins, removing free radicals produced by CLF, is assumed to be responsible for modulation of the...[cell damaging]...effect of CLF." [S011]

DEFICIENCY SYMPTOMS

- Anemia
- Bruising
- Capillary weakness
- Impaired digestion

- Loss of appetite
- Muscular weakness
- Nosebleeds
- Scurvy
- Skin hemorrhages
- Slow-healing wounds and fractures
- Soft and bleeding gums
- Swollen or painful joints
- Tooth decay

In a study of 80 reasonably healthy geriatric day hospital attenders, a progressive age-related decline in bone mass and ascorbic acid level was noted.[B010] In a 1993 study in Boston, older female patients were evaluated as to their bone density and bone mass, and relating these parameters to the use of certain nutrients, hormones and beverages. Vitamin C had a positive influence on bone density, whereas caffeine had a negative influence.[H072]

In a study of Danish pigs, "Depletion of vitamin C resulted in a pronounced decline in ascorbic acid concentration in most maternal and fetal organs as well as in plasma and embryonic fluids. No morphological malformations were found in the fetuses, but the ossification [conversion to bone] of the skeleton was severely deranged. With the naked eye one could see "...swelling of the costochondral junction [the place where the ribs and the catilage or grizzle meet], and separation of the epiphysial cartilage [the grizzle on the ends of the bone] ... in ribs and limb bones. Another characteristic finding was loosening of the periost [the thin membrane that wraps bones] from the cortex [the outer layer of the hard bone], often resulting in subperiosteal bleedings [into the space between these areas]. Microscopically normal osteoblasts were few and the formation of osteoid defective."[W05a]

In a rather cruel experiment, guinea pigs were fasted or made severely vitamin C deficient, and these circumstances produced substances which blocked the important developmental hormone IGF-1 (insulin growth factor 1). Vitamin C corrected these problems.[G082] It has been found that "...low tissue ascorbic acid levels in guinea pigs clearly alter the connective tissue composition of growing femur and skin...."[T073]

EFFECT OF SUPPLEMENTS OF VITAMIN C

Vitamin C intake in the form of supplements has been associated with a reduction in heart disease and cataracts. Linus Pauling, two time Nobel laureate was a strong believer in the effectiveness of vitamin C as an anti-aging compound. He credited it with extending his life span by 20 years and passed away at the age of 93 in 1994.[S160]

If osteoporosis keeps some Washington State ladies "Sleepless in Seattle", there is a reassuring study[L061] about the value of vitamin C Supplements. People with prolonged vitamin C supplementation had higher BMD, particularly noticeable in those women who were not even taking estrogen.

Vitamin C improves the metabolism and growth of chondrocytes, cartilage building cells.[V031] In another study[D023] performed in San Antonio, Texas, where I live, a combination of *beta-glycerophosphate* and vitamin C also showed bone building effects, and the production of proteins able to bind with minerals. In studies in chicken, vitamin C augmented the bone improvement that growth hormone can effect on young cells.[M221]

Vitamin C has been shown to increase the cells of the immune system, particularly in the elderly.

RECOMMENDED DOSAGE

Due to its solubility in water, Vitamin C is excreted from the body rapidly. Therefore a constant intake of this vitamin is necessary, in order to maintain the ideal levels of this anti-oxidant in the blood. The best way to ingest vitamin C is in a good diet with fresh fruits and vegetables, but this is usually insufficient, because environmental pollutants, cigarettes and other offenders may raise the body's demands of vitamin C many hundred fold. A supplement adds some insurance in people you are unable to monitor you intake or keep constant levels in your body through food.

Calcium ascorbate is a buffered (less acidic) form of vitamin C.
THE BEST DIETARY SOURCES OF VITAMIN C, listed from high to low are:

"FOOD	AMOUNT	MILLIGRAMS
Orange juice, fresh squeezed	1 cup	124
Green peppers, raw, chopped	1/2 cup	96

Grapefruit juice, fresh squeezed	1 cup	94
Papaya	1/2 medium	94
Brussel sprouts	4 sprouts	73
Broccoli, raw,chopped	1/2 cup	70
Orange	1 medium	70
Cantaloupe	1/4 melon	70
Turnip greens,cooked	1/4 cup	50
Cauliflower	1/4 cup	45
Strawberries	1/2 cup	42
Grapefruit	1/2 medium	41
Tomato juice	1 cup	39
Cabbage, raw, chopped	1/2 cup	15
Blackberries	1/2 cup	15
Spinach, raw, chopped	1/2 cup	14
Blueberries	1/2 cup	9" [C160]

Some potential side effects of Vitamin C in large doses:
- Diarrhea
- Dry nose
- Exacerbate the toxicity of iron in patients with *hemochromatosis* (an iron storage disease)
- Excess urination
- Heartburn
- Skin rashes

VITAMIN D

MAIN FUNCTIONS
- Absorption and utilization of calcium and phosphorous
- Bone and teeth formation
- Maintains a stable nervous system
- Normal heart action

DEFICIENCY
It revolves around the powerful influence of calcitriol on the metabolism of bone, whether growing or mature. A rapidly growing skeleton is partic-

ularly vulnerable to vitamin D deficiency: the more rapid the growth, the greater the risk.[S160]

DEFICIENCY SYMPTOMS

- Improper healing of fractures
- Inadequate absorption of calcium
- Lack of vigor
- Muscular weakness
- Retention of phosphorous in the kidneys
- Rickets
- Softening of bones
- Tooth decay

WHAT HAPPENS IN GROWING ANIMALS DEFICIENT IN VITAMIN D?

- Failure to mineralize osteoid and chondroid matrix at epiphyseal growth plates
- Failure to remove and remodel this matrix
- Retarded growth
- *Rickets* (may also be induced by a deficiency in phosphorous)
- Skeletal deformities
- Thickening of bones at fracture sites
- Thickening of bones at epiphyses
- Thickening of bones at diaphyses of long bones

EXCESS VITAMIN D

What happens in vitamin D overdosing? The major consequence is the induction of hypercalcaemia which results in hardening or mineralization (a kind of mummification) of many soft tissues:

- Endocardium (inner lining of the heart)
- Fibroelastic matrices in arterial walls (hardening of the arteries)
- Gastric mucosal cells (stomach lining)
- Myocardium (heart muscle)
- Pulmonary alveoli (small air cells in the lungs)
- Renal tubule cells (kidney)

These changes are referred to as *metastatic calcifications*.

In bone (hard tissues), it can cause:
■ Deposition of abnormal and characteristic osteoid matrix in the diaphyses of long bones
■ Deposition of abnormal and characteristic osteoid matrix in the metaphyses of long bones
■ Excessive new bone under the *periosteum* (bone lining membrane)
■ Excessive new bone in the medullary cavity
■ Thickening of long bone diaphyses

Other areas
■ Haemorrhages, especially gastric
■ "malaise", debilitation, lameness
■ Myocardial degeneration/necrosis
■ Renal failure
■ Renal tubular degeneration/necrosis
■ Sudden death

DIETARY SOURCES OF VITAMIN D
Vitamin D therapy has also been covered on page **143** of this book.
RDA's for adults 5-10 mcg.
THE BEST DIETARY SOURCES OF VITAMIN D are:

"FOOD	AMOUNT	MICROGRAMS (MCG)
Herring	3 ounces	35
Cod liver oil	1 tablespoon	34
Mackeral, fillet	3 ounces	8
Salmon, fillet	3 ounces	8
Tuna, Bluefin	3 ounces	4
Milk, fortified, whole	1 cup	2" [C160]

VITAMIN E
MAIN FUNCTIONS
■ Aids in bringing nourishment to cells
■ Alleviates fatigue
■ Helps prevent calcium deposits in blood vessel walls
■ Helps prevent sterility

- Helps prevent muscular dystrophy
- Helps prevent certain heart conditions
- Major anti-oxidant nutrient
- Prevents and dissolves blood clots
- Protects the red blood cells from destructive poisons
- Retards cellular aging due to oxidation
- Strengthens the capillary walls
- Supplies oxygen to the blood

DEFICIENCY SYMPTOMS

- Abnormal fat deposits in muscles
- Degenerative changes in the heart and other muscles
- Dry skin
- Lack of sexual vitality
- Loss of reproductive powers
- Rupture of red blood cells

Several types of Vitamin E are commercially available: **d-Alpha Tocopherol** (100% **natural**) is 4 times more potent in its biological activity than **dl-Alpha Tocopherol** (**synthetic**) Vitamin E: the biologic activity of 100 **international units** (**I.U.**) of d-Alpha (100% Natural) Vitamin E are equal to 400 I.U. dl-Alpha Tocopherol (Synthetic) vitamin E.[S160]

SOURCES OF VITAMIN E SUPPLEMENTS — DIETARY SOURCES

- Natural Vitamin E is derived from soybeans
- Synthetic vitamin E is a petroleum by-product

Since women on oral contraceptive therapy (a hormonal therapy) need more vitamin E than controls, a study was done on post-menopausal women receiving HRT (very similar in composition to many oral contraceptives), to see whether the same biologic variation was present. But, "Post-menopausal women did not have altered levels of vitamin E compared with pre-menopausal women. Similarly HRT has no effect on plasma vitamin E levels." HRT did not reduce vitamin E levels in a similar manner to oral contraceptives.[W100]

We may not like to think of ourselves as "chicken", but a 1996 study on chick cell cultures gives us good insight in the antioxidant protection provided by vitamin E: adding *linoleic acid* [unsaturated fatty acid—flax oil], and then creating more oxidation stress by adding iron, "...impaired *chondrocyte* [cells which form cartilage] cell function and caused cellular injury but ...vitamin E reversed these effects...vitamin E stimulated bone formation in chicks fed unsaturated fat, and the present findings in cultures of *epiphyseal chondrocytes* [cells which form cartilage on top of joint surfaces of bones] suggest that vitamin E is important for chondrocyte function in the presence of polyunsaturated fatty acids. vitamin E appears to be beneficial for growth cartilage biology and in optimizing bone growth."[W040] [emphasis added]. It reverses the harmful effects of free radicals.

You probably are familiar with the expression polyunsaturated fatty acids (PUFAs), the fats that are predominant found in vegetable oils, as opposed to saturated fats, mostly from animal sources. Vitamin E is the major fat-soluble antioxidant in human subjects and is crucial in protecting polyunsaturated fatty acids (PUFAS) against lipid peroxidation (oxidation). Dietary PUFA have been suggested to inhibit the absorption of vitamin E, yet a recent study performed with rats in The Netherlands showed that these substances lowered the presence of vitamin E in the body, but did not impair its absorption. If the results from the rat study apply to humans, people using a lot of vegetable oils should increase their intake of vitamin E.[T060]

Although this study was reported in a previous segment of the book, it is important to go over it again, under this heading. Antioxidants are important to avoid "free radical damage". In an interesting evaluation of the value of vitamin E, a study was done in Lucknow, India,[G050] on twenty heart failure patients. In these patients, damaging oxidizers were increased while the levels of antioxidants were decreased. These alterations were related to illness, not age or the cause of the condition. The addition of vitamin E in doses of 400 mgr. once a day orally for 4 weeks significantly reduced the damaging oxidizer levels and produced an elevation of the antioxidant enzymes. Thus, there is an apparent normalization of the indices of oxidative stress following treatment of heart failure and a markedly improved response on vitamin E supplementation which may be more beneficial.

What happens in growing animals deficient in Vitamin E and/or Selenium? Vitamin E and selenium are closely related in their nutritional biochemistry, and we see a similar close relationship in the diseases associated with their deficiency. The interactions between the two nutrients are complex and incompletely understood.

Since vitamin E and selenium constitute vital components of the mechanisms which protect cells from the constant threat of *oxidative* damage, a kind of biologic rusting, a deficiency, as studied in animals, adversely impacts on skeletal muscles. Normally, minerals flow in and out of cells in a well regulated manner; oxidative damage to the membranes of vulnerable cells destroys their ability to regulate this flow, particularly of calcium (which is central to muscle contraction and bone strength). Chaotic, imbalanced movements of calcium initiate severe cellular injury and lead to rapid cell death (*necrosis*).

As muscle fibers are elongated giant cells, the damage is often "segmental"; that is, it occurs in localized segments along the length of the fiber. In skeletal muscle, extensive segmental *necrosis* (cell death) occurs symmetrically in muscle groups in various regions, but seems to be most severe in muscles most actively being "used" at the time of peak vulnerability. In any particular muscle, the majority of fibers may be severely affected. In skeletal muscle the major effect is weakness.

Dehydroepiandrosterone (*DHEA*), an adrenal steroid, often taken to strengthen muscles and bones, unfortunately also induces "free radicals" and lipid peroxidation. Vitamin E doses of 400 mg/Kg in rats used in this study, decreased DHEA-induced intracellular lipid peroxidation. These results support the concept that alpha-tocopherol can protect against DHEA-induced lipid peroxidation and consequently against steroid-induced liver cell damage and, perhaps, also tumor development.[S240]

RDA for adults is 8-10 mg.
THE BEST DIETARY SOURCES OF VITAMIN E are:

"FOOD	AMOUNT	MILLIGRAMS
Wheat germ oil	1 tablespoon	37.2
Sunflower seeds	1/4 cup	26.8
Wheat germ, raw	1/4 cup	12.8
Almonds	1/4 cup	12.7
Pecan, halves	1/4 cup	12.5

Safflower oil	1 tablespoon	7.9
Peanuts	1/4 cup	4.9
Corn oil	1 tablespoon	4.8
Peanut butter	2 tablespoons	3.8
Soybean oil	1 tablespoon	3.5
Cod-liver-oil	1 tablespoon	3
Lobster	3 ounces	2.3
Salmon, fillet	3 ounces	0.6" [C160]

VITAMIN K

Could a natural tendency to bruising and/or blood-thinner therapy contribute to osteoporosis? Is this due to vitamin K deficiency?

Vitamin K is a fat soluble vitamin. Vitamin K is a substance found in green leafy vegetables, liver, tomatoes, egg yolks, and vegetable oils. It has a very important role in the clotting of blood after certain injuries. It is also synthesized in the intestine and liver. Vitamin K can be formed naturally by bacteria in the intestines. However, bacterial synthesis alone does not provide enough Vitamin K, dietary sources are needed.

Impaired vitamin K metabolism is associated with a biochemical irregularity of the protein osteocalcin, which is required for normal bone formation. Normally, the chemical group *carboxy* binds to osteocalcin in the bone. Post-menopausal women are afflicted with **under-carboxylation,** decreased binding of the chemical group *carboxy* to osteocalcin, which increases with age and is marked in the elderly. A similarly marked degree of the impaired biologic process occurs during a course with anticoagulant (preventative of clotting) substances, such as *coumarin* or *warfarin* (the popular blood *thinner Coumadin*, and a key question is whether this may lead to an accelerated loss of bone mass. A consistent trend for reduced BMD at all sites was observed in the *warfarin* treated patients.[P068] This was particularly marked in the cancellous bones of the wrist (9% reduction) and at the cancellous rich lumbar spine site (10.4% reduction). Because of the biochemical similarities between all of these substances related to the blood clotting process, this study provides a new lead on post-menopausal osteoporosis, and supports the hypothesis that impaired carboxylation of osteocalcin plays a role in bone loss in the elderly through deficiency in vitamin K metabolism.

Vitamin K is actually not one, but a group of three fat soluble vitamins of different sources:

- Vitamin *K1* (*phylloquinone*), from food sources
- Vitamin *K2* (*menaquinone*) formed by bacteria in the intestines
- Vitamin *K3* (*menaphthone* or *menadione*), which is synthetic

Vitamin K is used by the liver to make and transform proteins important to *blood clotting*. Whereas most people are aware of this function of vitamin K, it is a largely unknown that it is very important to bone and calcium metabolism.

EFFECTS ON BONE METABOLISM

The bone protein *osteocalcin*, which regulates the function of calcium in bone turnover and mineralization has to be changed (*converted*) from an inactive to an active form. Vitamin K is the "minister" that is in charge of this conversion. Since the presence of fats and bile in the gut is required in order for vitamin K to be absorbed, today's absurd diets, so low in fats, do nothing but compound the problems of osteoporosis.

From the point of view of calcium metabolism, Vitamin K is necessary for the production of a urinary protein involved in kidney function which inhibits the formation of *calcium oxalate* kidney stones. This may account for the fact that vegetarians, whose diets are often high in vitamin K, have low numbers of kidney stones.

VITAMIN K DEFICIENCY

It is rare. Signs of deficiency are:
- Bleeding from the gut
- Blood stained urine
- Bruising
- Easy bleeding
- Frequent nosebleeds
- Prolonged clotting time

It usually only occurs in people who are/have
- Elderly
- Malabsorption problems (*celiac disease* or *sprue* - tropical diarrhea-)

- Newborn
- Premature babies
- Prolonged diarrhea
- Serious illnesses
- Using antibiotics

DIETARY SOURCES OF VITAMIN K

RDA for adults is 60-80 mcg.
THE BEST DIETARY SOURCES OF VITAMIN K ARE:

"FOOD	AMOUNT	MICROGRAMS
Turnip greens, raw	1/2 cup	182
Spinach, frozen	1/2 cup	131
Liver, beef	3 ounces	104
Cauliflower, raw	1/2 cup	96
Soybean oil	1 tablespoon	76
Broccoli, raw	1/2 cup	58
Green cabbage, raw	1/2 cup	52
Tomato	1 medium	28
Egg yolk	1 large	25
Milk	1 cup	10
Corn oil	1 tablespoon	8" E001

Vitamin K is present in a wide variety of foods. Other sources of dietary vitamin K include: avocados, Brussels sprouts, cabbage, canola oil, carrots, cereals (small), cucumbers, dairy products, dark leafy greens, leeks, meats (small), olive oil, soybean oil, etc. Freezing foods may destroy vitamin K, but it remains stable when heated.

RECOMMENDED DIETARY ALLOWANCES

The RDA for vitamin K is 1 mcg per kg of body weight. It is assumed that at least half the necessary daily intake comes from the substance produced by the metabolism of intestinal bacteria (Men 80 mcg, Women 65 mcg), but estimates vary among the medical researchers of various countries. Vitamin K is available as a vitamin supplement. Alfalfa tablets are a good natural source of vitamin K.

TOXIC EFFECTS

These vary in seriousness, depending which product is used. Reports of toxic effects from natural vitamin K are rare. Large doses of the *synthetic* form of vitamin K, menadione may cause hemolytic anemia and liver damage.

SIDE EFFECTS

Accidental injection into a vein may cause problems, to include flushing, sweats, chest pain and constricted breathing. Intramuscular injection may cause pain and swelling. Since one of the many irrational practices is the injection of vitamin K into infants, there have been reports of a link between vitamin K injection and childhood cancer. This probably does not apply to adults.

VITAMIN K AND OSTEOPOROSIS

Large supplemental doses of vitamin K have been used to treat osteoporosis. Vitamin K may improve bone mineralization in post-menopausal women by boosting blood levels of the bone protein osteocalcin, possibly also by decreasing calcium excretion through the urine.

CAUSES OF DEFICIENCIES OF VITAMIN K

- Antibiotics, which kill the beneficial bacteria normally present in the human gut, which produce vitamin K
- Aspirin
- *Cholestyramine* (a cholesterol lowering drug)
- High intake of vitamin E (above 600 IU) may antagonize vitamin K action and lead to an increased risk of hemorrhage
- Mineral oil laxatives
- *Phenytoin* (*Dilantin*, an *antiepileptic* drug)
- X rays and radiation

All of the above can raise vitamin K requirements. as vitamin K can counteract the effects of these drugs. In technologically advanced societies vitamin deficiency results mainly from food faddism, misuse of drugs, chronic alcoholism, or prolonged intravenous (*parenteral*) feeding.

COENZYME Q10 (CO-Q-10, UBIQUINONE)
This is a vitamin-like substance, with high impact on cardiovascular functioning, immunity, allergies, asthma. It often makes patients feel energetic and healthy.

It is normally present in Mackerel, salmon and sardines.

MINERALS
Adam was fashioned from the earth, composed of *minerals*, or so the Bible tells us: when he dies, the dust shall return to dust. In these few but exacting words the information has come to us for the past six millennia: we are fashioned from the same minerals our planet is, everything mother earth is, we are. Minerals are the basic building materials for our organic and inorganic molecules. Biochemically, we are what our mineral makeup is, no more and no less.

Minerals are inorganic substances existing in our environment: calcium, magnesium, selenium, etc. Vitamins usually can not be assimilated without the aid of minerals. ALL MINERALS *MUST* come from the environment:

■   Directly, such as water and oxygen
■   Indirectly, in food, beverages or supplements

All tissues and internal fluids of our body contain varying quantities of minerals. Minerals are constituents of the bones, teeth, soft tissue, muscle, blood, and nerve cells. They are vital to overall mental and physical well-being. Minerals *can not* be synthesized in the human body: they *must* come from the earth that is our home, and packaged and processed in water, plants and animal products. If we tamper with the mineral equilibrium, we tread on dangerous ground. As Mexico City slid and quivered in those areas where its foundations were set on the soft bottom of lake Texcoco, so does our body give and weaken in the fault lines where wholesome bedrock has been replaced by abnormal substances.

The many varied elements, including the minerals of life, are catalogued in what we know as the *"periodic table of Mendelejeff"*. Although there are more than 100 substances in the periodic table of elements, human health only accepts up to number 50, the others being toxic. This apparently technical piece of information is to protect the individual about today's fraudulent hyping of "*colloidal* minerals", a brew of dirty water containing large numbers of toxic substances.

Minerals act as *catalysts* (activators or accelerators) for many biological reactions within the body:

- Digestion
- Muscle response
- Production of hormones
- Transmission of messages through the nervous system
- Utilization of nutrients in foods

According to the amounts in which they are present in our system, we can classify them into two groups

- *Macrominerals* (necessary in larger amounts)
- *Trace elements* (necessary in smaller amounts)

WATER

We have been brainwashed into oblivion, that, biochemically speaking, our body is largely water. Now let us remember that chemical formulas are just a code, an alphabet used for the symbolic representation of the structure of a substance. Whereas the abundance of hydrogen and oxygen molecules permits much of the body to be converted into water, saying that a complex chemical *is* water is as logic as stating that *boxes* of *Clorox*, and *oxygen* are mainly made from *oxen*, because the letters *o* and *x* are repeatedly found in the symbolic code (alphabet) used to write those words. But good part of the body *is* actually water and the salts dissolved in it. The predominant minerals are calcium, phosphorus and magnesium, main building blocks of the skeleton. Hair and skin are rich in sulphur and the rest of the tissues contain mainly iron (blood and muscle), copper, zinc, and the trace elements selenium, *molybdenum*, chromium, etc.

Since water is our main nutrient, either as a drink or as a solvent, pure and clean drinking water is essential to good health. The water our body uses is not only drank as such, but also comes from the metabolism of many nutrients that break down into *energy* and *water*.

We lose water in urine, stools, perspiration, breathing, etc. When we do not drink enough fluids, our bodies can not shed toxins properly. The urine can only concentrate solutes to a point; if we drink sodas, coffee, tea, or other drinks, they already carry a certain number of solids in solution, and are not as effective a cleanser as pure water. This is similar to what would happen if we were trying to pick up dirt and debris with wheelbarrows that are already partially filled with sand. Each would only be able to carry a few pounds of trash, and it would take more work, more men and more wheelbarrows to clean the area.

Our water supplies are now frequently contaminated. Aquifers that stored clean water for millennia, are now over-utilized and cannot be replenished at proper speed. The rainwater that fills them is often polluted. Recharge zones are sometimes too porous to properly filter and purify contaminated water. Contaminants are not only found in city water supplies, but also in sources far removed from civilization. Whereas disease producing germs used to be our greatest concern of yesteryear, toxins are today's most acute problem.

Water supplies are seldom tested for the presence of contaminating heavy metals or pesticides. To compound problems, recombinations of certain elements may result in new and unsuspected poisons. The very *chlorine* we use to kill harmful bacteria has been linked to the development of human cardiovascular problems and other illness. When organic matter and chlorine combine they can form gases similar to those used for anesthesia. *Trihalomethanes* (as these are called) also can form when *fluorine* is added to water supplies. *Artificial fluoridation* not only adds the potentially dangerous *fluorines*, but also trace amounts of lead, antimony, etc. The substances suspended or diluted in water concentrate as the aquifers are used up, and not properly replenished. Their levels can rapidly become a threat to health.

OPTIMAL HEALTH AND PURE WATER

Health conscious individuals are usually aware of the vital role clean drinking water plays in good nutrition, yet most are not aware of the insidious harmful potential of the water used to bathe in. Skin may not absorb water, but it absorbs other toxins with ease. While in the shower or in the tub, skin absorbency allows chlorine and other contaminants (algae, bacteria, *chloramine*, fluorine, fungus, hydrogen sulfide, iron, most heavy metals which some say, tongue in cheek, includes rock groups, **PCBs** (**poli-chlorinated-biphenyls**), and others, to be absorbed through the skin, and also inhaled as chlorine gas! It has been calculated that in just 15 minutes in a hot shower we absorb, through *osmosis* (the passage through a semi-permeable membrane), impurities equivalent to the ones derived from drinking 2 quarts of that same water!

CLEANSING THE CLEANSER

Distilled water has been both praised and criticized. The distillation processes commonly used (single distillation) do not always remove all substances dissolved in the water: often *petroleum derivatives* and *fluorine* distill <u>with</u> the water. A double distillation process is more effective. There are those who claim that demineralized, soft waters, are dangerous, and invite osteoporosis and debility. Others claim that natural minerals are deposited in the form of plaque and kidney stones. Whatever the dispute, it is clear that when people are only concentrate solutes to a point; if we drink sodas, coffee, tea, etc., although these are liquid, they already carry a certain number of solids in solution, and are not as effective a cleanser as pure water. This is similar to what would happen if we were trying to pick up dirt and debris with wheelbarrows that are already partially filled with sand. Each would only be able to carry a few pounds of trash, and it would take more work, more men and more wheelbarrows to clean the area.

Bottled spring and mineral waters are an interesting alternative, but not always guaranteed to be of the best quality. Some have a very high mineral content, and if used to excess, may overburden the body with the minerals they contain in solution. Probably, the best answer is to buy a home *water purifier* (three stage), and have your water checked periodically by a reliable laboratory. If you have fluoridated water you must buy a special module for the fluoride, because regular purifiers do not remove it.

Not all purifiers are made equal, and only very few protect the drinker from all contaminants. Since I have been often asked about adequate equipment, I have enclosed a page in the back of the book to request further information.

Water in the body is a giver of life, but may become a messenger of death if not properly distributed, pumped and used.

Contaminated Water May Be A Messenger of Death

If the heart or kidneys function improperly, if the diet generates an imbalance between sodium and potassium by faulty food habits, swelling (often referred to as *edema*) may occur. If instead of correcting the underlying problems patients rely on taking diuretics (fluid pills) to control such swelling, further harm is done, altering the metabolic balance. Waterlogged tissues are not only unsightly, but much more prone to foster the growth of harmful germs. Have you ever noticed how fruit jams are prepared gooey and thick, and how, when properly cooked they do not deteriorate easily, or how well dehydrated fruits keep? In food engineering it is well known, that the drier a product is, the less apt it will be to rot. The ability to fend off bacterial growth in a product depends on its being well concentrated. This relative concentration of solids vs. liquid is known as *water number*. In the body, waterlogged tissues are far more apt to foster the growth of germs, than properly balanced ones.

Water may not only be a giver of life, but the matrix of life itself. New and complicated European studies reveal a new world of structure and physics, where water (in a pyramidal structure) replaces RNA and DNA as the carrier of this elusive *life-force*. The philosophy behind this totally new world is complex and poorly known as of yet, but if these researchers are right, water way be able to "imprint" biochemical messages, transfer information, and forward "memory" to other locations.

If the heart or kidneys function improperly, if the diet generates an imbalance between sodium and potassium by faulty food habits, swelling (often referred to as *edema*) may occur. If instead of correcting the underlying problems patients rely on taking diuretics (fluid pills) to control such swelling, further harm is done, altering the metabolic balance. Waterlogged tissues are not only unsightly, but much more prone to foster the growth of harmful germs. Have you ever noticed how fruit jams are prepared gooey and thick, and how, when properly cooked they do not deteriorate easily, or how well dehydrated fruits keep? In food engineering it is well known, that the drier a product is, the less apt it will be to rot. The ability to fend off bacterial growth in a product depends on its being well concentrated. This relative concentration of solids vs. liquid is known as *water number*. In the body, waterlogged tissues are far more apt to foster the growth of germs, than properly balanced ones.

In this era of concern with contamination through body fluids, it behooves everybody to understand the various newly discovered roles of water.

The water that we bathe in, particularly in hot tubs, has been accused to transfer viruses that cause illness. This may be so, but a much less known, but certainly much more real risk is represented by the fact that these waters contain high concentrations of *chlorine*, *bromine* and other chemicals which are absorbed through the skin and create havoc inside the body's chemistry by their interactions with necessary minerals and processes, such as the utilization of iodine at thyroid level. I propose that all hot tubs should be protected by cleansing with ultraviolet lights that should turn themselves on intermittently so as to sterilize the liquid without harming the bathers. Harsh antiseptics commonly used in this process, may cause more harm than good, because they frequently wash off protective skin oils that are natural defenses.

WATER PURIFIERS

Water purifiers, devices to take toxins and bad flavors out of the water, may range form very high quality to very low standards. Many claims are made about various systems. There are reverse osmosis, magnetic, ultraviolet, etc., they may range form very high to very low quality, and are not standardized at present because no specific standardization mechanisms exist. Many *purifiers* have a problem of bacterial overgrowth. Others, leave harmful mineral residues in the filtered water. It takes a three stage purifier to give you real good, clean water. For further information, the reader may find a leaflet in the back of the book.

CALCIUM

Calcium is the most abundant mineral in the human body. The bulk of the body's calcium is contained in the skeleton. It is not only essential to build the mineral portion of bone, but it is necessary to the activity of muscles and nerves, it is involved in hormonal secretion and immune/oxidant response functions. It is involved in protective reactions against microbes, toxins and foreign substances.

ELEMENTAL CALCIUM

What is *elemental calcium*? The reader may have seen capsules or pills called *Calcium Gluconate* or *lactate*, or another amino acid form) 650 mgr. (100 mgr. elemental). This means that the molecule calcium *with* the protein complex represents 650 mgr. of the pill, but that this total amount only contains 100 mgr. of calcium (the element) itself, (the other 550 mgr. being the amino acid molecule to which it is bound). An *element* is each of the substances that exist uncombined in nature, such as iron, magnesium or hydrogen, which can enter into combinations.

Calcium is very important in the human body. Our bones contain large amounts of calcium which helps to make them firm and rigid. Calcium is also needed for many other tasks including nerve and muscle function and blood clotting.

Bone calcium is often used as a reservoir when biologic processes need more calcium than the diet can provide: when dietary calcium is too low, calcium will be lost from bone and used for other critical functions. Calcium in the blood is tightly controlled by the body's chemical balancing act known as *homeostasis*: blood will maintain the desirable level even under stressful circumstances, at the expense of bone losses. Total calcium status can therefore, not be fully assessed by measuring blood calcium levels alone.

ADEQUATE CALCIUM INTAKE

The opinions about the ultimate role of calcium nutrition in age-related bone loss are still controversial. Paradoxically, adequate calcium intake early in life, helping to achieve a peak bone mass, may be of greater importance to bone quality, than is calcium intake in later life. Calcium intake commonly declines with advancing age due to the changing food habits that are associated with social and technological change, also by the increasing concern about obesity in Western society. The trend is that women in particular, prefer to restrict their energy intake rather than increase their energy expenditure, to control weight. Thus, low energy intakes and the avoidance of dairy foods have contributed to the declining intakes of calcium and other minerals. Health educational programs designed to prevent osteoporosis and identify women who are most at risk of the disease, should provide sensible nutritional advice on an adequate calcium intake and regular weight-bearing exercise among other life-style changes.[A070]

In an American study about the consumption of calcium in the U.S., "Calcium intake [was] one of a number of factors that affect[ed] peak bone mass. Low bone mass is related to increased incidence of osteoporotic fractures. Data from the USDA [U.S. Department of Agriculture] 1987-88 Nationwide Food Consumption Survey were used to determine populations most at risk of less than optimal calcium intake and food sources of calcium intake. Mean per capita daily consumption of calcium for the total U.S. population was 737 mg and varied by region of the country, household income, ethnic group, sex, and age. For most groups of females, intake was substantially less than the RDA [Recommended Daily Amount]. About 50% of total dietary calcium was supplied by milk and milk products. Milk and cheese used as ingredients in meat, grain, and vegetable mixtures contributed another 20% of dietary calcium. The remaining 30% of calcium was provided by grains and grain products, meat, poultry, fish, vegetables, fruits, eggs, legumes, nuts, and seeds."[F041]

The commonly recommended daily allowance (RDA) intake of *elemental calcium* for most adults is 1000 mgr. The recommended total daily intake of elemental calcium for peri- and post-menopausal women is 1500 mgr.

For further information on calcium therapies, go to the section on minerals.

WHAT ABOUT CHELATED VS. INORGANIC CALCIUM

Personal perception about the adequacy of one's food intake is often biased, and inaccurate. Assimilation of various diets is very individual. It is the general consensus of opinion that one should not rely upon dietary calcium alone to satisfy the needs of osteoporotic individuals, unless a very detailed dietary history has been obtained, and one is absolutely certain that calcium intake is sufficient. Non-dairy dietary calcium INTAKE IN THE US, is generally less than 300 mgr. a day. Each glass of milk or ounce of cheese adds another 300 mgr. Patients with moderate to severe bone mineral density loss should receive 1500 mgr. of supplemental calcium, unless contraindicated by reason of personal or family history of calcium kidney stones, or the use of very high doses of vitamin D, in which case the dose can be lowered to achieve an estimated total elemental calcium intake from all sources of 1500 mgr. daily. In the opinion of the *Establishment*, it may be advisable to use *calcium citrate* instead of *calcium carbonate* whenever gastric acid is suspected of being low, spontaneously or as a result of anti-ulcer medications. (In the opinion of most alternative practitioners, calcium carbonate should not be used).

The general consensus of *Establishment* (not necessarily opposed by alternative), is that to enhance calcium absorption:

■ Calcium citrate should be given *between* meals
■ Calcium carbonate should be given *with* meals

Why is it so difficult to get clear and final answers about calcium supplements and their bio-availability? Many calcium absorption and utilization studies are done with rats, which have different nutritional requirements and metabolism, and the results obtained are often not equally applicable to humans.

Have we heard the last word on calcium supplements? Not yet...The effects of commercially available calcium supplements and milk, on calcium tissue levels and apparent absorption of calcium, magnesium, phosphorus, zinc, iron and copper[G100] were evaluated in two studies using defenseless rats. The supplements used as sole sources of calcium in nutritionally adequate diets, in this study, were:

■ Calcium phosphate dibasic
■ Calcium carbonate with and without supplemental iron and vitamins
■ Calcium lactate
■ Chelated calcium with and without chelated magnesium
■ Dolomite
■ Nonfat dry milk
■ Oyster shell preparations with and without supplemental magnesium

Rats fed calcium phosphate dibasic had enlarged kidneys with greater than 20-fold increases in calcium levels. The rats fed the three magnesium-fortified supplements had lower apparent absorption of calcium and iron and less accumulation of calcium in bone than rats fed milk. There were few differences in the utilization of calcium by rats fed milk or supplements containing only calcium lactate, chelated calcium, oyster shells and calcium carbonate, but magnesium retention in bone was greater among rats fed milk.[G110 C080]

The benefits of milk and milk derivatives are quite apparent: "Femoral Ca[lcium] and P[hosphorus] contents from rats fed **beta-CPP** [**casein phosphopeptides**, a substance similar to milk protein] tend...to be higher than those from control rats. These results suggest that beta CPP supplementation could have an effect on Ca[lcium] absorption...[if the rats are somewhat... Ca[lcium] deficien[t]. [T072]

Many calcium supplements are commercially available, and there has always existed a heated debate about which are more effective in being absorbed and helping form better bone.

How are the metabolisms of magnesium, calcium and phosphorus interconnected? In one study, excess dietary phosphorus and calcium decreased the apparent magnesium absorption ratios, and the concentrations of magnesium in the serum and femur, and increased the deposition of calcium in the kidney. When the effects of two supplements, calcium gluconate and calcium carbonate on the utilization of magnesium and **nephrocalcinosis** (calcification of the kidneys) in rats made magnesium-deficient by adding excess dietary phosphorus and calcium were compared, the low magnesium condition of the experimental animals aggravated the deposition of calcium.

The magnesium absorption and femur magnesium were dependent on calcium intake: concentration in the rats fed a calcium gluconate diet (with an equal number of molecules of calcium gluconate and calcium carbonate used as a source of calcium) were significantly higher than in the rats fed a calcium carbonate diet (only calcium carbonate was used as a source of calcium), irrespective of dietary magnesium concentration.

CALCIUM GLUCONATE SUPPLEMENTATION
IS MORE SATISFACTORY

Calcium gluconate supplementation gave more satisfactory results: Dietary calcium gluconate lessened the accumulation of calcium in the kidney and increased the serum magnesium concentration compared with dietary calcium carbonate, when the rats were fed the normal magnesium diet, but not the low magnesium diet.

> increase
< decrease

additional minerals	calcium in kidneys	calcium in bones	magnesium absorption and in bone
Excess Phosphorus and Calcium	>	<	
Ca Gluconate	<	>	>>>>
Ca carbonate	>	>	>
Low magnesium	>>		

One question that often arises is which commercial calcium product is better to take, and more effective in producing the desired results. Although we have already established that calcium gluconate is less harmful to the kidneys and helps the metabolism of magnesium, the calcium carbonate industry is often eager to produce other results. So, in 1992 they set out to determine which calcium tablets disintegrate (crumble easier in various imitation stomach juice solutions (none of which really represents the stomach juices), because the absorption of a pill often depends on how well this is dissolved in the stomach. A consumer test at the College of Pharmacy at Ann Arbor, Michigan, compared and standardized methods for measuring the breaking up of calcium tablets in the body. The results were compared to see how well they could predict the bioavailability (avail ability to the body) of calcium. The breakdown of 17 calcium supplement tablets immersed in various solutions, was studied.[M052] These liquids were:

- Distilled water

- Simulated Gastric Fluid Test Solution, USP (United States Pharmacopea), without pepsin

- White distilled vinegar

The tablets in the vinegar disintegrated faster on the average, but the results of these tests were so variable that no conclusions were definitely drawn.

THE ROLE OF CALCIUM IN BONE METABOLISM AND MENOPAUSE

The usual daily intake of elemental calcium in the United States, 450 mgr. to 550 mgr., falls well below the National Research Council's (*NRC*) recommended dietary allowance (*RDA*) of 800 mgr.; the RDA is designed to meet the needs of approximately 95% or more of the population. Calcium metabolic balance studies indicate a daily requirement of about 1,000 mgr. of calcium for pre-menopausal and estrogen-treated women. Since estrogen deficiency causes a yearly bone loss and calcium loss of a noticeable volume, post-menopausal women who are not treated with estrogen require about 1,500 mgr. daily for calcium balance, and even then will experience bone loss. Therefore, the RDA for calcium is evidently too low for post-menopausal women and may well be too low in elderly men.

In some studies, high dietary calcium suppresses age-related bone loss and reduces the fracture rate in patients with osteoporosis. It seems likely that an increase in calcium intake to 1,000 to 1,500 mgr. a day beginning well before the menopause will reduce the incidence of osteoporosis in postmenopausal women. Increased calcium intake may prevent age-related bone loss in men as well.

"Taking calcium pills does not prevent osteoporosis. Lack of calcium can cause osteoporosis, but taking extra calcium will not treat it. Bones do not pick up calcium effectively and incorporate it into their structure unless they have a stimulus from estrogen, testosterone, etidronate-like drugs or calcitonin. Several recent studies show that etidronate can prevent osteoporosis caused by diseases and medications that weaken bones, such as prednisone."[M211]

OPTIMAL CALCIUM INTAKE

Adequate vitamin D is essential for optimal calcium absorption. Dietary constituents, hormones, drugs, age, and genetic factors influence the amount of calcium required for optimal skeletal health. Calcium intake, up to a total intake of 2,000 mgr./day, appears to be safe in most individuals.[N070]

The *Establishment* would have it that the preferred sources of calcium are calcium-rich foods such as dairy products. This may be appropriate in an uncontaminated environment where animals are not fed toxic drugs, artificially fattened with anabolic steroids, exposed to environmental pollutants, fluoridated water sources and harmful fertilizers and pesticides. But in our real world, it is questionable whether anyone should ingest large amount of the white beverage laced with all manner of abominable chemicals, crushed by homogenization and denatured by pasteurization, we call milk.

The consensus panel's statement, summarized, is that calcium is an essential nutrient. Optimal calcium intake may vary according to a person's age, sex, and ethnicity. Other factors play a role in calcium intake, including vitamin D, which is needed for adequate calcium absorption. Many factors can negatively influence calcium availability, such as certain medications or food components. Optimal calcium intake may be achieved through diet, calcium-fortified foods, calcium supplements, or various combinations of these.

WHAT IS THE OPTIMAL AMOUNT OF CALCIUM INTAKE?

Optimal calcium (a major component of mineralized tissues) intake is the level of consumption necessary for the following:

■ Normal growth and development of the skeleton and teeth
■ To maximize peak adult bone mass
■ To maintain adult bone mass
■ To minimize bone loss in the later years

Calcium requirements vary throughout an individual's lifetime, with greater needs during the following:

■ Periods of rapid growth in childhood and adolescence
■ Pregnancy and lactation
■ In later adult life

Because 99% of total body calcium is found in bone, the need for calcium is largely determined by skeletal requirements. Most studies examining the efficacy of calcium intake on bone mass have used measurement of external calcium balance and bone densitometry.

CALCIUM IN FOOD

The major sources of calcium in the average U.S. diet are milk and dairy products. Each 8 ounce glass (240 ml.) of milk contains 275-300 mgr. calcium. But the *bioavailability* (the chance for the body to soak up this calcium) depends on many factors, including the chemical and physical form of the calcium, the presence of appropriate co-factors in the diet, the presence of certain enzymes. The silly habit of using skim or low fat milk to minimize fat intake, impairs the body's ability to absorb the calcium, a problem magnified by the fact that *pasteurized* milk has lost the enzyme *phosphatase,* essential for proper calcium absorption.

However, many non-dairy, high calcium foods are also high in fiber, and pass through the gut quite rapidly; it is questionable whether they really increase the bio-availability of calcium. For those unable to take in 1,000 mgr. to 1,500 mgr. of calcium through their diet, supplementation with calcium tablets (paying special attention to their elemental calcium content), is recommended both by the *Establishment* doctors and by the alternative therapists.

Calcium intake above this level could cause urinary tract stones in susceptible people. In my practice we always stressed that anyone with a history of *calcium oxalate* kidney stones should be well informed about how magnesium and vitamin B6, as well as an acidifying diet can help prevent these. Lately, I have learnt that cartilage proteins such as *glucosamine sulfate*, even *shark cartilage*, offer protection against kidney stones.

Normal levels of vitamin D are required for optimal calcium absorption. The requirement for vitamin D increases with age. The lack of daily sunlight exposure, as in those confined to home or to a nursing facility, adds a special risk for vitamin D deficiency.

VITAMIN D HAS SOME DANGEROUS EFFECTS AT HIGH DOSES

Vitamin D has dangerous effects at high doses. Although the toxic dose varies among individuals, toxicity has occurred at levels as low as 2,000-5,000 international units [I.U.] daily. Experts indicate that no one should consume more than 15 to 20 micrograms (600 to 800 units, twice the daily RDA) without a doctor's recommendation.

WHICH ARE THE BEST WAYS TO ATTAIN OPTIMAL CALCIUM INTAKE?

The simplest approach to attaining optimal calcium intake is through the daily diet. Additional strategies include the consumption of calcium fortified foods and calcium supplements. Many Americans consider that dairy products are the major contributors of dietary calcium because of their high calcium content (approximately 250-300 mgr./8 oz milk) and frequency of consumption. However, on the one hand, it may be necessary for individuals with lactose intolerance to limit or exclude liquid dairy foods, on the other, milk that has been pasteurized has lost then enzyme phosphatase, so that the absorption of calcium is uncertain. Adequate calcium intake (but not necessarily absorption) can be achieved through the use of low-lactose-containing dairy products, or addition of the enzyme *lactase* to the diet, through commercial preparations. Other foods also contain variable amounts of calcium, but again, the bioavailability of this mineral is affected buy many variables. High fiber foods and foods which contain antinutritional factors, such as *phytic acid*, contained in many grains, interfere with the absorption level.

NECESSARY INTAKE AND BEST DIETARY SOURCES

RDA for adults is 800-1200 mg.

THE BEST SOURCES OF DIETARY CALCIUM are:

"FOOD	AMOUNT	MICROGRAMS MG
Milk, evaporated skim	1 cup	580
Sardines, with bones	3 ounces	372
Collard greens, cooked	1 cup	355
Yogurt	1 cup	272
Turnip greens, cooked	1 cup	252
Milk, skim or 1%	1 cup	246
Milk, whole	1 cup	238
Buttermilk	1 cup	232
Salmon, with bones	3 ounces	167
Cottage cheese	1/2 cup	160
Broccoli	1 stalk	158
Almonds	2 ounces	132
Cheese, cheddar	1 cubic inch	129
Tofu	3.5 ounces	128
Tortilla, corn	1	120
Kidney beans	1 cup	115
Black beans	1 cup	105" [E001]

Calcium retention increases with increasing calcium intake up to a threshold, beyond which further calcium intake causes no additional increment in calcium retention.

WHAT DETERMINES THE QUALITY AND EFFECTIVENESS OF A CALCIUM PREPARATION?

bioavailability   calcium content
degree of ionization   solubility*

*A solid can be mixed into a liquid in various ways:

solution: small particles dissolve completely

suspension: particles sediment, has to be shaken up

In a study comparing *solutions* and *suspensions* of two different supplements, *citrate solution* and *lactogluconate/carbonate solution*, there was a significantly higher absorption from a *citrate* solution than from the *lactogluconate/carbonate* solution. But absorption from the *citrate* suspension was similar to that from the *lactogluconate/carbonate* solution. Vitamin D..., did not affect the absorption..." [H040]

COMPARING THE ABSORPTION OF VARIOUS SUPPLEMENTS OF CALCIUM & MAGNESIUM

Many calcium supplements contain only inexpensive, inorganic forms of calcium, such as *oxides* or *carbonates*. In general, most of these products are not worthwhile to take because most of the calcium is not well absorbed. Different individuals seem to be able to absorb different forms of calcium and magnesium, including *citrates*, *chelates*, *aspartates*, *gluconates*, *ascorbates*, *glycerophosphates*, *orotates* and *lactates*. It is advisable to use these instead of calcium carbonate, because the carbonate is almost non-absorbable, and has more side effects. To enhance absorption calcium citrate should be given between meals.

POORLY ABSORBED CALCIUM SUPPLEMENTS:

carbonates   oxides

WELL ABSORBED CALCIUM SUPPLEMENTS

ascorbates	aspartates
chelates	citrates
gluconates	glycerophosphates
lactates	orotates

absorption of citrate solution   >   *lactogluconate/carbonate* solution

absorption of *citrate* suspension   =   *lactogluconate/carbonate* solution

It is clear that calcium citrate in solution or suspension is superior as a supplement, calcium glucobionate/carbonate is of poor bioavailability.[M230]

Intravenous calcium gluconate is a very effective way to obtain good levels of this mineral. The intravenous injection must be given slowly to avoid unnecessary flushing or dizziness. The medication is available in the US, by prescription, in Mexico, over the counter.

MAIN FUNCTIONS OF A CALCIUM SUPPLEMENT

- Activates white blood cells
- Assists in normal blood clotting
- Builds and maintains bones and teeth
- Helps regulate the passage of nutrients in and out of the cell walls
- Helps maintain proper nerve and muscle function
- Important to normal kidney function
- Lowers blood pressure
- Promotes healthy sleep
- Reduces the incidence of colon cancer
- Reduces blood cholesterol levels
- Regulates heart rhythm

DEFICIENCY SYMPTOMS

- Arm and leg muscles spasms
- Back and leg cramps
- Brittle bones
- Depression
- Osteoporosis (a deterioration of the bones)

- Poor growth
- Rickets
- Softening of bones
- Tooth decay

Calcium also has important functions in physical comfort, electric conduction and control of pain. For instance, calcium ion concentration in **meridians** and **acupuncture points** in rabbits is significantly higher than that in non-meridian and non-acupuncture points.[G131] In the acupuncture treatment of **arrhythmias** (irregular heart beat), the curative effects of certain points are lost if calcium is removed by chelation at that point.[M161] Calcium is known to be part of the body messaging system, as intercellular messenger and determinant of the shape of developing body parts and various physiological functions.[S100] It contributes to the electric potential across cell membranes. Calcium waves can be elicited by electrical, mechanical or laser stimulation as well as chemical exposure, and propagate through **gap junctions**, or nerve connections.[C131 N041]

DOES BEING BREAST FED AFFECT HOW WELL YOUR BONES WILL DEVELOP, AND GIVE YOU PROTECTION FROM FUTURE OSTEOPOROSIS?

Because early calcium nutrition will determine later bone mass and performance, nourishing the infant will protect it from future osteoporosis. Calcium intake of infants **breast fed** exclusively during the first 6 months of life is in the range of 250-330 mgr./day, absorption being between 55% and 60% of that amount. Cow milk based formulas are less absorbable, about 40%. These formulas contain nearly twice the calcium content of human milk; this results in comparable calcium retentions of 150-200 mgr./day from both formula and breast milk. Net calcium absorption from **soy based** formulas is comparable to, or higher than, that of breast milk or cow milk formulas because of its considerably higher calcium content. However, soy formulas are usually inadequately supplied with essential fatty acids, and may alter vitamin D absorption, and other nutrients. Soy formulas may provide too much of a naturally occurring estrogen (**genistein**). For infants between the ages of 6 and 12 months, calcium intake ranges from 400 to 700 mgr./day. On the basis of balance data, the current RDAs for calcium, 400 mgr./day for infants from birth to 6 months and 600 mgr./day for those from 6 to 12 months, seem sufficient to provide optimal calcium intake. However, special circumstances such as low birth weight may require higher calcium intake.

Limited data from one recent study suggest that in children 6-10 years old, intake above 800 mgr./day may lead to increased rates of bone accumulation. Coupled with calcium balance data, this suggests that an intake of greater than 800 mgr./day may be optimal for this age group. It should also be noted that poor calcium nutrition in childhood may be related to the development of **enamel hypoplasia** and accelerated **dental caries**.

WHAT IS THE OPTIMAL AMOUNT OF CALCIUM INTAKE FOR CHILDREN AND YOUNG ADULTS (11-24 YEARS)

Calcium accumulation in bone during preadolescence is between 140 and 165 mgr./day and may be as high as 400-500 mgr./day in the pubertal period. Fractional intestinal absorption is very efficient and estimated to be approximately 40 %. Peak adult bone mass, depending on the skeletal site examined, is largely achieved by the age of 20, although important additional bone mass may accumulate through the third decade of life. Studies reveal a small but positive association between life-long calcium intake and adult bone mass. Therefore, optimal calcium intake in childhood and young adulthood is critical to achieving peak adult bone mass.

OPTIMAL CALCIUM INTAKE IN CHILDHOOD AND YOUNG ADULTHOOD IS CRITICAL TO ACHIEVING PEAK ADULT BONE MASS

Adding 500-1,000 mgr./day to calcium intake may, at least temporarily, increase bone accretion rates in preteen boys and girls; however, it is unclear whether the effect on bone accretion rates persists beyond the reported 18-month to 3-year periods of treatment and whether these increased rates of bone formation translate into higher peak adult bone mass. Calcium intake in the range of 1,200-1,500 mgr./day might result in higher peak adult bone mass. Population surveys of girls and young women 12-19 years of age show their average calcium intake to be less than 900 mgr./day, which is well below the calcium intake threshold. The consequences of low calcium intake during this crucial period of rapid skeletal growth may be serious.

WHAT HAPPENS TO BONE MASS IN FULLY GROWN ADULTS?

Once peak adult bone mass is reached, bone turnover is stable in men and women, so that bone formation and resorption are balanced. But in women, resorption rates increase and bone mass declines beginning with the fall in estrogen production, that is associated with the onset of menopause.

The decline in circulating *17-beta-estradiol* is the predominant factor in the accelerated bone loss that begins after the onset of menopause and continues for 6-8 years. Unlike hormone replacement therapy, supplemental calcium during this initial phase will not slow the decline in bone mass, which is due to estrogen deficiency.

> SUPPLEMENTAL CALCIUM WILL NOT SLOW THAT DECLINE IN BONE MASS
> THAT IS DUE TO ESTROGEN DEFICIENCY

WHEN, AFTER THE MENOPAUSE, IS CALCIUM SUPPLEMENTATION MOST BENEFICIAL?

According to various studies, the beneficial effects of calcium supplementation are more noticeable in post-menopausal women after the period when the effects of estrogen deficiency are no longer dominant (approximately 10 years after menopause), yet it is likely that the early post-menopausal years are also an important time to ensure optimal calcium intake. According to the National Institutes of Health (NIH) Osteoporosis *Consensus Statement*[N070] women between the ages of 25 and 50, who are otherwise healthy, should maintain a calcium intake of 1,000 mgr./day. For post-menopausal women who are receiving estrogen replacement therapy, a calcium intake of 1,000 mgr./day is recommended to maintain calcium balance and stabilize bone mass. For post-menopausal women who do not take estrogen, it is estimated that a calcium intake of 1,500 mgr./day may limit the loss of bone mass, *but should not be considered a replacement for estrogen.* Therefore, recommended calcium intake for post-menopausal women up to 65 years of age is 1,000 mgr./day in conjunction with hormonal replacement and 1,500 mgr./day in the absence of estrogen replacement.

(NIH) Osteoporosis *Consensus Statement* *Recommended Calcium Intake*

STAGE OF LIFE	MGR OF CALCIUM	ESTROGEN THERAPY
premenopause	1000	no
postmenopause	1,000	yes
postmenopause	1,500	no

A wonderful nutritional formula was developed in Italy, and rechecked by other Italian researchers:[B071]

Two matched groups of post-menopausal patients were treated with calcitonin or calcitonin and an *arginine-lysine-glycerophosphoric acid-lactose* formula. This latter was found to be the most effective in:

■ Exercising a direct action on osteoblasts
■ Exercising a direct action on the metabolism of bone matrix protein components
■ Improving intestinal absorption of calcium
■ Increasing bone density
■ Increasing plasma osteocalcin
■ Reducing analgesic intake
■ Reducing painful symptoms
■ Reducing serum levels of hydroxyproline
■ Reducing serum levels of parathoromone

CALCIUM INTAKE IN ADULTS (OLDER THAN 65 YEARS)

Low calcium intake and reduced absorption can translate into an accelerated rate of age-related bone loss in older individuals. In men and women 65 years of age and older, calcium intake of less than 600 mgr./day is common. Intestinal calcium absorption is often reduced because of the effects of estrogen deficiency in women and the age-related reduction in renal *1,25-dihydroxy- vitamin D* production. The calcium threshold for reducing bone loss may vary for different regions of the skeleton.

DO ADULT MEN ALSO HAVE OSTEOPOROTIC PROBLEMS, CONNECTED TO THEIR CALCIUM INTAKE?

They sustain fractures of the hip and vertebrae, although at a lower frequency than women. This has been found to be inversely correlated with calcium nutrition: inadequate calcium intake is associated with reduced bone mass and increased fracture risk. Optimal calcium intake among adult men has similar recommendations to that of women, namely 1,000 mgr./day.

The physiology of calcium *homeostasis* (balance of body levels) in aging men over 65 is similar to that of women with respect to these parameters:
■   Calcium absorption efficiency
■   Changes in markers of bone metabolism
■   Declining vitamin D levels
■   Rate of bone loss

It seems reasonable, therefore, to conclude that in aging men, as in aging women, prevailing calcium intakes are insufficient to prevent calcium-related erosion of bone mass. Thus, in women and in men over 65, calcium intake of 1,500 mgr./day seems prudent.

CALCIUM INTAKE OF PREGNANT AND LACTATING WOMEN
Young, pregnant women may one day be aged, osteoporotic women. The current RDA for calcium intake during pregnancy and lactation is 1,200 mgr./day. Pregnancy represents a significant physiological stress on the maternal skeleton. A full-term infant accumulates approximately 30 grams of calcium during gestation, most of which is assimilated into the fetal skeleton during the third trimester. Available data suggest that, with pregnancy, no permanent decline in body calcium occurs if recommended levels of dietary calcium intake are maintained. During lactation, 160-300 mgr./day of maternal calcium is lost through production of breast milk. Studies in otherwise healthy women demonstrate acute bone loss during lactation that is followed by rapid restoration of bone mass with weaning and the resumption of menses. Women who are lactating should ingest at least 1,200 mgr. of calcium per day. Lactating adolescents and young adults should ingest up to 1,500 mgr. of calcium per day.

EFFECTS OF CALCIUM INTAKE ON OTHER DISEASES
Appropriate calcium intake may protect more than bones. Low calcium intake has been implicated in *pre-eclampsia*, *colon cancer* and *hypertension*. In some recent epidemiological studies, higher calcium intake has been associated with a lower risk for the development of colon cancer. Systolic blood pressure levels appear to be reduced by calcium intake.

CO-FACTORS FOR CALCIUM ABSORPTION AND UTILIZATION

Does the malabsorption of calcium predispose to osteoporosis? Most certainly. "It is concluded that malabsorption of calcium is a significant risk factor for postmenopausal osteoporosis, probably because of a secondary increase in bone resorption to maintain serum calcium. The severity of the osteoporosis is directly related to the severity of the calcium malabsorption." [N01] Although calcium malabsorption is important in the development of osteoporosis, DHEA deficiency is not a factor in this malabsorption.

Several co-factors modify calcium balance and influence bone mass. These include:
■ Age
■ Dietary constituents
■ Drugs
■ Ethnic and genetic background
■ Gastrointestinal disorders (*malabsorption* and *post-gastrectomy* syndrome)
■ Hormones
■ Level of physical activity
■ Liver and renal disease
■ Unique host characteristics

CO-FACTORS THAT ENHANCE CALCIUM ABSORPTION

Vitamin D metabolites enhance calcium absorption. *1,25-Dihydroxyvitamin D*, the major metabolite, stimulates active transport of calcium in the small and large intestines. When there exists a deficiency of 1,25-dihydroxyvitamin D, no more than 10 % of dietary calcium may be absorbed; this is associated with an increased risk of fractures. It can be caused by the following:
■ Acquired resistance to vitamin D
■ Impaired activation of vitamin D
■ Impaired renal synthesis of 1,25-dihydroxyvitamin D
■ Inadequate dietary vitamin D
■ Inadequate exposure to sunlight

Elderly patients are at particular risk for vitamin D deficiency because of the following:
■ Impaired renal synthesis of 1,25-dihydroxyvitamin D

- Inadequate sunlight exposure, which is normally the major stimulus for internal vitamin D synthesis. This is especially evident in home bound or institutionalized individuals.

- Insufficient vitamin D intake from their diet

Supplementation of vitamin D intake to provide 600-800 IU/day has been shown to improve calcium balance and reduce fracture risk in these individuals. Also:

- Cod liver oil
- Fatty fish
- Sunlight
- Vitamin D-fortified liquid dairy products

Calcium and vitamin D need not be taken together to be effective, but if vitamin D is taken, calcium is a must! Vitamin D is easily overdosed, particularly because of the irrational commercial supplementation of various foods, done without any consideration of individual needs. Excessive doses of vitamin D may be risky, causing an excessive level of blood calcium, and urinary calcium loss.

INTERACTION BETWEEN HORMONES OTHER THAN ESTROGEN, AND CALCIUM

Although the ultimate meaning of these findings to human bone metabolism is not yet known, it is worth mentioning that certain hormones, such as FSH (follicle stimulating hormone, which produces the formation of sperm and egg-cells), prostaglandin E2, and prostaglandin F2 alpha, have distinct effects on calcium exchange in ovarian cells, indicating that this mineral and hormones are intimately interconnected.[V030]

DO MEDICATIONS AND COSMETICS ALTER CALCIUM AND VITAMIN D METABOLISM?

Do cats love milk?

Anticonvulsant medications, employed in the treatment of seizures, (such as *Dilantin®—phenitoin*) may alter both vitamin D and bone mineral metabolism, particularly in certain disorders, in the institutionalized, and in the elderly. Although symptomatic skeletal disease as a consequence of vitamin D deficiency is uncommon in non institutionalized settings, optimal calcium intake is advised by experts, for institutional residents using anti-convulsants.

FACTORS THAT DECREASE CALCIUM AVAILABILITY

Certain dietary and digestive factors increase calcium malabsorption and loss:

- Caffeine
- Calcium intake (account for only 25 % of the variance in calcium balance)
- Deficiency of bile
- Deficiency of stomach acid
- Fecal losses (diarrhea, maldigestion of fats)
- High *oxalate* and *phytate* in a limited number of foods
- Intestinal absorption
- Low fat diet
- Magnesium
- Phosphate
- Typical American diet consists of (high sodium, high animal protein, high fat diet)
- Urinary excretion (accounts for approximately 50%)
- Wheat bran

WHAT ABOUT GENETIC AND ETHNIC FACTORS?

They significantly influence many aspects of calcium and skeletal metabolism. Studies of twins indicate there is a marked influence of genetic factors on peak bone mass. *Environmental* factors appear to be more important in determining rates of bone loss in post-menopausal women. Racial and ethnic differences in bone mass and fracture incidence have been described, but these are not accounted for by differences in calcium intake. Whether there are genetic and ethnic differences in optimal calcium requirements needs to be determined.

BONE PARAMETERS	PREDOMINANT INFLUENCES
bone mass	genetic
bone loss	environmental

RISKS ASSOCIATED WITH INCREASED LEVELS
OF CALCIUM INTAKE

Excessive intake of calcium has several potential adverse effects, despite that percentile calcium absorption decreases as intake increases, providing a protective mechanism. This adaptive mechanism is limited, because it can be overcome by a calcium intake of greater than approximately 4 g/day (4,000 mgr./day).

People who take a lot of antacid medications containing *calcium carbonate*, accompanied by high dairy product intake, may develop an iatrogenic calcium toxicity known as *milk-alkali syndrome*, (high blood calcium levels, severe kidney damage, and *ectopic* (out of normal location) calcium deposition). Even at intake levels less than 4 g/day, otherwise healthy persons may be more susceptible to excess serum calcium or excess elimination of calcium in the urine. Subjects with mild or subclinical illnesses marked by dysregulation of 1,25-dihydroxyvitamin D synthesis such as *primary hyperparathyroidism* (a disease where the parathyroid glands overproduce their hormone), or *sarcoidosis* (a mysterious illness characterized by inflammatory knots in lungs and other areas), may be at increased risk from higher calcium intakes. Moderate supplementation up to 1,500 mgr./day has caused no problems. Actually, a higher intake of chelated calcium is often associated with a decreased risk of stone formation. Individuals who have a history of kidney stones must be careful, because high calcium intakes can increase urinary calcium excretion and might increase the risk of stone formation.

CAN CALCIUM INTAKE INTERFERE WITH THE ABSORPTION
OF OTHER SUBSTANCES?

It might interfere with the absorption of other nutrients, especially iron, which can be decreased by as much as 50% by many forms of calcium supplements, or also milk ingestion, but not by calcium that contains citrate and ascorbic acid: this actually enhances iron absorption. Thus, increased intakes of calcium carbonate (and others) might induce iron deficiency in individuals with marginal iron status. This is not a common or severe problem. Whether calcium supplements interfere with absorption of nutrients other than iron, has not been thoroughly studied. Calcium may also interfere with the absorption of certain medications, such as the antibiotic *tetracycline*.

> ## SOME CALCIUM SUPPLEMENTS,
> ### ALSO MILK INGESTION DECREASE IRON ABSORPTION

CAN CALCIUM SUPPLEMENTATION CAUSE UNDESIRABLE SYMPTOMS?

Gastrointestinal side effects of calcium supplements have been observed at relatively high dosages, with variable effects on *constipation*. The calcium ion stimulates the secretion of *gastrin* (a hormone which stimulates *gastric acid* secretion); this can produce a *rebound* hyperacidity—more acid is produced after, than before treatment—when calcium carbonate is used as an antacid. These side effects should not be major problems with a modest increase in calcium intake. Total calcium intake to approach or exceed 2,000 mgr./day seem more likely to produce adverse effects and should be monitored closely.

CAN THE CALCIUM YOU BUY BE CONTAMINATED WITH LEAD?

Although most commercial calcium preparations are tested to ensure that they do not contain significant heavy metal contamination, certain preparations derived from nature (e.g., *bone meal* and *dolomite*) can have significant contamination with lead and other heavy metals.

> ## SOME COMMERCIAL CALCIUM PREPARATIONS
> ## MAY BE CONTAMINATED WITH LEAD

COPPER

It is a nutritionally essential element, activator of many enzyme systems. It can be toxic if its presence is excessive.

MAIN FUNCTIONS

- Aids in the formation of red blood cells
- Helps proper bone formation and maintenance
- Helps oxidize vitamin C
- Necessary for the absorption and utilization of iron
- Works with vitamin C to form *elastin*, a chief component of elastic tissue (a support tissue which provides tone and suppleness to skin and other organs)

DEFICIENCY

"Copper is an essential trace element with a well established mechanism for maintaining balance of the metal in the body, which is controlled by at least two genes.....deficiency of available copper at the cellular level....results in abnormalities of collagen formation and brain maturation, leading to early death."[W000]

Basic cellular disturbances may be due to the impact of free radicals, since it is a component of the needed protective enzymes *superoxide dismutase* and *cytochrome oxidase.* Our main interest for the purpose of this book, lies in the fact that copper deficiency may cause osteoporosis (bone fragility), lameness, deformity, and anaemia. Bone pathology may be related to a defective cross-linking of collagen and elastin as the result of the role of the missing copper in the activity of the enzyme *lysyl oxidase.* This may be the basis of reduced production of osteoid protein in growing bones. Other symptoms are:

- General weakness
- Impaired respiration
- Skin sores

EXCESS INTAKE — TOXIC SYMPTOMS

The most common problem is the steady storage of copper in the liver, due to:

- Genetically-based tendency to store copper in the *lysosomes* of liver cells
- High dietary levels

Some types of copper preparations are more *bio-available* (absorbable into the body) than others. In a study performed on rats, preparations of *copper oxides* provided less mineral to the body than *copper-protein* or *chelated copper* compounds. Also, the effect of theses compounds reflected on the tissue absorption of *zinc in a proportionate manner.*[R090]

Rat liver cells are easily damaged by an excess of copper. Chelating (binding) the copper with a copper chelating substance, *2,3,2-tetramine*, had a partially protective effect, but exposure of the cell to the vitamin E product *D-alpha-tocopheryl succinate* could completely improve the situation. Vitamin E can protect against copper induced liver damage.[0s180]

It always holds true in biology, that the same substance that can help in smaller amounts, can cause a reverse effect in larger amounts. Copper is frequently used for the relief of arthritis, but "...accumulation of excess copper in the body, first in the liver leading to cirrhosis, and then in the brain giving rise to destruction of the centre [sic] of motor control and, frequently, changes in personality. Copper excess can also cause renal damage, osteoarticular changes and joint pains. If the renal lesion leads to calcium loss in the urine and other tubular defects, there may be osteoporosis or, occasionally, osteomalacia with **pathological fractures** [fractures due to preexisting illness, not accidents]. In this disease, the abnormal stores of copper can be mobilized [sic] with **chelating agents** or depleted by the administration of zinc salts or **thiomolybdate**. This usually, but not invariably, leads to improvement or even complete reversal of symptoms."[w000] [emphasis added]

NECESSARY INTAKE AND BEST DIETARY SOURCES
Estimated safe for adults 1.5-3.0 mcg (mg).
THE BEST FOOD SOURCES OF COPPER ARE:

"FOOD	AMOUNT	MICROGRAMS MG
Liver, beef	3 ounces	2.4
Oysters	3 ounces	2.3
Crab, canned	3 ounces	1.1
Kidney beans	1 cup	0.51
Potato, baked	1 medium	0.47
Pinto beans	1 cup	0.44
Black beans	1 cup	0.36
Spinach, cooked	1 cup	0.31
Almonds	1/4 cup	0.27
Shrimp	3 ounces	0.26
Wheat germ	1/4 cup	0.23" [E001]

IRON
It is a nutritionally essential substance, the basis of blood pigment and breathing ability.

MAIN FUNCTIONS

- Builds up the quality of the blood
- Combines with protein and copper in making (red blood pigment)
- Formation of *myoglobin*, a protein which is found only in muscle tissue
- Increases resistance to stress and disease
- Prevents fatigue and promotes good skin tone

BOTH IRON DEFICIENCY AND EXCESS ARE HARMFUL

Iron deficiencies not only cause low oxygen supply to tissues, but also poor muscle development. Athletic training often causes *iron* deficiencies in individuals who exercise to excess in proportion to the iron in their diet. Low body stores of iron weaken the T-cells, decreasing their normally highly active responses.

Children who are iron deficient, are frequently the victims of recurrent infections. Their vitality is low and can be aided by the supplementation of *iron*.

DEFICIENCY

- Anemia
- Constipation
- Paleness of skin
- Weakness

EXCESS INTAKE—TOXIC SYMPTOMS

Excess *iron* intake, on the other hand, may also cause problems. Several researchers have expressed concern about the damage that this practice could do. The *iron* transport system in the human body depends on certain substances of the protein family: *lactoferrin* and *transferrin*. They pick up the *iron* atoms as a ski lift does with skiers, to carry them to the proper location, when the environmental conditions are right. Some "chairs" are usually left open not to overtax the system and for emergency availability. The "empty" lift chairs (unsaturated enzymes) then are available in the event of contamination as they are able to scavenge iron molecules away from the germs and in this fashion, destroy them. A person oversaturated with iron has no empty chairs (enzymes) for these emergencies.

The American diet is inappropriately, and usually excessively, supplied with large amounts of iron in the form of the substance *ferrous fumarate* (an iron salt) added to various grain, flour and other food products. *Dietary iron overload* is linked not only to heart disease, but also to cancer, diabetes, osteoporosis, arthritis, and possibly other disorders. Plasma concentrations of several antioxidants are decreased in the presence of dietary iron overload disease. Inappropriate iron overload occurs due to the imbalanced addition of this substance to flour and other foods. Cast iron cookware may be an unsuspected source of excessive iron, as are many vitamin and mineral supplements. This is compounded by the fact that absorption of iron is enhanced by the intake of certain "enhancers": *citric acid* (used as a preservative in many products), and *ascorbic acid*, both abundantly represented in the diet. Iron overload may be the most important common causative factor in the development of the diseases mentioned; therefore, the synergistic combination of citric and ascorbic acids may play a major role in our worsening disease statistics.[141] On the other hand, *tannins*, contained in green tea and certain vegetable sources, are protective against this excess, and when taken on a regular basis will prevent this problem.

NECESSARY INTAKE AND BEST DIETARY SOURCES
RDA for adults is 10-15 mg.
THE BEST DIETARY SOURCES OF IRON are:

"FOOD	AMOUNT	MILLIGRAMS
Liver, pork, cooked	3 ounces	24.7
Cereal, 100% fortified	3/4 cup	18
Cream of wheat, cooked	1/2 cup	9
Liver, chicken, cooked	3 ounces	7.2
Prune juice	1/2 cup	5.3
Navy beans, cooked	1 cup	5
Lima beans	1 cup	4.9
Spinach,cooked	1 cup	4.3
Black-eyed peas	1 cup	4.3
Oysters	4	3.6
Roast beef	3 ounces	3.1
Blackstrap molasses	1 tablespoon	2.3

Watermelon	4 x 8 inch wedge	2.1
Dried apricots	12 halves	2
Dried prunes	10	2
Kale, cooked	1 cup	1.8
Collard greens, cooked	1 cup	1.5
Egg	1 whole	1.3" E001

MAGNESIUM

This mineral is an important enzymatic activator. Probably as many as 70% of all enzymes are activated by *magnesium* (*Mg*).

In one study, rats were subjected to a chronic deficiency of magnesium, under experimental conditions. Their white blood cell count *increased*, especially at the expense of the *eosinophils*, the cells involved in allergic conditions. However, this increase in number was not indicative of an increase of immune function: to the contrary, magnesium deficient animals were functionally immunodeficient, producing increased amounts of the amino acid *histamine*, which triggers allergic reactions, and they were prone to developing a form of leukemia.

Globulin (the protein that carries immune antibodies) levels drop when experimental subjects are made *magnesium* deficient. Cell membranes, important in controlling what enters and leaves the cells, become unstable when magnesium is deficient. Magnesium is also important in a balance with calcium in promoting certain electromagnetic equilibrium.

Since magnesium is an essential component of *chlorophyll* (the green pigment of plants), fulfilling a function equivalent to iron in blood, any fresh green foods contain abundant magnesium. Chlorophyll is a natural deodorant and antiseptic. Junk food diets have very little fresh vegetables in them, and magnesium may be undersupplied.

MAIN FUNCTIONS
- Converts blood sugar into energy
- Maintains normal heart rhythm
- Necessary for proper vitamin C metabolism
- Necessary for proper calcium metabolism
- Regulates the neuromuscular activity of the heart

DEFICIENCY SYMPTOMS

- Calcium depletion
- Confusion
- Heart spasms
- Kidney stones
- Muscular excitability
- Nervousness

Magnesium (Mg) deficiency occurs frequently in chronic alcoholism and may contribute to the increased incidence of osteoporosis and cardiovascular disease seen in this population. Mg deficiency is primarily due to:

- Dietary Mg deprivation
- Gastrointestinal losses with diarrhea or vomiting
- Renal Mg wasting
- Use of drugs such as *diuretics* and *aminoglycosides* (certain antibiotics)

TOXIC SYMPTOMS

Not a cause for worry, excepting in people with damaged kidney function.

NECESSARY INTAKE AND BEST DIETARY SOURCES

RDA for adults is 280-350 mg.
THE BEST SOURCES OF DIETARY MAGNESIUM are:

"FOOD	AMOUNT	MILLIGRAMS
Brown rice	1 cup	265
Spinach, cooked	1 cup	157
Black beans	1 cup	121
Pinto beans	1 cup	95
Halibut, broiled	3 ounces	91
Almonds	1/4 cup	85
Wheat germ	1 cup	69
Oatmeal, cooked	1 cup	56
Peanuts	1 ounce	53
Pistachios	1 ounce	45

Shrimp	3 ounces	35
Banana	1 medium	33
Milk, whole	1 cup	33" E(0)1

POTASSIUM

It is one of the important *electrolyte elements* which control the flow of electricity in and out of cells, as well as an activator of some enzymes.

This mineral is amply distributed in nature in vegetables and other foods; it is the most abundant mineral of the intracellular (the body fluids inside the cells). It is essential to establish normal body electrical balance by interacting with sodium, and to prevent tissues from getting waterlogged. Insulin is not effective in the proper metabolism of carbohydrate, if potassium is deficient, fostering the occurrence, or the worsening of diabetes. *Potassium* loss may occur due to mechanisms that eliminate it from body reservoirs, such as stress, fluid pill intake, improper diet, vomiting and diarrhea. Excess table salt intake causes an imbalance between sodium and *potassium*. Weather changes cause *potassium* drops, particularly in weather sensitive individuals. *Licorice*, used in candy and as a flavoring agent of tobacco, also depletes potassium.

> **MUCUS MAY BE MORE IMPORTANT TO YOUR HEALTH,
> AND MORE CONNECTED TO YOUR POTASSIUM METABOLISM,
> THAN YOU'D THINK**

People seem to be forever worrying about having too much mucus in their sinuses or colon, and mucus-free diets are often heavily advocated. They never consider that mucus has its very important role in protecting the body's membranes, and that low body *potassium* levels cause sluggish bile flow. This, in turn, will cause *mucin*, the protein component of mucus, to be destroyed excessively and leave delicate membranes in an unprotected state.

MAIN FUNCTIONS

- Activates insulin
- Aids in clear thinking by sending oxygen to the brain
- Assists in reducing high blood pressure
- Balances out sodium

- Normalizes heart rhythm
- Preserves proper alkalinity of body fluids
- Promotes healthy skin
- Regulates the body's waste balance
- Stimulates the kidneys to eliminate poisonous body wastes

American diets are often too low in **potassium**, or imbalanced between **potassium** and table salt. Areas with high **potassium** content in their drinking water have shown a statistical association with less incidence of cancer.

DEFICIENCY
- Cardiac arrest in a limp heart (*diastole*)
- Fluid retention (*edema*)
- Muscle damage
- Nervous disorders
- Poor muscular reflexes
- Respiratory failure

EXCESS INTAKE — TOXIC SYMPTOMS
- Cardiac arrest in contraction of the heart (*systole*)

NECESSARY INTAKE AND BEST DIETARY SOURCES
Estimated safe intake for adults is 3500 mg.
THE BEST DIETARY SOURCES OF POTASSIUM ARE:

"FOOD	AMOUNT	MILLIGRAMS
Prunes	8 large	940
Raisins	1/2 cup	575
Potato, white, boiled	1 small	407
Milk, skim	1 cup	406
Spinach, raw	3 ounces	403
Banana	1 small	370
Pork, cooked	3 ounces	334
Beef, lean round, cooked	3 ounces	317
Artichoke, cooked	1 bud	300
Cauliflower, raw	1 cup	295

Lettuce, iceberg	1/4 head	264
Cantaloupe	1/4 fruit	251
Apricots, dried	4 halves	244
Tomato	1 small	244
Chicken, cooked	3 ounces	242
Orange	1 medium	237" E(X)I

PHOSPHORUS

Major dietary sources of Phosphorus include most foods, especially fish, meat, poultry, dairy products, eggs, peas, legumes (dried beans) and nuts.

MAIN FUNCTIONS

It is required for the formation of healthy bones and teeth. It is also necessary for energy metabolism.

DEFICIENCY SYMPTOMS

- Bone loss
- Fatigue
- Loss of appetite (*anorexia*)
- Pain
- Weakness

EXCESSIVE INTAKE AND TOXICITY

- Interferes with Calcium utilization
- Interferes with Iron utilization

BEST DIETARY SOURCES: RDA for adults is 800-1200 mg.
THE BEST SOURCES are:

"FOOD	AMOUNT	MILLIGRAMS
Liver, beef	3 ounces	395
Salmon, canned, with bone	3 ounces	279
Pinto beans	1 cup	273
Milk, skim	1 cup	247
Halibut	3 ounces	242
Black beans	1 cup	241

Milk, whole	1 cup	228
Tenderloin, beef	3 ounces	194
Ham	3 ounces	192
Almonds	1 ounce	148
Ground beef, lean	3 ounces	141
Peanuts	1 ounce	105
Egg	1	86" E001

SODIUM

Sodium is a mineral. We extensively deal with salt in another part of this book, and most of the information on salt overlaps with sodium. Major dietary sources of sodium include table salt, soy sauce, monosodium glutamate, cheese, smoked and cured meats, processed and canned foods.

MAIN FUNCTIONS:

- Electrolyte—helps maintain acid-base balance
- Helps regulate blood pressure and water balance in cells
- Muscle contraction and nerve impulse transmission

DEFICIENCY SYMPTOMS

Deficiency is rarely caused by inadequate dietary intake, but by excessive sweating, some kidney problems (*salt losing nephritis*), fluid pills, etc. Major symptoms are:

- Headaches
- Muscle cramps
- Shock
- Weakness

EXCESSIVE INTAKE AND TOXICITY

- Edema (fluid retention)
- Hypertension (high blood pressure) in salt sensitive people

"FOOD	AMOUNT	MILLIGRAMS MG
Bacon, beef	3 slices	766
Bologna, beef	1 slice	226

Cheese, American	1 ounce	406
Cheese, cheddar	1 ounce	176
Cottage cheese, 1% fat	1 cup	918
Green beans,canned, low salt	1/2 cup	109
Ham, lean (5% fat)	1 slice	405
Hot dog, beef	1	585
Peas and carrots,canned	1/2 cup	277
Potato chips	1 ounce	168
Pretzels	1 ounce	486
Soy sauce	1 tablespoon	920
Soy sauce, lite	1 tablespoon	605
Table salt (sodium chloride)	1 teaspoon	2,132
Tomato juice	6 ounces	658
Tomato juice, no added salt	6 ounces	18
Turkey salami	1 slice	244
V-8 juice	6 ounces	553
V-8 juice, no added salt	6 ounces	42" E001

TRACE ELEMENTS

Trace Elements are essential for normal growth and development of skeletons in humans and animals. Although they are minor building components in teeth and bone, they play important functional roles in bone metabolism and bone turnover.[0039] TRACE MINERALS are minerals that are necessary, but only needed in tiny amounts, or traces. They play a major role in the body, since even minute portions of them can powerfully affect health. They are essential in the assimilation and utilization of vitamins and other nutrients. They aid in digestion and provide the catalyst for many hormones, enzymes and essential body functions and reactions. they also aid in replacing electrolytes lost through heavy perspiration or extended diarrhea and protects against toxic reaction and heavy metal poisoning.

- ■ Aluminum impairs bone formation by inhibiting bone building cells (osteoblasts).

- ■ Copper induces low bone turnover, suppressing of osteoblastic and osteoclastic functions.

- Fluoride accumulates in new bone formation sites and results in a net gain in bone mass (but this bone is hard and brittle).
- Gallium suppresses bone turnover in malignancy.
- Iodine is part of the thyroid hormones *thyroxine* and *triiodothyronine*; it enhances bone turnover.
- Magnesium enhances bone turnover; it stimulates cells that break down old bone (osteoclasts).
- Zinc regulates secretion of calcitonin from the thyroid gland.

Repeating something stated before: "Among the trace elements in bone and hair, significant differences were found in the contents of zinc, copper and manganese between normal subjects and osteoporotic patients. However, exact involvements of the trace elements in osteoporosis have not yet been clarified.[0050]

The Japanese studied the "effect of essential trace metals on bone metabolism...in the *femoral-metaphyseal* [shaft of the femur] tissues obtained from *skeletal-unloaded* rats [they actually mean: poor critters suspended by their hind legs].[Y008] After four days they exposed the bones, obviously after killing the rodents, to certain trace elements: "nickel, manganese, cobalt, copper, zinc, or *zinc-chelating dipeptide (beta-alanyl-L-histidinato zinc; AHZ*) [a substance that binds zinc]...." The cruel *off their feet situation* damaged the bone metabolism, but the addition of zinc or zinc compounds improved the readings of bone related activity. "This effect was not seen by nickel, manganese, cobalt and copper.

The bone tissues feed on *glucose* (simple sugar) "This consumption was inhibited by nickel, manganese, or copper..., while cobalt, zinc, and AHZ had no effect. DNA content in the bone tissues was significantly increased by all metal compounds. This "... study demonstrates that, of various essential trace metals, zinc compounds have an unique anabolic [tissue building] effect on bone metabolism in the femoral-metaphyseal [shaft of the thigh bone] tissues of rats with skeletal unloading [cruelly taken off their normal weight-bearing—this may be a situation similar to that of very inactive humans]. *Zinc-chelating dipeptide* [a molecule of zinc bound to two amino acids] may stimulate bone protein synthesis.[Y008]

Since the toxic levels for many trace elements, copper, manganese, fluoride, chromium and molybdenum, may be only several times usual intakes, the upper RDA (recommended daily allowance) levels for these trace elements should not be habitually exceeded, and close monitoring can be accomplished with yearly hair analyzes.

CHROMIUM

It is an essential element, necessary to proper fat metabolism and the utilization of sugar and insulin.

MAIN FUNCTIONS

- Cleans the arteries
- Helps transport amino acids to where the body needs them
- Helps control the appetite
- Protective effect against diabetes
- Protective effect against heart problems
- Protective effect against cancer
- Reduces Cholesterol and Triglyceride levels
- Stabilizes blood sugar levels
- Works with insulin in the metabolism of sugar

DEFICIENCY SYMPTOMS

- Atherosclerosis
- Depressed growth
- Glucose intolerance in diabetics
- Heart disease
- Obesity
- Tiredness

USES OF CHROMIUM PICOLINATE

Chromium picolinate, an insulin-sensitizing nutrient has been found to reduce urinary excretion of hydroxyproline (a bone amino acid) and calcium in post-menopausal women, a lab value presumably indicative of a reduced rate of bone resorption. This nutrient also raised serum levels of *dehydroepiandrosterone-sulfate* (*DHEA*), a body building, male type hormone, which may play a physiological role in the preservation of post-menopausal bone density. The impact of chromium picolinate (alone or in conjunction with calcium and other micronutrients) on bone metabolism and bone density, may be very important because this substance can be easily found in stores.

Effects of chromium picolinate
- Insulin-sensitizing (glucose tolerance factor)
- Raises serum levels of *dehydroepiandrosterone-sulfate* (*DHEA*)
- Reduces rate of bone resorption in post-menopausal women
- Reduces urinary excretion of calcium in post-menopausal women
- Reduces urinary excretion of hydroxyproline (a bone amino acid) in post-menopausal women

Estimated safe intake for adults are 50-200 mcg (μg).
THE BEST FOOD SOURCES OF CHROMIUM are:

"FOOD	AMOUNT	MICROGRAMS MG
Apple	1 medium	15
Cheese, American	1 ounce	48
Chicken breast	3 ounces	22
Mushrooms	1 cup	20
Peanut butter	1 tablespoon	41
Spinach, cooked	1 cup	36
Wheat bread	1 slice	16" [E001]

GALLIUM

What is new in the nutritional mineral world? Another mineral similar in atomic structure is *gallium*, a metal, liquid at room temperature. Gallium, in considerable excess of aluminum, effectively competes with aluminum for absorption in bone and beneficially displaces aluminum. Elemental gallium and its various compounds are potent inhibitors of bone resorption that act to maintain and restore bone mass in vertebrate species. By virtue of these biological effects, gallium compounds are useful treatments for a variety of human diseases that are characterized by accelerated bone loss, including cancer-related hypercalcemia (including *multiple myeloma*, a usually fatal bone marrow cancer which destroys the bone itself, and breast cancer), bone metastases, Paget's disease, and post menopausal osteoporosis in older women.[W010] Since gallium is a mineral, it is considered to be a "dietary supplement" under the U. S. Dietary Supplement Health and Education Act of 1994.

Certain gallium compounds (*gallium nitrate solutions* for example) in appropriate dosages are considered safe and highly effective agents in reducing accelerated bone loss in both cancer and metabolic bone disease, and in restoration of bone mass. Gallium compounds converts blood hypercalcemia into hypocalcemia, resulting in a marked reduction in urinary calcium. Gallium enhances mineralization of newly forming bone rather than simply acting to decrease physiologic resorption. Gallium concentrates in the metabolically active end of bones along with calcium, restoring bone strength.[W010]

IODINE
A mineral which forms part of thyroid hormones.

MAIN FUNCTIONS
- Condition of the hair, skin, and teeth
- Development and functioning of the thyroid gland
- Develops and impacts on mentality
- Develops and impacts on speech
- Helps burn excess fat by stimulating the rate of metabolism
- Regulates the body's production of energy

DEFICIENCY SYMPTOMS
- Cold intolerance
- Dry skin and hair
- Enlarged thyroid gland
- Infertility
- Irregular menstrual periods
- Loss of physical and mental vigor
- Low back pain
- Mixedema
- Slow mental reaction
- Weight gain

Excessive iodine intake, due to dietary and other factors, is common. It is a common contaminant of table salt (purported to be a nutritional plus—which is fraudulent excepting in geographic areas that are naturally severely deficient—), and an additive (allegedly *inert* or non-reactive), to antiseptics and tablets.

TABLE SALT IS CONTAMINATED WITH IODINE

Undue exposure to toxic levels of iodine happens on a daily basis, by the indiscriminate use of the highly toxic substance *betadine*, (*povidone-iodine*), a brown, nauseating smelling antimicrobial and antiseptic, available in solutions, creams, pre-treated pads, etc.[H170]

In a study of how high the blood levels of iodine of burn patients, treated with this abominable substance would rise, it was noticed that "peak serum iodine levels in patients treated within 24 hours of injury ranged from 595 to 4,900 micrograms per dL. The amount of iodine absorbed was directly related to the size of the burn. Serum iodine levels continued to rise until the drug was discontinued and remained elevated for as long as 7 days after discontinuance. Iodine excretion was directly related to renal function. The highest serum and lowest urinary iodine levels were present in patients who developed renal failure...serum levels of this inorganic ion imply potential toxicity, but clinical evidence of cell or organ toxicity is as yet undetermined."[H170]

Although the 1980 article reported no thyroid disease, the prolonged chronic use of the substance must surely be harmful as is any chronic iodine intake. Unfortunately, *povidone-iodine* is not only contained in antiseptic medications, but is a very common component of oral tablets of any kind (quantity not labeled). There is a permanent question in my mind of how much of this dangerous thyroid suppressant is ingested daily by people who may take 20 or 30 medication tables a day!

As early as 1982, the fact that iodine on the skin is toxic was clearly spelt out, when comparing iodine to an antibiotic: "Irrigation of a contaminated wound with a solution of povidone-iodine was *no more effective* than the use of *cefazolin* (an antibiotic) powder but may be associated with significant toxicity."[S060] [emphasis added]

As this book is undergoing its final revision, a study about adverse effects of povidone-iodine used in infants was published in a medical weekly, warning about the damage done to the thyroid and other organs by this unsafe practice.   Dr. Siegfried of the Pediatrics and Dermatology Departments at Saint Louis University Health Sciences Centers is quoted as saying that "'You have to err on the side of caution, and that's well illustrated by what has happened in the past. Clinicians have historically overlooked the potential for percutaneous [through the skin] poisoning in recommending therapy [with povidone-iodine] for infants.'"[B181]

TOXIC SYMPTOMS

Because of excessive iodine's depressing effect on thyroid hormone production, it may be a co-factor in the development of osteoporosis. See under *iodization of salt* and other products.

RDA for adults is 150 mcg.
THE BEST DIETARY SOURCES OF IODINE are:

"FOOD	AMOUNT	MICROGRAMS
Cheese, American	1 ounce	16
Cheese, cheddar	1 ounce	14
Egg, boiled hard	1	24
Milk, whole	1 cup	88
Shrimp	3 ounces	31" [E001]

LITHIUM

In our times, *lithium* is used as a pharmaceutical, in the form of *lithium carbonate,* allegedly as a therapeutic agent for the treatment of *bipolar or manic-depressive* disorders. Despite much evidence as to the worthlessness and danger of this therapy, and to the fact that similar, and much better results can be achieved with the use of diets to control hypoglycemia, the barbarous practice continues, fanned by the healthy dollars that this "sick" abuse produces. Who has ever seen a victim of lithium poisoning, with the darkened, rough and swollen (*myxedematous*) patches of skin, bloated from kidney damage, and almost "zombified", will never forget what the prostitution of modern psychiatry does. In statistical and laboratory studies *lithium* therapy has been shown to promote a higher incidence of malignancy, an indication of immune incompetence. I personally know an attorney who lost his family, career, and health, due to lithium poisoning, and is at present suing the manufacturer.

One common way to find over the counter *lithium* preparations is as a cream against herpes, used directly on the surface of a lesion or when it is taken in as a nutrient. Herpes researchers have found lithium creams to be beneficial to the patient in the treatment of the herpes lesions.

Lithium deficiency predisposes to depression and mental illness. Chelated lithium can be obtained at the health food store.

TOXIC SYMPTOMS

Excesses of *lithium*, however, or imbalances between *lithium* and iodine may have harmful effects on the thyroid function, and impact on protein synthesis in osteoporosis, indirectly damaging bone which needs proteins for healthy structure.

Problems with *lithium* may occur due to its chemical characteristic of being a *halogen*. These are substances that easily form salts (*halogens*). *Chlorine, fluorine, bromine* and *iodine* are also halogens. Mutual interference, especially with thyroid hormone, may have serious effects on the metabolism of proteins, immune reactions, etc., and therefore impact adversely on osteoporosis.

MANGANESE

This mineral trace element is indispensable to enzymatic processes, the synthesis of certain proteins, and to brain as well as hormonal functions. In animal experiments, rats born of *manganese* deprived mothers became diabetic even without a genetic history of that illness. We have previously elaborated on the connections between diabetes and osteoporosis.

MAIN FUNCTIONS
- Activates various enzymes active in the proper digestion and utilization of foods
- Antioxidant nutrient
- Catalyst in the breakdown of fats and cholesterol
- Helps nourish the nerves and brain
- Important in the blood breakdown of amino acids
- Maintains sex hormone production
- Necessary for the metabolism of Vitamin B-1
- Necessary for the metabolism of Vitamin E
- Necessary for normal skeletal development
- Production of energy

DEFICIENCY SYMPTOMS

- Allergies—severe
- *Ataxia* (loss of spatial perception, as seen when a person takes a drunken driving test)
- Blindness and deafness in infants
- Bone metabolism problems
- Convulsions
- Digestive problems
- Dizziness
- Fatigue
- Infertility
- Inflammation
- Loss of hearing
- Paralysis
- Physical endurance decreased
- Skin problems
- Slow growth of hair
- Slow growth of fingernails

TOXIC SYMPTOMS

We must remind ourselves that manganese poisoning is becoming more common because of the addition of manganese to gasolines to replace lead. Excess manganese, can cause anomalies in various animal glands, including testicles, pituitaries and *pancreatic beta cells* (where insulin is produced). Excess manganese is linked to brain and mental disturbances. Manganese also may act as a calcium channel blocker causing as of yet unknown problems when interacting with these medications.

DIETARY SOURCES OF MANGANESE

Estimated safe for adults 2.0-5.0 mg.
THE BEST SOURCES OF DIETARY MANGANESE are:

"FOOD	AMOUNT	MILLIGRAMS
Almonds	1/4 cup	0.65
Black beans	1 cup	0.76
Brewed tea	1 cup	0.52
Brown rice	1 cup	6.93
Kale, cooked	1 cup	0.54

Liver, beef	3 ounces	0.36
Oatmeal, cooked	1 cup	0.95
Spinach, cooked	1 cup	1.68
Strawberries	1 cup	0.43 E001
Wheat germ	1/4 cup	3.83"

MOLYBDENUM

Molybdenum is a trace mineral. Major dietary sources of Molybdenum include milk, whole grains, liver, legumes (dried beans) and dark green leafy vegetables.

MAJOR BODY FUNCTIONS
- Activates certain enzymes in the body (xanthine oxidase inhibitors)
- Aids in blood, cartilage and bone formation (where it links up with osteoporosis)
- Necessary in energy metabolism

DEFICIENCY SYMPTOMS
Deficiency symptoms include:
- Amino acid intolerance
- Irritability

Although not commonly known, in our practice we have had excellent results in treating gout with molybdenum as the only therapy, in addition to a vitamin program.

TOXICITY SYMPTOMS
- Gout like symptoms
- May interfere with copper absorption

DIETARY SOURCES OF MOLYBDENUM
RDA's for adults are 75-250 mg.
THE BEST DIETARY SOURCES OF MOLYBDENUM are:

FOOD	AMOUNT	MICROGRAMS MG
Beef, sirloin, cooked	3 ounces	6
Halibut	3 ounces	3

Milk, whole	1 cup	17
Spinach, cooked	1 cup	46
Strawberries	1 cup	20

SELENIUM

Selenium is a member of the powerful *antioxidant* patrol, in conjunction with vitamins A and E, C, the amino acid products *GS* (*Glutathion-reductase*), *reduced glutathion*, and the fatty acid *GABA*.

Supplementation of *selenium* in small quantities can correct oxidation problems. If *selenium* is permitted to become deficient, vitamin E can temporarily take over and improve the condition. If the defense mechanisms of experimental animals are damaged by the intake of *cadmium*, a powerful protoplasmic poison, mere supplementation of *selenium* can improve the condition and help counteract the cadmium. Since most damage to biological processes is caused by free radicals, and *selenium* is part of the antioxidants (the first line of attack against these substances), proper *selenium* nutrition can not be emphasized enough.

MAIN FUNCTIONS
- Decreases the risk of breast, colon, lung and prostate cancer
- Helps in the treatment and prevention of dandruff (Selsun shampoo)
- Major antioxidant nutrient
- Preserves tissue elasticity
- Prevents free radical generation
- Protects cell membranes
- Slows down the aging and hardening of tissues through oxidation

DEFICIENCY SYMPTOMS
- Dandruff
- Heart disease
- Loose skin, premature aging

TOXIC SYMPTOMS
- Nausea, abdominal pain and diarrhea
- Peripheral neuropathy, fatigue and irritability

IMPORTANCE IN OSTEOPOROSIS

Since it has a protective effect against cancer, supplementation is very important in a disease where hormones linked to cancer production may have to be administered.

Selenium is an especially important antioxidant. The wide latitude of its effects is due to selenium's activity in the cellular and sub-cellular levels, where it prevents the destruction and decay of cellular functions. Selenium is a mineral vital for the body's antioxidant defense system. It is a part of an enzyme, known as *glutathione peroxidase*, which works with vitamin E to protect body tissues from oxidation [biologic rusting]. Actually, the most common form of selenium in the body is *selenocysteine*, a compound of selenium with the *sulphur* containing amino acid *cysteine.* The metabolic functions of glutathione peroxidase are part of the mechanism responsible for the detoxification of oxygen. These agents also alleviate the toxic effects of drugs and antibiotics, as well as experimental chemical carcinogens.

Selenium is not only an antioxidant, it's the most important of a group of intracellular antioxidants. It is an important component of cells that acts as a *substrate* (substance acted upon by an enzyme) for other enzymes, which decrease the effects of oxygen-free radicals. Its various effects are:

- Helps or prevents arthritis
- Improves the energy levels and affects fertility and sex drive
- Inhibitory effect on a variety of carcinogens
- Lower risk of miscarriage in the first three months of pregnancy, to women with sufficient selenium levels
- Prevention and relief of skin disease(s), psoriasis, etc.)
- Prevention of cardiovascular diseases
- Preventive agent in many forms of cancer
- Slowing down of some of the symptoms of aging (skin condition, cataracts, etc.)
- Strengthens the immune system

Selenium deficiency has been found in patients with or without diarrhea and malabsorption. Cancer patients are usually selenium deficient. Infection and increased metabolic rates compound the loss of selenium. Selenium deficiency is associated with heart disease and with anemia.

Keeping a person's immune system and other functions healthy with selenium, will reduce their need to take drugs which may worsen osteoporosis.

DIETARY SOURCES OF SELENIUM
RDA for adults is 55-70 mcg.
THE BEST DIETARY SOURCES OF SELENIUM are:

"FOOD	AMOUNT	MICROGRAMS
Chicken breast	3 ounces	23
Crab, cooked	3 ounces	19
Egg, hard boiled	1	12
Halibut	3 ounces	51
Kidney beans	1 cup	9
Liver, beef	3 ounces	48
Oatmeal, cooked	1 cup	20
Sardines, canned	3 ounces	29
Shrimp	3 ounces	27
Wheat bread	1 slice	11" [E001]

STRONTIUM

"Prolonged administration of *strontium* to postmenopausal osteoporotic women resulted in...a[n] increase in the lumbar spine bone mineral density of treated subjects."[R031] [emphasis added]

SULPHUR

Sulphur, a yellow element of strong odor, resembling the smell of burnt eggs or boiling cauliflower, has often been called *the forgotten mineral*. Sulphur is necessary in the diet, as part of the sulphur containing amino acids *cystine*, *cysteine*, and *methionine*. It is also an element in cauliflower, cabbage, garlic, etc. It is not to be confused with *Sulfa* drugs, to which some people are allergic.

Sulphur is a component of the very therapeutic and detoxifying *DMSO*, and serves to antidote mercury, protecting the tissues from toxicity.

MSM is *Methyl Sulfonyl Methane*, a nutritional form of sulfur. It is a naturally occurring, vital nutrient which is often lost through the processing of our food. MSM is not a drug, herb, or stimulant. It is completely safe, odorless, and non-toxic. It has been tested and proven to provide relief from many ailments. It is intended as a food supplement only. It is not a medicine or drug. Studies have shown that MSM works well in conjunction with Vitamin C.

Sulphur is frequently found in hot, thermal waters, which come from under the ground. These are usually favorable therapies to treat people with arthritis and a host of skin ailments, and can be found in many world-famous spas.

VANADIUM

In a study in India on the effects of the trace element vanadium on hormones, the levels of progesterone "were stimulated with low concentrations of vanadyl sulphate and were inhibited at higher concentrations. Vanadyl sulphate, when it was added with *hCG* [human Chorionic Gonadotrophin, a placental hormone], and a certain enzyme,...caused inhibition of the normally hCG induced progesterone biosynthesis."[R011] We glean that this very scarce trace element possibly has important hormone modulatory functions which we are just now becoming acquainted with. [emphasis added]

VANADIUM AND MANGANESE

Vanadium compounds and manganese compounds such as *forskolin* activate or deactivate certain hormones, especially LH, FSH, depending on their dosage. Manganese activates cyclic AMP at low doses, but abolishes it at high doses. The effect of *vanadyl* ion was very similar to that of Mn2+. *Vanadate* anion on the contrary was without effect on FSH stimulation.[T050] [emphasis added]

ZINC

It is an essential mineral, which acts as a co-factor or activator in several enzyme systems. It is absorbed in the small intestine, where competition may occur with copper and iron.

MAIN FUNCTIONS

- Aids in the digestion and metabolism of alcohol
- Aids in the digestion and metabolism of phosphorus
- Antioxidant nutrient (*superoxide-dismutase,* an antioxidant, activator)
- Governs the contractility of muscles
- Helps in normal tissue function
- Important for blood stability
- Maintains the body's alkaline balance
- Necessary for protein synthesis
- Vital for the development of prostate functions and male hormone activity
- Vital for the development of the reproductive organs
- Wound healing

A Japanese study on—cruelly—immobilized rats, revealed that, "... of various essential trace metals, zinc compounds have an unique...[protein building] effect on bone metabolism in the femoral-metaphyseal [shaft of the femur or thigh bone] tissues of rats with *skeletal unloading* [they really mean, immobilized and suspended]. [This may be a situation similar to that of very inactive humans. Zinc-chelating dipeptide may stimulate bone protein synthesis]....[2009]

DEFICIENCY SYMPTOMS

- *Ageusia* (inability to taste)
- *Alopecia* (hair loss)
- Apathy
- Anemia
- Anorexia
- *Anosmia* (inability to smell)
- Decreased alertness
- Delayed healing
- Delayed sexual maturity
- Depression
- Diabetes
- Diarrhea
- Fatigue
- Hypochlorhydria (low stomach acid)
- Night blindness which is resistant to therapy with vitamin A

- Prolonged healing of wounds
- Retarded growth
- Rough and dry skin
- Sexual dysfunction (especially in males)
- Stretch marks
- Susceptibility to infections
- Underdeveloped sex organs
- White spots on finger nails

In a certain study on copper and zinc, the absorption and retention of zinc, was not affected by whether this zinc was or was not chelated, but the simultaneous administration of copper improved the zinc levels for those taking the chelated copper.[R090]

WHAT DISEASE STATES OCCUR WITH A DEFICIENCY OF ZINC?

The nutritional biochemistry of Zinc has its major biological role via **metalloenzymes** (enzymes bound to a metal atom), which are involved in nucleic acids (RNA, DNA) metabolism. A deficiency

- Disturbs **keratinization** (the full maturation of epithelial or surface cells), most obviously in the epidermis and its appendages, but also in the upper alimentary tract
- Disturbs inflammatory and immune mechanisms
- Disturbs tissue growth
- Disturbs tissue maturation
- Disturbs tissue repair
- Interferes with food utilization
- Retards growth
- Suppresses appetite
- Suppresses fertility
- Suppresses immune function
- Suppresses wound-healing

The situation is complex, and the diseases are sometimes referred to more as **zinc-responsive** conditions than zinc deficiency conditions: the central problem can be one of availability.

Is estrogen therapy favorable to people who are chronically low in Zinc? "Estrogen replacement therapy reduced excretion [loss] of zinc, magnesium, and hydroxyproline in... [women who were losing these nutrients.] Zinc excretion decreased 35% after 3 months and 26% after 1 year of treatment.... This change was more pronounced in women with osteoporosis and elevated zinc excretion. Because zinc excretion is almost uninfluenced by variation in diet, it may be used as an additional marker of changes in bone metabolism."[H072] [emphasis added]

BASIC SYMPTOMS OF ZINC DEFICIENCY IN ANIMALS

In animal studies, several cellular disturbances are noticed, especially interference with the process of keratinization in the epidermis and upper alimentary epithelium. The normal maturation and transformation of surface cells is to orderly, protective, toughened (*keratinized*) layers of scaly, hardened tissue (the skin we often see flake off). When Zn is deficient, there is accumulation of an adherent layer of partially-keratinized cellular remnants on the epithelial surface, somewhat similar to what we call *psoriasis* (a skin condition with disorderly growth of layers) in humans. Some breeds of cattle, who have a genetic defect which prevents the absorption of $Zn2+$ from the intestine, have typical excessively dried and hardened skin changes, what we often see as calluses and hard skin (*hyperkeratosis*), but also suffer from underdeveloped thymus glands and severe immune deficiency, and die at an early age.

EXCESSIVE ZINC

The symptoms include gastrointestinal problems and others:

- Blurred vision
- Diarrhea
- Fast heart beat
- Low body temperature
- Nausea
- Sweating
- Vomiting

WHAT HAPPENS IF ANIMALS HAVE AN EXCESS OF ZINC?

Excessive concentrations of zinc are indeed toxic, and several entities are described, although by and large there is little information currently available in standard textbooks.

RDA's for adults 12-15 mg.
THE BEST DIETARY SOURCES OF ZINC are:

FOOD	AMOUNT	MICROGRAMS
Almonds	1 ounce	1.4
Collard greens, cooked	1 cup	1.2
Crab, cooked	3 ounces	3.6
Garbanzo beans	1 cup	2.5
Ground beef, lean	3 ounces	4.4
Kidney bans	1 cup	1.5
Liver, beef	3 ounces	5.1
Pacific oysters, steamed/boiled	3 ounces	28.2
Pumpkin seeds	1 ounce	2.1
Raisin bran cereal	3/4 cup	3.8
Special K cereal	1 1/3 cup	3.7
Tenderloin, beef	3 ounces	4.5
Wheat germ	1/4 cup	4.7

ANTI-OXIDANTS AND VITAMIN SUPPLEMENTS

WHAT IS FREE RADICAL FORMATION?

If you are scared of chemistry, only skim over this one!

Free radicals can be formed by environmental pollution, solar and cosmetic radiation, smoking, toxins and for the purpose of this discussion, by metabolic processes in the body. We represent these radicals by the initials of the substance with a superscripted dot, for example $HO^\bullet$ for *hydroxil*.

Many substances in the body are metabolized or processed by substances called *oxydases*, which may add an electron to an oxygen molecule. For example, *electron transport chains oxidases* (e.g., *NADPH*, amino acids, *xanthine*, etc.), *redox cycling* (*quinones*), and *cytochrome P-450* can yield the superoxide oxygen radical ($O2^{*-}$). Although this radical is a poorly reactive one, it can again react with hydrogen to form hydrogen peroxide ($H2O2$) + O2. These molecules can again react with hydrogen to yield O2, H2O, and the fearsomely-reactive radical, a *hydroxyl radical* (*HO**).

In a cell, there is genetic material, DNA molecules, made from *sugars* attached to *bases*, of which there are several kinds. When these are altered or changed, *mutations* may occur. Hydroxyl (HO*) radicals (memory help: *hide-rock-sill*) will react with anything they are next to, "stealing" their favorite treat, an electron. If one is next to a DNA molecule, harm leading to mutations (disease) may occur. This, in turn, can lead to cancer. For example, a hydroxyl radical may react with a base called *guanine* *(one-in)* to yield *8-hydroxyguanine* and other products which are associated with cancer incidence.

WHAT ARE ANTIOXIDANTS?

They are common nutrients and other substances which have become very popular in the nineties. You have probably been exposed to this word from every medium around you. We are not seeing anything new, but a reclassification of certain nutrients, food factors and chemicals by one of their important functions.

In a humorous parallel to the political radicals who are always saying they need just one more thing to be happy, free radical molecules have the main problem of being one electron short on their outer orbit. Another molecule (like a politician who uses other people's money) could donate this electron to them, and here, to help, instead of "Uncle Sam"comes a molecule called "Auntie Oxi Dent" (*anti-oxidant*), to the rescue. These anti-oxidants are molecules that prevent free radicals from doing harm to our DNA, proteins, and cells by donating an electron. Studies show that antioxidants can

- Help prevent certain diseases such as arteriosclerosis brought on by free radicals oxidizing the *low-density lipoprotein* (*LDL*) cholesterol damaging the artery lining
- Help prevent damaging affects of visible light on the retina and the lens epithelium
- Help prevent (maybe) cancer by stopping the attack of *hydroxyl radicals* on *purine* and *pyrimidines* which can then lead to mutations

Anti-oxidants protect the body from *free radical* damage, like rust protectors prevent metal from rusting. Free radicals form naturally, being byproducts of the cellular breathing process, but if their production is unbridled can be damaging to your other body cells. Free radicals have been linked to a number of serious, even terminal diseases. Adding an anti-oxidant supplement as part of a healthy lifestyle for disease prevention is the prudent way to receive those protective levels of key vitamins, so you can help to protect your body against the maladies that result from insufficient levels of protection.

Antioxidants are not only beneficial to prevent lipid peroxidation, harmful biologic rusting, but to lower blood pressure. As demonstrated in Leeds, England, a combination of antioxidants (200 mgr. of zinc sulphate, 500 mgr. of ascorbic acid, 600 mgr. of alpha-tocopherol (sodium succinate salt) and 30 mgr. of beta-carotene daily) lowered the blood pressure of their test subjects.[G010]

French studies showed the effectiveness of the trace element *selenium* (*Se*), and the selenium molecule *selenomethionine* (*Sm*), in decreasing undesirable blood clotting. Sm associated with vitamin E was efficient to prevent oxidative damage of platelet membranes (platelets are clotting particles) in diabetics, and thus, to modify platelet membrane hyperactivity, decreasing clumping.[D080]

Does diet affect free radical formation? Diet has a definitive impact on free radical formation. In a study where people were fed a diet high in fat and meat, and poor in fiber, free radical production was increased in the *colon* or large intestine. *Dimethylsulfoxide* [*DMSO*] was used as the free radical scavenger. Oxidation or biologic rusting increased remarkably with the test diet: "The mean hydroxyl radical production was 13 times greater in...[stools]...of subjects when they consumed the diet rich in fat and poor in dietary fiber...than when they consumed the diet poor in fat and rich in dietary fiber..." This difference was associated with a 42% higher fecal iron concentration ...when they consumed the first diet than when they consumed the second...The results of this study confirm that diets high in fat and meat and low in fiber markedly increase the potential for hydroxyl radical formation..."[B049] [emphasis added]

Some metals invite the formation of free radicals. Rat liver cells, even human liver cells, are easily damaged by an excess of copper. *Chelating* (binding) the copper with a copper binder or chelator (*2,3,2-tetramine*), had a partial protective effect, but exposure of the cells to the vitamin E derivative **D-alpha-tocopheryl succinate** completely improved the situation. Vitamin E can protect against copper induced liver damage.[S180]

NATURAL ESTROGEN SUPPLEMENTS

GLANDULARS OR PROTOMORPHOGENS

A **glandular or Protomorphogen** is a small fragment of gland tissue or organ taken from beef (bovine glandular) or pork (porcine glandular) that supplies biologically active hormones, hormone precursors, enzymes, vitamins, minerals, soluble proteins, and natural lipid factors. Scientific research has demonstrated that glandulars have tissue specific activity and exert significant biological effects in humans; thus bovine liver tissue has a biological effect on human liver, porcine pancreas tissue has a biological effect on human pancreas, and so forth. Glandulars offer a diversity of hormones and hormone related substances in a natural, non-toxic quantity for therapeutic, rejuvenative and preventive health care. They are usually available in tablet, drop or capsule forms.

HERBS

FOODS AND HERBS WITH ESTROGENIC QUALITIES

Many individuals are forever looking for a safe and effective food or herbal substitute for pharmaceuticals. I am enclosing a small list of substances recommended by nutritionists and herbologists, but *making no claim* that these will effectively *treat* osteoporosis.

Any natural substance which is thought to exert an estrogen-like effect, is referred to by natural therapists as "estrogenic". This activity is found in many plants, and the active substances are called **phyto-estrogens**. **Phyto-estrogens** include several classes of naturally occurring chemical compounds (i.e., **isoflavones, coumestans**, and **lignans**) which are structurally similar to endogenous [internal] estrogens. In the body, they exert estrogenic, and also antiestrogenic effects, "...and may reduce the risk of developing certain types of hormonally related diseases."[H140] These substances have variable effects, from very powerful to very weak ones.

PHYTO-OESTROGENS IN FOODSTUFFS

alfalfa	green beans	rhubarb
aniseeds	hops	rice
apples	licorice	rye
barley	lime flowers	potato
carrots	oats	sage
cinnamon	peas	sesame seeds
cherries	plums	sunflower seeds
elder flowers	pomegranate	soya beans
fennel seeds	parsley root	wheat
french beans	red clover	yeast
garlic	red beans	

Many commonly eaten foods contain natural estrogens. It is still being studied how effective these foods are in reducing symptoms of menopause or osteoporosis. In some individuals, intestinal bacteria denature plant estrogens and render them inactive. These women will experience no benefits from increased intake. Despite this, there is some historical and cultural evidence pointing to desirable effects, as well as a few serious clinical studies..

A study at the Royal Hospital for Women, New South Wales, Australia, in 1995-96, reviewed the sources, metabolism, potencies, and clinical effects of phyto-estrogens on humans. "All studies concurred that phytoestrogens [sic] are biologically active in humans or animals. These compounds inhibit the growth of different cancer *cell lines* [cells grown in dishes generation after generation, and derived from each other], in cell culture and animal models. Human epidemiologic evidence supports the hypothesis that phytoestrogens [sic] inhibit cancer formation and growth in humans. Foods containing phytoestrogens [sic] reduce cholesterol levels in humans, and cell line, animal, and human data show benefit in treating osteoporosis."[K092]

HUMAN DATA SHOW BENEFITS OF INGESTING PHYTO-ESTROGENS IN TREATING OSTEOPOROSIS

"This review suggests that phyto-estrogens are among the dietary factors affording protection against cancer and heart disease in vegetarians. With this epidemiologic and cell line evidence, intervention studies are now an appropriate consideration to assess the clinical effects of phytoestrogens [sic] because of the potentially important health benefits associated with the consumption of foods containing these compounds."[K092]

The most important thing to remember about plant estrogens is that they may not exert the same effect on the body as does synthetic estrogen. Nor are they traditionally ever prescribed in the same way, that is for life or for very long periods. As well, there has been no research on the ability of plant estrogens to improve bone density, and women with osteoporosis would need to take other precautions to adequately address this condition.[T071]

In a study concerning the availability of plant estrogens to various populations, it was concluded that "...little information is available on population differences in exposure to phyto-estrogens. To examine racial/ethnic differences in urinary phytoestrogen [sic] levels, 50 young women (ages 20-40 years) were randomly selected from participants in a previous epidemiological study in which 24-h urine specimens and a dietary assessment were obtained. Subjects were members of the Kaiser Permanente Medical Care Program of northern California. Selection was stratified on race/ethnicity. Urinary levels of seven phyto-estrogens were measured using high-performance liquid chromatography-mass spectrometry. Substantial variation in phytoestrogen levels was observed and racial/ethnic differences are described. The highest levels of coumestrol and the lignans [other estrogenic substances] were observed in white women and the lowest levels in Latina and African American women. Genistein levels, however, were highest in Latina women; other isoflavone levels did not differ significantly by race/ethnicity."[H140]

One of these phyto-estrogens, "...coumestrol[,] is a unique substance in that it inhibits bone resorption and, at the same time, stimulates bone mineralization. Coumestrol exhibited less estrogenic activity than 17 beta-estradiol as estimated by the increase in uterine weight of ovariectomized rats. As coumestrol has less estrogenic activity than 17 beta-estradiol, it may prove to be a more potent drug against bone diseases including osteoporosis."[T081]

A study in Atlanta, Georgia, showed that what is good for the goose is not always good for the gander. And, watch out, McDonald's, it also showed that there are differences in sexual behavior according to diet, even in rats. "The effect of phyto-estrogens on the sexual differentiation [normally induced in infant animals by]...*gonadotropin* [a hormone that stimulates ovaries and testicles] function was examined by neonatal exposure of pups [to these phyto-estrogens] through milk of rat dams fed [either] a:

- coumestrol (100 micrograms/g)
- control, or
- chow diet

during the 'critical period' of the first 10 postnatal days or throughout the 21 days of lactation. In females, exposure to coumestrol throughout the period of lactation produced growth suppression and an *acyclic* [no cycles of heat] condition in early adulthood resembling the premature *anovulatory syndrome* [no egg-cell production]. When the period of treatment was restricted to the first...10 days [after birth], however, no effects on vaginal cyclicity were seen. The 10-day exposure period produced more marked effects in males, resulting in transitory reductions in body weight in weanling males and reductions in mount and ejaculation frequency and a prolongation of the latencies [time in between episodes] to mount and ejaculate. Testicular weights and plasma testosterone levels did not differ among treatment groups, suggesting that the deficits in male sexual behavior were not due to deficits in adult gonadal function [hormone production]. Few effects of chow treatment were observed. However, significant differences from controls were apparent for weight at vaginal opening in females, and mount rate for chow-treated males was intermediate between that of controls and that of the coumestrol-treated group. These data provide evidence that lactational exposure to phytoestrogen [sic] diets can alter *neuroendocrine* [nervous system and glands] development in both female and male rats."[W062] [emphasis added]

"Evaluation of the potential benefits and risks offered by naturally occurring plant estrogens requires investigation of their potency and sites of action when consumed at natural dietary concentrations....investigations have examined the effects of a range of natural dietary concentrations of the most potent plant isoflavonoid, *coumestrol*, using a rat model and a variety of estrogen-dependent tissues and end points. Treatments of immature females demonstrated ...[helping or enhancing]...action in the repro-

ductive tract, brain, and pituitary at natural dietary concentrations....
coumestrol did suppress *estrous* [going into heat] cycles in adult females."
[emphasis added] The effects on the young "...were examined by neonatal
exposure of pups through milk of rat dams fed a coumestrol, control, or
commercial soy-based diet during the critical period of the first 10 postnatal days or throughout the 21 days of lactation. The 10-day treatment did
not significantly alter adult ...[cycles]..., but the 21-day treatment produced a persistent *estrus* [heat] state in coumestrol-treated females by 132
days of age. In contrast, the 10-day coumestrol treatments produced significant deficits in the sexual behavior of male offspring. These findings
illustrate the broad range of actions of these natural estrogens and the variability in potency across end points. This variability argues for the importance of fully characterizing each phytoestrogen in terms of its sites of
action, balance of...[enhancing and suppressing]..., natural potency, and
short-term and long-term effects.[W061]

The humble soy bean is listed in ancient herbals, as useful in counteracting
the ageing process. It contains active hormonal substances, the *triterpenes*,
which are also found in *Ginseng*, one of the major tonic and longevity herbs.
Fermentation of soy decreased the isoflavone content of the product fed but
increased the urinary isoflavonoid recovery. This finding suggests that fermentation increases availability of isoflavones in soy.[H180]

A study in N.C. followed ninety-seven postmenopausal women, who were
divided into two groups, one of which had soy foods added to their diet.
To determine hormonal effects, the characteristics of their vaginal lining
cells were used. Vaginal cells, easy to test as a part of a Papp smear, have
different shapes which can tell the doctors what the hormonal status of the
patient is. The percentage of vaginal *superficial* cells [cells which attest to
high estrogen levels] increased 19% in those eating the soy diet, compared
with 8% increase in controls.   The urinary isoflavone concentrations
increased, but no other major findings were made..[B009]

The *common pea* is also considered estrogenic: it has been found to contain a contraceptive principle, which is effective only after *repeated and
excessive* consumption. This has been observed in Tibet, where peas and
barley form the staples of the diet: their population has remained stable
for the past 200 years. Whether this effect is due only to the estrogenic
principle or other agents in the pea is yet to be established, but a clear hormonal influence has been demonstrated.

Alfalfa, which is also a member of the pea family, also contains *phyto-estrogens*. Research has shown that, when estrogen levels are low, the phyto-estrogens exert some hormonal activity; they occupy estrogen receptor sites. In a laboratory experiment, where rats were fed massive doses of estradiol, those that were concurrently fed alfalfa were protected from the blocking of ovarian function normally caused by those massive doses of estradiol (ovarian inhibition). Other research on stock animals, however, has shown that infertility and altered cycles of *going into heat* will occur if an animal is fed too much alfalfa.

The *pomegranate* is an ancient symbol of fertility and has been found to contain an estrogen which is identical, chemically, to estrogen (1.7 mg/100gm.) In fact, even though the pomegranate is remembered as a fertility symbol, its most common use world wide has been as a contraceptive agent or *abortifacient* [an agent to induce a miscarriage]. Again, whether the plant is a fertility enhancer, a contraceptive or an abortifacient is possibly dose dependent.

The common garden *rhubarb* has been investigated and found to contain a hormonal component which has been identified as estrogenic. It is used by some European doctors in a herbal extract with *hops* for menopausal complaints, with good results.

Sage is an old menopausal remedy, since it stops women's hormone induced sweating, and contains estrogenic principles.

ARE HERBS FREE FROM SIDE EFFECTS?

Most estrogenic herbal remedies have a higher hormonal content or index than estrogenic foods, such as soy, which also means that they are prone to a greater degree of risks and possible undesirable effects that can be experienced if they are incorrectly selected, given over an excessive time frame, or are taken in the wrong doses.

THERE IS NO CONCEPT OF *SIDE EFFECTS* IN ALTERNATIVE MEDICINE:
SUBSTANCES HAVE A RANGE OF EFFECTS,
ALL OF WHICH ARE TO BE TAKEN INTO ACCOUNT WHEN THEY ARE USED

It is also useful to note that there is no concept of *side effects* in alternative medicine. Substances have a range of effects, all of which are to be taken into account when they are used. If undesirable effects are experienced by the recipient, this would be considered to be caused by incorrect choices which failed to take into account all of the effects of that herb. Only effects which are positive, indicate that the right choice has been made. Those who regularly self prescribe, need to take this piece of information into account.[T071]

ARE ALCOHOLIC BEVERAGES A SOURCE OF ESTROGENIC SUBSTANCES?

Feminizing changes are often seen in male alcoholics: this is considered to occur due to substances present in the alcoholic beverages, because when measured, the alcoholics' internally produced hormones are not really very elevated. Yet, I do not think that this should prompt us to make alcohol an option for therapy![G021]

KANGGUSONG

Chinese are master herbalists. This strange sounding concoction is the result of a Chinese study, which extols the beneficial effects of a traditional herbal remedy compounded from 8 herbs (**Kanggusong**, or **KGS**), evaluated on rats that were made to suffer from osteoporosis. Although we may be encouraged by the promise of this remedy, we can not help but be disturbed about some new information that derived from the experimental design of the study: the osteoporosis was induced in the rats, not by an exotic drug, but by *retinoic acid*, the active principle in some widely used *anti-wrinkle creams*![W090]

The mechanisms of action of KGS might be:
- Activating osteoblasts
- Increasing the blood concentration of calcium and estrogen
- Positive balance of bone metabolism
- Protecting against the injury of sex glands by retinoic acid
- Suppressing osteoclasts

NUTRITION

FOODS, IN GENERAL

For the purpose of this book, and as a definition of the author, *foods* are all of those substances we can eat or take in, in amounts of one cup or larger, and which the body can process in that quantity without suffering any harm. Milk is a food, by this definition, so is spinach, or beef. Those substances which are of an appealing flavor, but can not be tolerated in quantities of one or more cups, such as pepper or pure lemon juice, we call *condiments*. Brewed coffee, by this definition, is a food, but powdered coffee is not. Substances which are not tolerated in even small amounts, without causing marked manifestations in the body, or which can be used in the correction of undesirable problems or symptoms, are either *medicinal herbs*, or *toxins*.

BENEFITS OF A "HEALTHY DIET"

How does diet impact on health?

Certain substances produced inside the body, and usually associated with the occurrence of inflammation, are grouped under the technical name: *multifunctional cytokines* (substances which induce certain actions in cells). You may have noticed how, after you sustain a scratch or prick yourself with a thorn, the skin reddens, swells, hurts. *Interleukin-6 (IL-6)*, remember as "isle 6", a cytokine, of which you will probably hear more in the future, is proving to be a major contributor to this acute phase inflammatory response. When checked by lab tests, IL-6 is normally low and serum levels are usually non detectable in normal young subjects. What happens in older people? There is an increase with advancing age, *even if no inflammation is present.* IL-6 may contribute to the development of several diseases that are common in late-life.[E060]

Interleukin-6 (IL-6 or isle 6) related illnesses are some of the monster plagues of our days:

- *Alzheimer's* disease (a dementia)
- *Lymphoma* (tumor of the lymph glands)
- Osteoporosis

This chemical aging process is largely preventable by life span-extending dietary restrictions.

THE EFFECTS OF DIET IN PROTECTING AGAINST CANCER AND OSTEOPOROSIS

Summarizing the conclusions from many health practitioners, and my own from the days I was in practice, we conclude that whenever cancer is a concern, as it is with the public—whether justified or not—in estrogen replacement therapy for osteoporosis, preventive and protective measures are of great interest to the patients. The best protective measure would have been prevention: never to receive cancer genes—*oncogenes*, (in the form of vaccines and biologicals), but short of reversing time, we must resort to the manipulation of our environment. The internal environment is best affected by our diets.

Much controversy has arisen about what foods are good to eat. We label them as American diets, junk food diets, diabetic diets, vegetarian diets, etc., etc. Some individuals make of their eating habits, a religion. No foods are free from contaminants, some are safer than others.

I had over twenty years of clinical experience in medicine, thirty years with nutrition. In these years I dealt with many osteoporotic patients. My conclusions were that there was no need to remember exotic herbs or very specific recipes for the purpose of being healthy, conserving quality bone, etc. A varied supply of nutritional staples would do, keeping in mind that neither excessive protein or fiber are good for the bones. Small amounts of meats, chicken and fish at least once a day, eggs several times a week, and milk, one cup, at least once a day. Coffee, tea and soft drinks only occasionally. Sweets sparingly, once or twice a week.

One pretty good rule was that meat should never be ground, for all the booty of toxic chemicals is in the fat. Even in the Bible, we read: "Speak unto the children of Israel, saying, Ye shall eat no manner of fat, of ox, or of sheep, or of goat."[B141] Steaks should be well manicured to remove the fat, chicken and other oven cooked meats placed on a rack, so that much of the fat can drain off. Women who for some reason or another do not want to take hormones or raw ovary, a product that can be bought in health food stores, should eat plenty of soy, particularly fermented soy.

Commercial salt should be avoided, and that means avoiding commercial foods cooked with that salt. Health conscious individuals should use every opportunity to tell owners of restaurants and packing facilities that they would prefer they would use non-iodized, and, if possible, sea salt.

Most packaged food is amply supplied with a feast of harmful or unproven chemicals. Food should be fresh, from the counter.

MILK

Each serving of milk or milk products on this list contains about 12 grams of carbohydrate and 8 grams of protein. The amount of fat in milk is measured in percent (%) of butterfat. The calories vary, depending on what kind of milk you choose. The list is divided into three parts based on the amount of fat and calories: skim/very low fat milk, low fat milk, and whole milk. One serving (one milk exchange) of each of these include:

TYPE	Carbohydrate	Protein	Fat	Calories
Skim/Very Lowfat 1/2% 1%	12	8	trace	9
Lowfat 2%	12	8	6	120
Whole 4%	12	8	8	150

Skim and Very Lowfat Milk (1 cup)	Lowfat buttermilk (1 cup)
Lowfat Milk (1 cup)	Evaporated skim milk (1/2 cup)
Skim milk (1 cup)	Dry nonfat milk (1/3 cup)
1/2% milk (1 cup)	Plain nonfat yogurt (8 oz)
1% milk (1 cup)	2% milk (1 cup)

plain low fat yogurt (with added nonfat milk solids) (8 oz)

WHAT ARE THE RISKS OF INGESTING DAIRY FOODS?

The *Establishment*, which at present has placed saturated fat in the nutritional dog house, expresses concern that increasing the intake of dairy products increases the intake of saturated fat. However, under nutritionally appropriate conditions, no type of food substance is harmful. It is the pollutants, the agricultural hormones, the fertilizers and antibiotics which represent a problem, because they are largely dissolved in the otherwise harmless fat! Although reduced-fat or no-fat dairy products contain as much calcium per serving size as high-fat dairy product they still carry harmful stowaway chemicals. People who are sensitive to milk products may have *lactose intolerance* and *allergic* problems. *Lactose reduced* milk is available.

RECOMBINANT BOVINE SOMATOTROPIN (RBST)

This rather specialized subject is covered in detail in this book, because osteoporotic women who are taking estrogen replacements, should be aware of as much information as possible about a substance often present in the cow's milk they drink. Milk contains many natural and artificial chemicals, some directly derived from the cow's metabolism, some a result of technology and biotechnology. Individuals in all conditions of health and disease are exposed to these, and as a result may suffer adverse consequences. One substance of great concern is *Recombinant Bovine Growth Hormone (rBGH)*, also known as *Recombinant Bovine Somatotropin (rBST)*.[U151] It is a genetically engineered drug, the first to be widely marketed through the food supply. It is administered to increase milk production in dairy cows by ten to twenty percent. Its commercial name is *Posilac*. Many environmentalists and consumer advocates are deeply suspicious about the safety of this substance, although on November 5,1993, Recombinant Bovine Somatotropin was declared to be "safe" by the Food and Drug Administration.[U210] Its manufacturer, Monsanto Corporation of St. Louis, Missouri[D021] is recognized as the producer of many substances of large distribution but questionable safety: *Agent Orange*, *PCB's*, *Saccharin*, *Nutrasweet®* and most recently *"Roundup Ready" Soybeans (RRS)®*.[F040] Laws concerning labeling which differentiates milk from rBST-treated cows from milk from rBST-free cows have been a highly controversial topic. Currently (in a 1996 article), voluntary labeling is permitted as a help to those customers who might want to avoid purchasing milk from cows injected with the drug, despite Monsanto's attempts to prohibit this voluntary labeling.[M222]

I often wonder whether these hormones may actually exert a beneficial effect on protein synthesis, (I use the mnemonic rule **RoBuST**), but, on the other hand, in people who have cancer genes or a cancer in any stage, they may accelerate its growth. By the nature of the recombinant process, cancer producing genes are *adventitious* [they are supplied with the product, not added] to these products, a euphemistic way of saying "contaminated", and although one would not hesitate in administering them to someone gravely ill with Alzheimers or Parkinsonism, it is a folly to expose children and people of any age to this risk in an indiscriminate manner.

Another family of proteins found in milk, both bovine and human, is *Insulin-like Growth Factors* (*IGF*), a hormone produced in the liver, induced by the stimulatory effects of the growth hormone. IGF-1 has been linked to gastrointestinal and breast cancer. The concentration of IGF-1 in rBST milk is 25 to 70 percent above the amount in milk from untreated cows. Epstein, a researcher in this field, also insists that pasteurization increases IGF-1 content by 70 percent. He links IGF-1 to gastrointestinal cancer by arguing that IGF-1 is different from other proteins in that it doesn't get digested and broken down in the digestive tract. Based on this premise, he states that IGF-1 is active in the intestine by stimulating the proliferation of intestinal cells. Ultimately, a high IGF-1 concentration may result in gastrointestinal cancer due to the division and multiplication of any cancerous cells of the intestine. Evidence of its involvement in breast cancer comes from reports that blood and malignant tissue of breast cancer patients have high concentrations of IGF-1.

Even if there were no direct human safety risks from rBST treated milk, issues related to the health of the treated cow may ultimately have an indirect effect on the health and safety of humans. The drug increases udder infections (*mastitis*), and, consequently, these cows leak blood and puss into the milk, and get more antibiotics which find their way into the milk. The increased presence of antibiotics in the milk we consume leads to an increased prevalence of these antibiotics which make it into the human body through ingestion. The fear is that the body is subjected to additional antibiotics which could impair the development of the immune system in children as well as cause the growth of resistant strains of bacteria and viruses which may lead to serious health problems later in life.

Even if the milk is tested for antibiotics, it is not tested for all of them, and amounts that may not harm one person, could hurt another. Any illness which derives from milk would probably not be recognized by physicians who don't even know that a problem exists with its consumption.

Despite FDA's conclusion that products from cows treated with BST are safe for human consumption,[viii] there continues to be skepticism and suspicion amongst the public. There have been many claims made accusing the FDA of a flawed and manipulated study. Whether they are true or not, falsified data, internal pull from former Monsanto employees, and concealed data about proven cancer links to BST are just some of the accusations FDA and Monsanto Corporation are facing. It becomes a case of "who to believe?"— Should the U.S. public put blind faith in the government and its relationship with a corporation giant or rather take the word of consumer activist groups which have the reputation of fighting for the well-being of the people? Currently, the decision is up to the consumer. I hope the right for the consumer to choose for themselves will not be taken from our grasps by the power and money possessed by America's super-corporations.[Ull1]

SOY FOODS

Although all foods are important, the majority of readers probably are better acquainted with chicken, beef or milk, than with soy. Because of its many beneficial features, especially for osteoporotic women, several pages are devoted to this interesting food.

WHAT IS SOY?

Soybeans belong to the family of plants called *legumes* (beans, peas, lentils etc.). Soybeans differ from other legumes in some important ways. Although they are high in complex carbohydrates, they contain much less than other beans. They also contain quite a bit more protein and fat than other legumes.

CONTENT OF NUTRIENTS IN SOY COMPARED TO OTHER LEGUMES

Proteins	higher (+)
Fats	higher (+)
Carbohydrates	lower (-)

Foods DERIVED from soy are a very nutritious, high in many vitamins and minerals; their high protein content is unusual in plant foods. Soybeans derive about 35 to 38% of their calories from protein, compared to approximately 20 to 30% in other legumes.

SOY PROTEIN

Proteins are composed of smaller parts called amino acids. In a human, eight of these are "essential" (the human body can not make them). PROTEINS WHICH CONTAIN THIS PROPER ASSORTMENT ARE

CALLED "COMPLETE". The most unique feature is that soy protein is "complete", being the only vegetable derived protein that is. Although the amount of protein in a food is important, the quality of that protein is paramount. "Quality" refers to how well suited a particular type of protein is to human physiological needs. Soy protein is of the highest quality. Under new guidelines that have been adopted by the Food and Drug Administration and the World Health Organization for evaluating protein quality for children and adults, soy protein isolate receives a rating of 1, which is the highest possible score. This means that the quality of soy protein is equal to that of meat and milk proteins.

SOY FAT

Soybeans, and many soy foods, are unusual because of their relatively high fat content. Approximately 40% of the calories in soy come from fat while most legumes (with the exception of peanuts) contain between two and 14% fat. The fat portion of the soybean is used extensively both in the food industry and directly by consumers. Soy oil is a common cooking oil; cooking oils sold generally as "vegetable oil" are usually soy oil. Most of the fat in soybeans is unsaturated. Soybeans are one of the few plant sources of *omega-3 fatty acids*. Omega-3 fatty acids may be essential nutrients for infants, and they may also help to reduce risk of both heart disease and cancer.

SOY FIBER

All whole, unprocessed plant foods contain dietary fiber. A fiber-rich diet is very important to reduce the risk of certain types of cancer and heart disease. One serving of soybeans provides approximately eight grams of dietary fiber. However, many soy foods are processed in ways that decrease their fiber content significantly.

OTHER NUTRIENTS IN SOY

Many soy foods are high in calcium. Soy foods are high in both *oxalates* and *phytate*, two compounds that inhibit calcium absorption, yet the calcium from soy is reported to be as well absorbed as the calcium from milk. The calcium content of tofu is quite high, it ranges from 120 to 750 mgr. per serving, depending on how the tofu was processed.[E022]

Trypsin inhibitor (TI), *tannin*, *phytate*, *phytic acid* affect nutrient digestibility and absorption in many legumes. However, these legumes may pose no serious problems to populations consuming them especially when heat treatment is applied before consumption.[M151]

SOY FOODS MAY PROTECT AGAINST OSTEOPOROSIS

Soybeans and some *soy foods* include *soy flour*, *soybeans* and some *tofu*; they are a good source of calcium that is easily absorbed by the body. In addition, laboratory studies with animals have shown the consumption of soy protein not only delayed the onset of the age-related increase in bone loss, but the total amount of bone loss was significantly less. In human subjects, the soy protein, or the fact that soy contains the hormone like substance genistein (*Jenny Stein*), favorably impacts on calcium metabolism. You will hear more of this in the future.

> **SOY PROTEIN NOT ONLY DELAYS THE ONSET OF THE AGE-RELATED INCREASE IN BONE LOSS, BUT THE TOTAL AMOUNT OF BONE LOSS IS SIGNIFICANTLY LESS AS WELL**

TEXTURED SOY PROTEIN

Textured soy protein, *TSP* or *TVP*® (a registered trademark of the Archer Daniels Midland Company), is used as a nutritious "extender" in a variety of food products. It is soy flour compressed until the structure of protein fibers changes. When it is rehydrated with boiling water, TSP has a texture similar to ground beef. Another type, available in chunk-sized pieces, takes on the consistency of stew meat when rehydrated, before it is used in recipes. (Use 7/8 of a cup of boiling water for each cup of soy protein. For the granules, just pour the water over the TSP. The chunks need to be simmered for a few minutes).

Soy protein is rich in protein and extremely low in both fat and sodium. It is also a good source of fiber.

One cup of prepared soy protein provides:

Calcium 170 mgr.	Fat 0.2 g	Sodium 7 mgr.
Calories 120 g	Iron 4 mgr.	Zinc 2.7 mgr.
Carbohydrate 14 g	Protein 22 g	

Source: Composition of Foods: Legume and Legume Products. United States Department of Agriculture, Human Nutrition Information Service, Agriculture Handbook, Number 8-16. Revised December 1986.

SOY FLOUR

Soy flour is made from roasted soybeans that have been ground into a fine powder. Rich in high-quality protein and other nutrients, soy flour also adds a pleasant texture and flavor to a variety of products. Two kinds of soy flour are available:[U060]

■ Natural or full-fat soy flour contains the natural oils found in soybeans.

■ Defatted soy flour has the oils removed during processing.

MISO

Miso is a rich, salty condiment, it is the essence of Japanese cooking. Many Japanese begin their day with a fortifying bowl of miso soup, and also use miso to flavor a variety of foods. Making miso is a household art in Asian countries, comparable to the American practice of canning foods. To make miso, soybeans, and sometimes rice or another grain, are combined with salt and mold culture. The mixture is then aged in cedar vats for one to three years. Most miso made in western countries is produced in a similar manner. Quick miso (also available) is generally inferior in taste to traditionally aged miso.

Miso is actually a group of condiments. The addition of different ingredients, and variations in the duration of aging produce different types of miso that vary greatly in flavor, texture, color, and aroma. In Japan, different types of miso are prepared and evaluated in much the same way Westerners judge fine wine and cheese.

TOFU

Tofu, also known as soybean curd, is a soft, cheese-like food made by using a clotting agent (*coagulant*) or acidic liquids such as lemon juice or vinegar, on fresh hot soy milk. Traditionally, the curdling agent used to make tofu is *nigari* — a compound found naturally in ocean water—or calcium sulfate. Normally, these curds are then pressed into a solid block.

OSTEOPOROSIS: THE ALTERNATIVES

Tofu was first used in China around 200 B.C., but the discovery of the process for making tofu is lost to the ages. According to Chinese legend, the first batch of tofu was created by accident. A Chinese cook used nigari to flavor a batch of pureed, cooked soybeans and the combination produced the curd we know today as tofu.

Tofu is a dietary staple throughout Asia, made fresh daily in small tofu shops, and usually sold on the street. Cubes of firm tofu can be added to any casserole or soup. Tofu acts like a sponge. It has the miraculous ability to soak up any flavor added to it. Crumbled into a pot of spicy sauce, it tastes like chili. Blended with cocoa and sweetener it becomes a double for chocolate cream pie filling.

There are three main types of tofu, and they are available in American grocery stores.
- **Firm tofu** is dense and solid. It holds up well in stir fry dishes, soups, on the grill, or anywhere it needs to maintain its shape. Firm tofu is higher in protein, fat, and calcium than other forms of tofu.
- **Soft tofu** is a good choice for recipes that call for blended tofu or in Oriental soups.
- **Silken tofu** is made by a slightly different process that produces this creamy, custard-like product. Silken tofu works well in pureed or blended dishes. In Japan, silken tofu is enjoyed as is, seasoned with soy sauce and topped with chopped scallions.

SOME OF THE NUTRITIONAL VALUES OF TOFU:
- B-vitamins
- Calcium (when the curdling agent is calcium salt)
- Fat (while 50% of the calories in tofu come from fat, a 4-ounce serving contains just 6 grams. It is low in saturated fat and contains no cholesterol. Generally, the softer the tofu, the lower the fat content. For low-fat diets, reduced fat or "lite" tofu is available.)
- High-quality protein
- Iron
- Sodium: (very low in it, making it a perfect food for people on sodium restricted diets.)

SOY MILK

Soy milk is the rich, creamy product of whole soybeans. With its unique, nutty flavor and rich nutrition, soy milk can be used in a variety of ways. Soy milk is free of the milk sugar lactose, making it a smart option for people who are lactose intolerant. It's also a good alternative for those who are allergic to cow's milk.

In China and Japan, fresh *soy milk* is made daily using a simple, centuries-old process. Dissolved soy milk is extracted from cooked and soaked soybeans, by compression. In these countries, soy milk is sold by street vendors or in cafés. It is served hot or cold, often sweetened for a delightful beverage, or flavored with soy sauce, onions, and vegetables to produce a spicy soup.

Soy milk is available as a plain, unflavored beverage or in a variety of flavors including chocolate, vanilla, carob, and almond. With the growing interest in lower-fat food products, a number of light soy milks with a reduced fat content are appearing on the market.

TEMPEH

Tempeh (pronounced 'tem-pay') is a traditional Indonesian food. This chunky, tender cake of soybeans is consumed daily in Indonesia, with rice as a part of the main meal, or sometimes by itself, as a snack. In Indonesia, tempeh making is an art that varies somewhat from home to home. Whole soybeans are usually mixed with a grain such as rice or millet. A "starter", usually a piece of tempeh from a previous batch, is added to begin the fermentation process. In traditional home-based tempeh making, the mixture is wrapped in banana leaves and left to ferment for 18 to 24 hours. In western factories, commercial starters are often used to produce tempeh, where the fermentation process takes place under more carefully controlled conditions. Whatever process is used, the result is a cake of soybeans with a rich flavor sometimes described as smoky or nutty. The flavor has also been compared to that of mushrooms.

Since tempeh is made from whole soybeans, it's a fiber-rich food. It's also a generous source of many nutrients such as calcium, B-vitamins, and iron.[U070]

GENISTEIN, THE GENIE IN SOY PRODUCTS

As stated on page 254, soybeans and some soy foods include soy flour, soybeans and some tofu; they are a good source of calcium that is easily absorbed by the body. It has also been found that laboratory studies with animals have shown that the consumption of soy protein not only delayed the onset of the age-related increase in bone loss, but the total amount of bone loss was significantly less. In human subjects, the fact that soy contains the hormone like substance genistein has invited many studies:

It has been postulated for a long time, that soy is not only a substance which benefits menopausal and osteoporotic women, relieving their symptoms, but that it also reduces the incidence and development of malignancy. This is of great interest to those who by virtue of their condition must rely on supplemental estrogen. These effects are attributed to a family of natural chemicals called *isoflavones* (eyes of lay bones). You will also hear of these.[A090]

In an interesting study on non-vegetarian women, the effects of regular diets, diets enriched with soy containing natural amounts of isoflavones, and soy deprived of isoflavones were compared. Hormonal changes occurred in all women consuming the natural soy, irrespective of whether the diet was or was not vegetarian, favoring an increase in estrogen part of the cycle.[P010]

BENEFITS OF SOY IN REDUCING CANCER

The low incidence of breast cancer in countries with a *flavonoid*-rich (rich in certain natural chemicals known as *flavones* or *isoflavones*) *soy-based* diet, mostly in the Orient, has always puzzled researchers. To see what the consumption of these substances, or, at least, one of their ingredients, can do for laboratory animals, genistein, a natural *isoflavonoid phyto-estrogen*, was given to them. Protection against experimental mammary tumors in rats by soy-derived products, was remarkable, which suggests that genistein and other isoflavonoid compounds may exert an anti-tumor activity, counteracting tumor stimulators. Incidentally one of these stimulators, is insulin.[F070]

Experimental and epidemiologic studies support the view that soy foods prevent cancer as well as diseases and symptoms associated with estrogen deficiency. Recent research suggests that the isoflavonoid genistein, a phytoestrogen found in abundance in soy foods, may be one of the principal molecular components responsible for these health benefits. In this study...[the researchers]...investigated the effects of a broad physiologically relevant concentration range of genistein on [certain cancer markers:]...estrogen receptor (ER) binding, induction of the estro- gen-regulated antigen *pS2*, and cell proliferation rate in ER(+) and ER(-) human breast cancer cells grown *in vitro* [the test tube]. Dose response to genistein was compared with that of estradiol, *tamoxifen*, and several other structurally similar iso- and bioflavonoids (e.g., *equol*, *kaempferol*, and *quercetin*). Our results revealed that genistein has potent estrogen *agonist* [works *with* estrogen] and cell growth-inhibitory actions over a physiologically achievable concentration range (10 nM-20 microM). Other flavonoids over the same concentration range were good estrogen agonists and poor cell growth inhibitors (*equol*) or poor estrogen agonists and potent growth inhibitors (*kaempferol* and *quercetin*). The growth-inhibitory actions of flavonoids were distinctly different from those of *triphenyl antiestrogens* like tamoxifen. In summary, ...[their]...results reveal that genistein is unique among the flavonoids tested, in that it has potent estrogen agonist and cell growth-inhibitory actions over a physiologically relevant concentration range.[Z000]

A tumor, like a plant, needs to be irrigated to grow and prosper, so it needs a good supply of blood and has to have its own set of new blood vessels. Preventing new blood vessel formation prevents tumor growth. A study performed in Italy confirmed that the consumption of a plant-based diet can prevent the development of new blood vessels and therefore, the progression of chronic diseases that are associated with this. The active substance, and the most potent in this diet proved to be the isoflavonoid genistein. This same substance manifested a protective effect against chemically induced mammary cancer even in rats which are genetically cancer-prone.[L030]

Surprisingly enough, even when chemotherapy is deemed necessary, genistein improves the effectiveness of this treatment.[M240]

Studies have indicated a correlation between a high level of genistein measured in urine, a high level of the lignan *enterolactone* (another plant chemical), and a low incidence of hormone-dependent cancers, such as breast and prostate cancer. Previously it has been observed that a vegetarian diet is associated with high plasma levels of **sex hormone-binding globulin (SHBG)**, reducing clearance of sex hormones and probably risk of breast and prostate cancer.[M260]

On the basis of these and other studies, the researchers suspect that the **Western** diet, compared with an **Eastern**, vegetarian or semi-vegetarian diet, may alter hormone production, metabolism or action at the cellular level. This does not appear to be limited to soy products, but include also other sources of the protective genistein and lignans. The precursors of the biologically active compounds originate also in whole grain cereals, seeds, probably berries and nuts (mainly lignans). The plant lignans and isoflavonoids are converted to hormone-like compounds with weak estrogenic and antioxidative activity by intestinal bacteria, although some intestinal metabolisms may also destroy them. They have now been shown to influence:

- **Angiogenesis** (formation of new blood vessels)
- Growth factor action
- Intracellular enzymes
- Malignant cell reproduction
- Malignant cell **differentiation** (becoming more mature and less invasive)
- Protein synthesis
- Sex hormone metabolism and biological activity

All of these features make them strong candidates for a role as natural cancer protective compounds. The highest levels of intake of these compounds are found in countries or regions with low cancer incidence.[A030]

Although soybean milk isoflavones (genistein, **daidzein,** enterolactone) seem to be 85% broken down in the intestine, their availability, especially of daidzein, may be sufficient to exert some health-protective effects.[X020] Data suggest that this isoflavone stabilizes protein-linked DNA and prevents strand breakage (this breaking of DNA—genetic material or chromosomes—is the first step in permitting abnormal rearrangements or recombinations, fostering disease).[N090]

SOY SAPONINS AS ANTI-CARCINOGENS
Other substances present in soy are **saponins**, they are present also in other plants. They are soap-like, detergent-like substances.[R010]

NUTRITIONAL SUPPLEMENTS

A scientifically balanced regimen of nutritional supplements reinforces the body's antioxidant defenses and should include vitamins E, C, B1, B2, B3, B6, B12, pantothenate, PABA, and Vitamin A. A balanced program of mineral and trace element supplementation should include magnesium, zinc, selenium, manganese and chromium. The exact prescription for nutritional supplements is determined individually for each patient, based on nutritional assessment and laboratory testing.

EXERCISE

> IF IT'S PHYSICAL, IT'S THERAPY!

What are the effects of the patient's level of physical activity?

Inactivity leads to bone loss. Some recent studies suggest that *weight bearing* exercises may reduce bone loss. Modest weight-bearing exercise, such as walking, is usually recommended. But, is all exercise equally beneficial?

In a study of 40 international top ranked, high performance athletes of different disciplines (28 weight-lifters, 6 sports-boxers and 6 bicycle-racers) bone density measurements of the lumbar spine and the left hip were performed by dual-photon absorptiometry (DEXA; QDR 2000, Siemens) and evaluated by an interactive software-programme (Hologic Inc.). It came as no surprise that in the high performance weight lifters there was an increase of bone density of 23%, compared to the control individuals. The sports-boxers had an increase up to 17% in the low back (lumbar spine), 9% in the hip, and 7% over all. But it was an absolutely unexpected finding, that in the third athletes group (*Tour de France*-bikers) BMD was decreased 10% in the lumbar spine, 14% in the hip, and 17% over all.[S010] The final conclusions were that while:

- Training programs stressing axial loads (weight bearing) of the skeletal system may lead to an increase of BMD in the spine and the hip of young individuals

- The BMD of endurance athletes may decrease

Reasonable amounts of physical exercise are generally very wholesome.

Even a brisk 45-minute walk several times per week will help maintain health benefits and improve circulation, this resulting from the dilation of blood vessels and natural chelation. (Lactic acid normally builds up in tissues during sustained exercise and lactate is a natural chelator. Also, and probably the most important factor, is that exercise induces the secretion of **HGH**, (**human growth hormone**).

Back extensor strengthening exercises are highly recommended for management of back pain, especially back pain related to osteoporosis.[S140] It:
- Decreased thoracic kyphosis
- Increased lumbar lordosis
- Increased sacral tilt

Bone mineral density and physical activity score did not show any significant correlations with the radiographic factors. The results indicate that the stronger the back extensor, the smaller the thoracic kyphosis and the larger the lumbar *lordosis* (the curvature that causes the scooped area between the back and the buttocks), and pelvic tilt. Back extensor strength is an important determinant of posture in healthy women. However, prescribing back extensor strengthening exercises alone may also increase lumbar lordosis, which is not desirable.

"Osteoporosis has obvious physical and functional consequences such as kyphosis, restricted range of motion, and pain. What are not so obvious are the psychosocial sequels that result from this metabolic bone disease. Many patients in the initial phases of the disease express substantial anxiety, especially about the possibility of future fractures and physical deformity. As the disease progresses, depression can become profound for those who experience hip or multiple vertebral fractures. The effects of the chronicity of osteoporosis, its disabling and disfiguring aspects, and the chronic postural pain that develops as time passes challenge even the most stable individuals. In addition, osteoporosis has substantial impact on interpersonal relationships and social roles. The dependency created by this disease affects close relationships, because the patient with osteoporosis cannot reciprocate in social support. Today's older women find the restrictions of the disease socially devastating. These women, unlikely to work in the labor force, took pride in their roles of housekeeper and cook. Unfortunately, severe osteoporosis can force women to relinquish even these social roles, leaving them with no source of self-esteem or accomplishment. In all, osteoporosis is devastating both psychologically and socially.[MG070]

The effects and benefits of certain exercises (for 60 minutes, three times a week, over a period of 12 months) were evaluated in a study of 124 post-menopausal women with low bone mass, aged between 50 and 70, who were living in Sherbrooke, Quebec, at the time of the survey.[B190] These exercises were:

■ Aerobic dancing
■ Flexibility exercises
■ Weight-bearing exercises (walking, stepping up and down from benches)

The effects were:

TEST GROUP	CONTROL GROUP
Spinal BMD stabilized	Spinal BMD decreased
Femoral BMD unchanged	Femoral BMD unchanged
Functional fitness improved	Functional fitness unchanged
Flexibility improved	Flexibility unchanged
Agility improved	Agility unchanged
Strength improved	Strength unchanged
Endurance improved	Endurance unchanged
Well-being improved	Well-being unchanged
Back pain decreased	Back pain unchanged
Self-perceived health increased	Self-perceived health unchanged

Menopause and osteoporosis are problems of older people. "Advancing age is associated with profound changes in body composition, including increased fat mass, decreased fat-free mass (particularly muscle), decreased total body water and decreased bone density. However, the capacity to increase muscle mass through high resistance exercise is pre-served even in the oldest subject. Even up to the age of 96 years, men and women can respond to resistance training with a substantial (greater than 200%) increase in strength and muscle size."[E070] Remember the adage "No pain, no gain!" The most peculiar finding in this study was that muscle damage might actually be the primary stimulus for muscle enlargement, by stimulating increased rates of muscle breakdown and repair. The effects were not to be sneezed at!

And now, the final question!

THE EFFECTS OF MIND AND SPIRIT

The Chinese say that our lifestyle affects how the "life Energy they call *Qi* circulates in our body. If we frequently feel ill, especially mentally, we might need a change of lifestyle. How we think and how we coordinate the *Qi* pattern in our body with the natural *Qi* is very important for health. Whenever the *Qi* circulation opposes the *"Dao"* (nature), we will be sick. Walking for an hour or doing *Qigong* exercises every morning is recommended by Oriental practitioners of the healing arts.

ATTITUDE AND PERFORMANCE IN LIFE: THEY IMPACT ON OSTEOPOROSIS AND FRACTURES

A California group of researchers was able to correlate mood and attitude with fractures. "Osteoporosis and its sequels have been associated with many factors...pathologic osteoporotic hip fractures [occur] in elderly females with major *depression*."[V020] [emphasis added].

We all have heard about the value of positive thinking and attitude. Maybe a practice of these virtues would help osteoporotic people regain functionality.

Is there a physical and psychological predisposition to developing osteoporosis, and getting broken bones? Do older women without fractures function better than those who do have them? In a 1993 study of elderly females, without taking in consideration their condition prior to sustaining fractures, in Durham, North Carolina, it was determined that "Vertebral compression fractures are associated with significant performance impairments in physical, functional, and psychosocial domains in older women."[L150] They were judged according to certain parameters: the "Functional Status Index". Subjects of this study were not significantly different in "age, weight, number of current illnesses, number of prescribed medications, number of pain medications, ratings of lumbar spine degenerative disc disease, or lumbar spine facet joint arthritis. Activity levels and exercise participation were similar in both groups. Control subjects had no vertebral fractures, whereas fracture subjects had 4.2 +/- 2.6 fractures (range: 2 to 10). **Thoracic kyphosis** was increased **and lumbar lordosis** was reduced in fracture subjects."[L150] Fracture subjects had:

- 6-minute walk test
- Functional reach
- Mobility skills
- Reduced maximal trunk *extension torque* (stretch twisting)
- Thoracic and lumbar spine sagittal plane motion (lateral movements)

The Functional Status Index showed reduced levels of functional performance in fracture subjects compared with controls, [with need for] increased levels of assistance, pain with activity, and difficulty in activities. Psychosocial performance was limited in fracture subjects with increased psychiatric symptoms, increased pain, and greater perception of problems caused by health."[L150] [emphasis added]

If we postulate that the severity of typical menopausal complaints (hot flushes and vaginal dryness) are related to hormone imbalances which can lead to osteoporosis, then it must follow that these must be worse in hysterectomized women (one or both ovaries present) than in women whose uterus and both ovaries are present, and who have reached menopause. "Hysterectomized women, especially those aged 39 to 41 years, report significantly more vasomotor complaints, vaginal dryness, and atypical complaints than do normal climacteric women of the same age. The higher prevalence of typical climacteric complaints in hysterectomized women largely explains their higher level of atypical complaints...the literature indicates that hysterectomized women with ovarian conservation are over-represented with regard to osteoporosis, cardiovascular disease, osteoarthritis, depression, and sexual problems."[0040] [emphasis added]

THE EFFECTS OF CLOTHING

Enzyme action and protein synthesis are temperature dependent. Viruses can only replicate at low temperatures. What we wear affects our body. In the winter we must stay warm, and especially protect our joints. Many man-made fibers can adversely affect us. For example, polyester can accumulate a considerable charge of static electricity in the winter. This builds up an electromagnetic field, which causes static discharges when we kiss, touch a car, etc. Many people are electrically sensitive, and synthetic clothing makes them irritable or hurt. Natural fibers seem to foster better health, and lamb's wool often appears to have soothing effects.

THE EFFECTS OF SEXUAL ACTIVITY

It is reported that sexual activity can stimulate the adrenal glands to produce more corticosteroid, a hormone that reduces joint inflammation and pain. It is believed that sexual activity may also trigger the release of endorphins, a naturally occurring painkilling substance. (*7)

THE EFFECTS OF OUR ENVIRONMENT

The physical environment can affect the body: this can impact adversely on the comfort of osteoporosis sufferers, especially if they are also afflicted with other aches and pains, and arthritis. If the climate where you live is too damp or too cold, or you live near high tension power lines it may be affecting your general well being. It has recently been discovered that our bodies can be significantly affected by the electromagnetic fields generated by modern technology which has given rise to the long known concept of "sick houses", which are associated with some forms of cancer. Perhaps similar environmental effects on osteoporosis or arthritis will be found.

THE EFFECTS OF UNIVERSAL HARMONY IN OUR ENVIRONMENT

FENG SHUI

"Feng Shui (pronounced 'phong schway' and meaning literally 'wind water') is part of an ancient Chinese philosophy of nature. Feng shui is often identified as a form of geomancy, divination by geographic features, but it is mainly concerned with understanding the relationships between ourselves and nature so that we might live in harmony within our environment.

"Feng shui is related to the very sensible notion that living with, rather than against nature, benefits both humans and our environment. It is also related to the equally sensible notion that our lives are deeply affected by our physical and emotional environs. If we surround ourselves with symbols of death, contempt and indifference toward life and nature, with noise and various forms of ugliness, we will corrupt ourselves in the process. If we surround ourselves with beauty, gentleness, kindness, sympathy, music and various expressions of the sweetness of life, we ennoble ourselves as well as our environment."[C020] [emphasis added]

Without attempting to pass judgment on the way the craft is practiced, this seems to be excellent advice to remind us that we largely create the reality that we live, attracting that which befalls us through our thoughts and action.

THE WONDERFUL THERAPIES

THERAPIES THAT ESTABLISHMENT CHOOSES TO TOTALLY IGNORE

There are wonderful therapies out there, of which you may have never heard, or that your doctor may pooh-pooh. However, *Establishment* gradually, but surely is opening up to alternatives. Just this month, November 1997, "Alternative Medicine: What works, and what do you tell your patients,"[H141] a mini-course in alternatives was published in a popular continuing education magazine. But, remember, until you yourself try it, you won't really know, for the proof of the pudding is in the eating, and the might of the gigantic medical and pharmaceutical industries, does not make right!

CHELATION THERAPY

Calcium belongs in bones and nails, but when its metabolism is abnormal, it deposits in soft tissue: an example is plaque in arteries. This is called *metastatic* calcium. Chelation mainly consists in removing metastatic (out of place) calcium, and some toxic minerals from their location in the human body, to create a healthier state of being. The main mechanism by which this is accomplished is by preventing the *free radical* damage that toxic substances may cause.

WHAT IS EDTA CHELATION THERAPY?

Chelation therapy uses, *Ethylene-diamino-tetraacetic acid* (*EDTA*), in combination with vitamins and minerals as an intravenous drip. EDTA is a synthetic amino acid (a building block of proteins) that originated from the German *ersatz* (substitute) research from WWII Europe, and was compounded to replace *citric acid* in the fabric dying industry. It was useful because it could scavenge undesirable minerals contained in the water, and prevent them from staining fabrics undergoing the dying process.

Its therapeutic applications were eventually recognized: It reduces abnormal production of *free radical molecules* (molecules which react destructively with others, causing the oxidizing of fats - *lipid peroxidation* - in cell membranes). This protects DNA, enzyme systems and lipoproteins and allows the body's natural healing mechanisms to take over, and often reverse disease processes. It was first used in the 1940's for the treatment of heavy metal poisoning, and is widely recognized as effective for that use. Also, it is the emergency treatment of choice for *hypercalcemia* and the control of *ventricular arrhythmias* from *digitalis* (a heart drug) toxicity. In the late 1960's the National Academy of Sciences/National Research Council indicated that EDTA was considered possibly effective in the treatment of occlusive vascular disorders caused by arteriosclerosis. In the human body, EDTA binds *ionic metal catalysts* and removes them.

It is a therapy mainly used in the treatment of occlusive vascular disease and other degenerative illnesses associated with aging. It consistently improves blood flow. It relieves symptoms in most of the patients treated, and has been safely and effectively utilized by physicians throughout the nation and hundreds of thousands of patients have received demonstrable benefit from it.

By solubilizing the inert calcium that is occupying undesirable locations in the body, it promotes a better calcium pool to remineralize osteoporotic bone.

CONTROVERSIES

This therapy has been heatedly under attack by the *Establishment*. Although accepted at first, the advent of profitable surgical procedures and the sustained benefit of keeping people enslaved by lifelong dependence on worthless drugs, added to the fact that the product has long lost its patent, put it in the *Establishment's* doghouse. The technique is not illegal, but physicians who help their patients using this technique are harassed and persecuted, often losing their licenses under false pretexts of the licensing boards.

> CHELATION THERAPY IS USED IN TREATING
> DEGENERATIVE DISEASES ASSOCIATED WITH AGING

A free radical is defined as any atom or molecule in a particular state of activation, with *one* electron in the *outer orbit* of the atom remaining unpaired. The conversion of normal molecular oxygen to toxic oxygen radicals occurs by the transfer of a single electron by the *mitochondrial* or *microsomal electron transport chain* (located in small pockets inside the cell, called *mitochondria),* or through *oxidant enzyme systems (xanthine oxidase, aldehyde oxidase, flavin dehydrogenase, amine oxidase, cycloxygenase,* and *lipooxygenase).*[H100] This article also refers to the implications of oxygen-derived free radicals in atherosclerosis and other diseases.

BACKGROUND INFORMATION TO UNDERSTAND CHELATION

(if this is too technical for you, you may skip it)

"In order to appreciate the truly remarkable potentials of chelation therapy it is necessary to examine briefly some of the chemical processes involved in the natural phenomena of chelation and free radical activity." [C040]

Since everything is made from combinations of elements, the smallest unit of which is the atom, we must know a little about these. "Each atom consists of a central nucleus, made up of *protons*, positively (+) electrically charged. The number of protons in an atom determines what the element is. In the case of hydrogen, for example, there is just one proton, whereas carbon has 6 protons, sodium 11, calcium 20 and uranium 92.

"Spinning around the central core of protons—in orbit, so to speak—are precisely the same number of negatively (-) charged electrons, or, in the case of hydrogen, one electron. Electrons are much smaller than protons; by weight it actually takes 1835 electrons to equal one proton. Despite this imbalance in weight, the negative electrical charge of one electron is just as powerful as the positive electrical charge of one proton. Thus in a stable, electrically neutral atom, the electrical charge of the proton(s) is precisely in balance with that of the electron(s).

"Electrons (much like people) have a natural tendency to find partners so that they can become paired. When this does not happen, as during radiation or certain chemical processes, a 'free radical' or a molecule (combination of atoms) with an unpaired electron may evolve (see below for more on these miniscule troublemakers)."[C040]

Under natural conditions, the electrons are arranged in layers, or 'shells', orbiting like planets The inner shell has two electrons, there are eight electrons in the next. In some instances electrons are shared by more than one atom.

Some atoms can gain or lose from one to three electrons from the outer layer, thus turning into *ions* (an atom or group of atoms which has lost or gained one or more of these orbiting electrons, becoming able to conduct electricity).

There are two kinds of *ions*:
- *Anion* is an ion which is negatively charged, which has gained one or more electrons
- *Cation* is an ion with a positive electrical charge, which has lost one or more electrons

Chlorine (Cl) has 17 protons and 17 electrons. Again the 'shell' system demands two electrons in the inner layer, eight in the next and in chlorine an unbalanced seven electrons (remember eight is the ideal) are found in the outer 'shell'. When sodium and chlorine are brought together, the 'odd' electron in sodium latches on to the seven in the chlorine to create a perfect 'shell' of eight electrons.

This process of combination creates a salt in which sodium and chlorine are bound together (in this case as table salt, NaCI) in a crystalline form. The sodium which has lost its free spinning electron (see above) is therefore now a positive ion, and this is expressed as sodium (Na+), while the chlorine which has gained an electron has become a negative ion, expressed chlorine (Cl-).

WHAT IS CHELATION

Chelation (pronounced key-lay-shin) is an interaction between an organic compound which has two or more *available attachment points* or *reactive sites* in its outer shell, with which it links with a metal that has two free electrons in its outer shell. A true chelation reaction has two or more such bonds or links. Together, the organic compound (chelating agent) and the metal form a stable ring-like structure when they combine. The word *chelate* is derived from the Greek word χηελα (claw) and refers to the way we theorize that EDTA binds plaque, toxins and calcium deposits from arteries, veins and the body at large. The red pigment in blood which carries oxygen, is a chelate of iron. Chlorophyll, the green pigment of plants, is similar in structure to , and a chelate of magnesium. Bone is a chelate of ostein, calcium, magnesium and phosphate.

The natural processes of chelation can go both ways: if, when you eat iron rich food at a meal, you drink tea at the same time, the *tannin* (a substance like the ones used to tan hides of animals) in the tea will chelate with the iron (forming insoluble *iron tannate*) before it gets a chance to be absorbed, thus depriving your body of the iron. If you take PUFAs or eat vitamin C-rich food at the same meal as an iron-rich food, this will chelate with the iron and actually enhance and speed up its absorption. The iron, once in the bloodstream, is released from the proteins with which it was chelated for transportation, and can recombine (another chelating process) with *transferrin* which is then stored for later use.

A water softener chelates calcium (and other minerals) out of the water. A detergent, in washing clothes or dishes chelates the minerals in the "dirt" allowing the solubilized compounds to be washed away by water.

The chelation that we do *artificially* is similar to the natural process, using a synthetic chemical (EDTA) instead of the natural chemicals of the body (actually, EDTA is a *polymer*, a multiple molecule of four vinegar molecules). The purpose of the therapeutic chelating substance is not to keep the mineral as part of the body, but to make it soluble and have the kidneys eliminate it. EDTA, electrically charged in opposition to the charge the body does accept is used: therefore it is kicked out in a hurry. Chelation is one of the mechanisms by which such common substances as aspirin, antibiotics, vitamins, minerals, and trace elements work in the body.

HOW IS IT DONE?

Chelation therapy, as practiced today, consists of slow intravenous (IV) drip injection of EDTA (ethylenediamine tetraacetic acid), a synthetic amino acid. The EDTA in solution bonds with metals in the body, and helps eliminate them in the urine. In most cases it is an outpatient treatment available in a physician's office or clinic. It is so simple and safe that during my practice I have often encouraged individuals to learn to mix the solutions, insert the needles and do it at home. They have done great!

WHY IS IT NOT BETTER KNOWN?

There are healing techniques that the general population knows nothing about because the traditional medical doctors aren't aware they exist, having this knowledge suppressed over the years by various powerful organizations. Critics of the therapy in the AMA and the FDA claim that there is no good scientific evidence to back up the extravagant claims of advocates. Defenders of the therapy claim that the medical establishment has engaged in a half-century of deceit and conspiracy to suppress chelation because of fear it would cut into the profits made by drug therapy and surgery. Advocates claim that chelation is about 10 times cheaper than a coronary bypass with equal or better results. They also claim that scientific medicine does not decide to use certain treatments because they have been shown to be effective in controlled studies. Instead, the advocates of alternative therapies, such as chelation, maintain that these decisions are mainly political and economic.

Chelation therapy used for the treatment of chronic degenerative disease, is not covered by Medicare nor will most insurance companies pay for it. The American Heart Association's Task Force on New and Unestablished Therapies reviewed the available literature on the use of chelation in treating arteriosclerotic heart disease and claimed they found no scientific evidence to demonstrate any benefit from this form of therapy. They chose to ignore the very positive findings of the Office for Technology Assessment.

Although it has been tested and proven to be an effective treatment of vascular diseases, skeptics, which includes the American Medical Association and the American Heart Association, deny that studies support any such claims. There have not been any *double blind* trials, the yardstick by which so much in *Establishment* medicine is judged. Halstead states: "It is impossible to administer EDTA blindly (i.e. vitamin C so that neither the doctor nor the patient knows whether real EDTA or a substitute is being used), because it can be readily differentiated from an innocuous placebo by even one unacquainted with the compound." [emphasis added] It does, however, not require double-blind control studies, to show that people are actually getting better, and show steady improvement in their functions, better muscular coordination, the disappearance of angina pain, etc. This is particularly true in many patients who are slated to undergo bypass surgery, and this brings us close to the real reasons for its rejection: the medical *Establishment* is more interested in making money than they are in curing diseases. "Bypass surgery and drug treatment of the conditions which chelation so often effectively deals with are very big business indeed. In the USA alone, $4 billion is the current turnover per annum of the bypass industry. A lesser, but nevertheless enormous, sum is involved in medication for conditions which the relatively cheap (and now out of patent) substance EDTA can be shown to help. "After surgery patients remain hostage to hundreds of dollars in medications, laboratory tests, medical evaluations and future hospitalization and surgery. Such vested interests should not be underestimated when it comes to the lengths to which they will go to try to discredit methods which threaten their stranglehold on the 'market'. Chelation therapy continues to grow, however, as public awareness and knowledge increases of this safe alternative to surgery and drugs, many of which are of questionable safety and value." However hard this may be to believe, the American medical *Establishment* systematically suppresses evidence and persecutes anyone who challenges their monopoly. The conspiracy theory is argued at length in James Carter's excellent book, as well as in "Murder by Injection", and "Medical Monopoly", among others."[C040]

WHAT IS CHELATION AS A MEDICAL TREATMENT, IS IT DONE JUST ONCE?

On the contrary, chelation therapy is a course of treatments which usually consists of anywhere from 20 to 50 separate infusions, depending on each patient's individual status. I developed a rule of thumb to determine the number of treatments using parameters such as age, clinical history, toxins in the hair test, etc. Some patients eventually receive more than 100 infusions. It is usually the patients who insists in taking more and more treatments, because they recognize the growing benefits. Each treatment takes from three to four hours or longer in most practices, based on certain assumptions that they work more effectively if they are done slower. Not having made that experience, we reduced them to usually no more than two hours. Patients normally receive one or more treatments each week. Over a period of time, this halts the progress of the free radical disorders and many other degenerative diseases of aging. After several months these injections bring profound improvement to many metabolic and physiologic processes in the body. The body's regulation of calcium and cholesterol is improved by normalizing the internal chemistry of cells. Osteoporotic bone growth receives new impetus thanks to chelation related benefits:

- Better circulation
- Corrected free radical pathology
- Elimination of lead
- Improved metabolism
- Solubilization of metastatic calcium

DOES IT HURT? WHAT DOES IT FEEL LIKE TO BE CHELATED?

Being "chelated" is quite a different experience from other medical treatments. There is no pain, and in most cases, very little discomfort. Patients are seated in reclining chairs and can read, nap, watch television, do needlework or chat with other patients while the fluid containing the EDTA flows into their veins. If necessary, patients can walk around. They can visit the restroom, eat and drink as they desire, or make telephone calls, being careful not to dislodge the needle attached to the intravenous infusion they carry with them.

ARE THERE RISKS OR UNPLEASANT SIDE EFFECTS?

EDTA is relatively non-toxic and risk-free, especially when compared with other treatments. The risk of serious side effects, when properly administered, is less than 1 in 10,000 patients treated. By comparison, the overall death rate as a direct result of bypass is approximately 3 out of every 100 patients undergoing surgery, varying with the hospital and the operating team. The incidence of other serious complications following surgery is much higher, including heart attacks, strokes, blood clots, permanent brain damage with personality changes and prolonged pain. Chelation is more than 300 times safer than bypass surgery.

If EDTA is given too rapidly or in too large a dose, it may cause harmful side effects, just as an overdose of any other medicine can be dangerous. A few reports of serious and even rare fatal complications in the early treatments of the 1950s, have stemmed from using excessive doses of EDTA (maybe 8 times what we usually give), improperly administered.

Occasionally, patients may suffer minor discomfort at the site where the needle enters the vein, or along the path of the fluid, all of which is easily correctable. Some may experience mild nausea, dizziness, or headache for a little while. When properly administered, chelation is as safe as taking aspirin. My youngest child often asks for a chelation therapy before a

Karate competition (he is a black belt champion), because he feels his performance is enhanced after an infusion.

A FAVORITE ANTI-CHELATION LIE

Considering that the side effects of most drugs occupy many columns of the PDR, where in very small print we read of the disastrous consequences of most therapies, it seems presumptuous that the *Establishment* attacks the innocuous chelation by stating that EDTA therapy is damaging to the kidneys. This is totally inaccurate: one study of kidney function done on 383 chelation patients, before and after treatment with EDTA for chronic degenerative diseases indicates the reverse is often true. There is significant improvement in kidney function following chelation. In my own practice we did an informal review of at least 100 patients who had been chelated, and our results showed excellent function in all, with improved function in those who had been having a weak elimination. We tend to agree that treatments must be given more slowly and less frequently if kidney function is not normal, and patients with some types of <u>severe</u> kidney problems (not common kidney infections) should maybe not receive EDTA. In my own experience, we have seen people who already were on *dialysis* (kidney machine), start putting out urine by themselves after very slow and light chelation therapies.

IS CHELATION THERAPY NEW?

Not at all. Its earliest application with humans was during World War II when the British used the chelating agent *British Anti-Lewesite* (*BAL*) as a poison gas antidote. BAL is still used today in medicine.

Dr. Leon Chaitow, from Greece, reports that EDTA was first introduced into medicine in the United States in 1948 as a treatment for industrial workers suffering from lead poisoning in a battery factory. The U.S. Navy advocated chelation therapy for sailors who had absorbed lead while painting government ships and dock facilities. Lead poisoned adults receiving EDTA chelation treatments, who had also had atherosclerosis, experienced additional health improvements–diminished angina, better memory, sight, hearing, sense of smell and increased vigor. Encouraged by these serendipitous discoveries, a number of physicians began to treat individuals suffering from vascular conditions with chelation therapy and reported consistent improvements.

Chelation therapy remains the undisputed treatment of choice for lead poisoning, even in children with toxic accumulations of lead in their bodies as a result of eating leaded paint from toys, cribs or walls. It is also the treatment of choice for digitalis (a heart medicine) poisoning. Insurance and third party payors will pay for these indications.

But from 1964 on, despite continued documentation of its benefits and the development of refined treatment methods, the use of chelation for the treatment of arterial disease has been the subject of controversy.

IS IT LEGAL?
Absolutely. There is no legal prohibition against a licensed physician using chelation therapy for whatever conditions he deems it to be appropriate, even though the drug involved, EDTA, does not yet have atherosclerosis listed as an indication on the FDA-approved package insert. The FDA does not regulate the practice of medicine, but merely approves marketing, labeling and advertising claims for drugs and devices in interstate commerce.

It costs millions of dollars to perform the required research and to provide the FDA with documentation for a new drug claim, or even to add a new use to marketing brochures of a long-established medicine like EDTA. Physicians routinely prescribe medicines for conditions not yet included on FDA approved advertising and marketing literature. This is known as an "off-label" indication.

IS WITHHOLDING LIFE SAVING INFORMATION A CRIME?
On the question of legality, the interpretation of laws pertaining to "informed consent" is evolving in the courts and it is now possible that a physician who withholds information about the availability of other treatment choices, such as chelation therapy, prior to performing vascular surgery (along with all other treatment modalities) could be found legally liable. Withholding information about a different form of treatment may be tantamount to medical malpractice, if as a result, a patient is deprived of possible benefits. Thus, it is the doctors who refuse to recognize and inform their patients of chelations who are risking legal liability—not those chelating physicians who provide an innovative treatment which they feel to be the safest, the most effective and the least expensive for many of their patients.

WHAT PROOF EXISTS THAT CHELATION WORKS?

Physicians with extensive experience in the use of chelation therapy observe dramatic improvement in the vast majority of their patients. Since it is most often prescribed for cardiovascular problems, they see angina routinely relieved: patients who suffered searing chest pains when walking only a short distance are frequently able to return to normal, productive living after undergoing chelation. Far more dramatic, but equally common, is seeing diabetic ulcers and gangrenous feet heal. Many individuals who had been told that their limbs would have to be amputated because of gangrene are thrilled to watch their feet heal with chelation. In an informal study performed in our office during the 1980s, densimetry radiography of patients before and after was surprisingly improved. These patients had not only received chelation but other alternative modalities. Quality of life and relief of symptoms are far more important than the results of laboratory tests.

WHAT DOES IT COST?

A course of treatment generally requires from six weeks to six months. It may cost up to $3,000 or more for 30 treatments. This is considerably less than bypass surgery, which often costs over $35,000. A person who receives fewer treatments for preventive benefits can expect to pay approximately $60-$100 for each treatment. There are, of course, the costs of tests prior to, during, and after therapy. Insurance companies usually only cover chelation therapy if there is heavy metal toxicity found prior to therapy.

HOW DOES IT WORK?

Is it true that chelation therapy combats atherosclerosis by acting like a "liquid plumber" – by leeching calcium out of the atherosclerotic plaque?

Not exactly. It used to be hypothesized that EDTA chelation therapy had its major beneficial effect on calcium metabolism–that it stripped away the excess calcium from the plaque, restoring arteries to their pliable, pre-calcified (before they harden) state. This frequently offered explanation — the so-called "roto-rooter" concept — is not the only reason. The fact that EDTA does remove some abnormally accumulated, distributed, *metastatic* calcium is now felt to be one of the less prominent aspects of its benefits. It is considered more important that EDTA binds substances which could act as potent catalysts of excessive free radical reactions: the so-called transition metals, iron and copper, and the related toxic metals, lead, mercury, cadmium and others. A leading American physician, Elmer Cranton, MD, states his expert view of the importance of using EDTA to counteract the free radical scourge (Cranton and Frackelton 1982): "Two essential nutritional elements, iron and copper, are the most potent catalysts of lipid peroxidation [the degradation of fats by free radicals]. Catalytic iron and copper accumulate near *phospholipid* [fats bound to phosphorus] cell membranes, in joint fluid, and in *cerebrospinal* [of the brain and spine] fluid with age, and are released into tissue fluids following trauma or *ischaemia* [lack of oxygen supply due to circulatory inefficiency]. These unbound extracellular iron and copper ions have been shown to potentiate free radical tissue damage." What is the importance of this? Phospholipid cell membranes play a definitive role in the development of Alzheimer's disease, a condition which may be of concern in the osteoporotic group.

Free radical pathology, is now believed to be the underlying process triggering the development of most age-related ailments, including cancer, dementia and arthritis, as well as atherosclerosis.

HOW DOES EDTA AFFECT PROCESSES OF AGING?

EDTA's primary benefit is that it greatly reduces the production of free radicals. It does so by removing accumulations of metallic catalysts that accumulate at abnormal sites in the body as a person grows older speeding the *aging process by free radical pathology*. This is the process which triggers:

- Arthritis
- Atherosclerosis
- Cancer
- Dementia

This is a greatly oversimplified explanation of what actually occurs. For those of you with a decided interest in the scientific technicalities, you can send for the manuscript entitled "Free Radical Pathology in Age-Associated Diseases: Treatment with EDTA, Nutrition and Antioxidant'" by Doctors Elmer M. Cranton and James P. Frackelton. For a fuller explanation of the many issues involved, written in popular form for the general public, you might enjoy reading "Bypassing Bypass" by Dr. Elmer M. Cranton and Arline Brecher. Both publications, as well as others, are available from the American College of Advancement in Medicine, 23121 Verdugo Drive Suite 204, Laguna Hills CA 92653, (714) 583-7666. Telephone before ordering to find out costs, or you may purchase them from our office or in the bookstore. A new book, "FORTY SOMETHING FOREVER", by Arlene Brecher, is a wonderful addition to many already great publications.

SHOULD YOU ASK YOUR AMA DOCTOR ABOUT CHELATION THERAPY? WOULD YOU ASK THE AYATOLLAH ABOUT WOMENS' LIB?

Chelation therapy for cardiovascular disease or osteoporosis is not taught in medical school, and the average physician has, at best, only heard about it, read nothing about it, and all his information is false and negative. However, if you want to talk to him or her, after you get a negative answer, ask the doctor how many hours he has devoted to the study of the subject, and whether he can provide you with any documentation to support his views, one way or another.

A LITTLE PHYSICS TO UNDERSTAND FREE RADICALS

In order to appreciate the truly remarkable potentials of chelation therapy it is necessary to briefly examine some of the chemical processes involved in the natural phenomena of chelation and free radical activity.

Our entire universe is made up of atoms of various elements. Each atom consists of a central nucleus, made up of **protons**, with a positive electrical charge. The number of protons in an atom determines what the element is. In the case of hydrogen, for example, there is just one proton, whereas carbon has 6 protons, sodium, 11, calcium, 20 and uranium, 92.[U142]

Spinning around the central core of positively charged protons—in orbit, so to speak—are the same number of negatively charged **electrons**; in the case of hydrogen, only one electron. Electrons are much smaller than protons: by weight it actually takes 1835 electrons to equal one proton. It has been said: "One man, one vote, one particle, one charge": despite this imbalance in weight, the negative electrical charge of one electron is just as powerful as the positive electrical charge of one proton. Thus in a stable, electrically neutral atom, the electrical charge of the proton(s) is precisely in balance with that of the electron(s).

IT TAKES TWO TO KEEP MOLECULES FROM TURNING RADICAL

Electrons (much like people) have a natural tendency to find partners so that they can become paired. When this does not happen, as during radiation or certain chemical processes, they become "frustrated", and lose not only their composure, but an electron of their outer shell: a *free radical* (a molecule - combination of atoms - with an unpaired electron) may evolve.

The electrons which spin in orbit around the protons are arranged in such a way as to form concentric *shells,* that resemble the layers of an onion, each such shell being placed just a little further out from the nucleus than the previous one . The arrangement of electrons in each shell or layer is always the same, with only two electrons in the inner shell and eight electrons in the subsequent shells. In some instances atoms actually share electrons with other atoms.

This is the way *molecules* (combinations of atoms) are formed, allowing, for example, the two gases hydrogen and oxygen to combine to form water. Some atoms can gain or lose anywhere from one to three electrons when necessary, thus turning themselves into *ions*. Molecules, after losing the orbiting electrons, become capable of conducting electricity.

Ions can be:
- *Anions* (negatively charged, having gained one or more electrons
- *Cations* (positively charged after losing one or more electrons

WHAT CAUSES FREE RADICALS TO FORM?

What kicks an electron out of an orbit, or puts an extra one into it? One way in which free radicals are created, is as a result of *radiation*, often described as *ionizing radiation*. This is because radiation is able to dislodge individual electrons, leaving unpaired electrons behind. Some molecules with unpaired electrons are extremely dangerous and can have very damaging effects on body tissues. Another way is by *oxidation*. Hydrogen peroxide ($H2O2$) does its damage to tissue by free radical action. An example of free radical action is the effects of hydrogen peroxide on hair, which we call "bleaching".

Factors that cause free radicals:
- Drinking alcohol
- Hydrogen peroxide

- Many chemicals
- Pollutants
- Radiation (ionizing radiation)
- Smoking
- Too much sun, even
- Too much fat in your diet
- Too much exercise

When your body produces too many free radicals, the "extra" free radicals prey on healthy molecules. Free radicals have actually a beneficial purpose. There is an almost continuous production of free radicals by the defense cells of the body, used as a means of destroying invading microorganisms or cancer cells.

This is a natural process which is going on all the time in the body; there are also control mechanisms to prevent undesirable consequences from free radicals on healthy body cells when we are in good health.

Just as iron rusts, and an exposed apple or potato will turn brown when its surface meets the air, so do our bodies endure oxidation (ageing), for all of these are examples involving free radical activity. Placing of lemon juice on an apple will stop it from turning brown by 'mopping up' the unpaired electrons, thanks to the antioxidant vitamin C in the juice. In similar fashion, our body contains numerous antioxidant and free radical deactivating substances (specific enzymes, amino acids, vitamins, minerals, uric acid, etc.). The body can protect itself when it is well nourished with these substances, by quenching those free radicals which it produces itself, or which are created by radiation or from other sources.

Some antioxidants are synthetic. You are probably familiar with their acronyms from the labels of commercial products; they include: *butylated hydoxytoluene (BHT)*, *butylated hydroxyanisole (BHA)*, and *propyl gallate*. These antioxidants have been chemically manipulated to play significant roles in the production of cosmetics (especially those designed to prevent the aging of skin), plastics, rubber, and probably most importantly, to prevent diseases such as some cancers and heart disease.

A SIMPLE CHELATION DEMONSTRATION YOU CAN DO AT HOME
Maybe you can catch more flies with sugar, than with vinegar, but who

wants more flies, anyhow? But vinegar can do something else: scavenge more calcium, as one can see by doing a small experiment "in the privacy of your home", and show how some of the effects of chelation take place. To perform this inexpensive but really earthshaking demonstration, we use a little water, vinegar and some eggshells, all of which we place in a bowl. Over several days, the eggshells will become increasingly thin, as the vinegar progressively chelates the calcium out of the shell. With enough time and vinegar, the shell will eventually have all of its calcium removed, which now will be in solution in the liquid. The biologic membrane, in turn, will be clear, pliable, and baby soft.

WILL THE CALCIUM BINDING OF EDTA DAMAGE BONES AND TEETH?

EDTA only chelates ionic, unbound, calcium. It will not leach calcium out of the normal bound sites such as the bones and teeth. When the free calcium from the bloodstream is removed, and the calcium level drops, this decrease triggers parathyroid hormone to be released, which in turn unbinds metastatic (out of normal locations) calcium, such as seen in plaque deposits in the blood vessels. Soluble calcium becomes available for various purposes, including bone repair.

                    triggers   unbinds
calcium level drop ———> parathyroid hormone release ———> metastatic calcium

OTHER BENEFITS FROM EDTA INFUSION

Just as the use of EDTA in treating lead poisoning revealed its ability to remove unwanted calcium, so additional benefits were discovered when circulatory conditions were being treated. Many patients with osteoarthritic and similar problems reported relief of symptoms and an improved range of movement in previously restricted joints. It seems that obstructive calcium deposits in these areas were also being removed during chelation treatment.

SAFETY

The safety aspect of the use of EDTA in therapy has been phenomenal, with hardly any serious reactions being recorded amongst the host of seriously ill people to whom chelation therapy has been correctly applied. By 1980 it was estimated by Bruce Halstead, MD, (Halstead 1979) that there had been over 2 million applications of EDTA therapy involving some 100 million infusions, with not a single fatality, in the US alone. I have personally overseen more than 60,000 infusions, at least. The most effective use of EDTA chelation therapy has, over the 30 years of its successful application, been consistently found to be related to those diseases in which heavy metal or calcium deposits are major factors.

REJUVENATION: THE POSSIBLE DREAM

Several substances have become commercially available, that can be used to give more stamina, encourage tissue regeneration, and actually return the body and mind to a younger, more effective and healthy state. These substances are hormones which are normally produced in the body in high amounts at a younger age, and have become depleted or non-existent. It is, ultimately, the deficiency of these hormones, which causes the degenerative condition known as aging.

These rejuvenating hormones include the ones previously mentioned, and also, and primarily

- DHEA
- HGH

DHEA (DEHYDRO-EPI-ANDROSTERONE)

"Dehydroepiandrosterone (DHEA, prasterone—not to be confused with progesterone) is a major adrenal hormone with no well characterized function. In both animals and humans, low DHEA levels occur with the development of a number of the problems of aging: *immunosenesence* [aging of the immune system], increased mortality, increased incidence of several cancers, loss of sleep, decreased feelings of well-being, osteoporosis and atherosclerosis. DHEA replacement in aged mice significantly normalized [sic] immunosenescence, suggesting that this hormone plays a key role in aging and immune regulation in mice. Similarly, osteoclasts and lymphoid cells were stimulated by DHEA replacement, an effect that may delay osteoporosis."[W050] [emphasis added]

- Atherosclerosis
- *Immunosenesence* (aging of the immune system)
- Osteoporosis
- Decreased feelings of well-being

- Increased incidence of several cancers
- Increased mortality
- Loss of sleep

DHEA replacement in aged mice significantly normalized immunosenescence, suggesting that this hormone plays a key role in aging and immune regulation in mice. Similarly, osteoclasts and lymphoid cells were stimulated by DHEA replacement, an effect that may delay osteoporosis.

"...the insulin-sensitizing nutrient chromium picolinate [which] has been found to reduce urinary excretion of hydroxyproline [a bone amino acid related to bone destruction] and calcium in postmenopausal women, presumably indicative of a reduced rate of bone resorption...[has]...also raised serum levels of dehydroepiandrosterone-sulfate, which may play a physiological role in the preservation of postmenopausal bone density."[M090]

A recent study was done to evaluate hormone levels and bone density on pre-menopausal and peri-menopausal women. The menopausal condition was classified according to their levels of the *follicle stimulating hormone (FSH)* (less than 12 U/L in pre-menopausal, equal or more than 12 U/L in menopausal or peri-menopausal women. Some research data suggested that women who were still menstruating had relative deficiencies in both estrogen and testosterone, with reduced bone densities as a consequence.[S211] Low serum DH[E]A appears to represent a further risk factor, either because of its role as estrogen precursor or (possibly) because it promotes bone formation. However, the severity of the osteoporosis...[is]...not related to the serum DH[E]A level and only weakly to the DH[E]A...[to cortisol]...ratio.[N091]

Studies from Hershey, Pennsylvania "...emphasize the association of declining adrenal sex steroid production [DHEA] with declining bone density during the process of aging."[W063]

Long-term oral administration of the adrenal substance, *dehydroepiandrosterone (DHEA)*, a steroid in structure, has previously been shown to inhibit the development of spontaneous breast cancer and chemically induced lung and colon tumors in various mouse strains. The synthetic steroid, *3 beta-methylandrost-5-en-17-one*, which, unlike DHEA, is not demonstrably estrogenic in the rat, also inhibits genital warts (*papilloma*) development.[P040]

In a rat study in Canada, DHEA combined with an anti-estrogen drug (EM-800), proved to protect the rats from the development of cancer, and two animals that did get cancer had their tumors disappear after some time. Certain markers of health and illness were favorably influenced by the combination therapy "The combination of the two drugs had important inhibitory effects on the urinary excretion of calcium and phosphorus as well as on the urinary hydroxyproline/creatinine ratio. Serum total alkaline phosphatase was stimulated by DHEA. Treatment with EM-800 decreased both serum triglyceride and cholesterol levels, whereas DHEA had an inhibitory effect on serum triglycerides...."[L131] It is a well established fact that the substance DMBA (di-methyl-benz-anthracene) induces many cancers. In this study "The present data show the additive inhibitory effects of DHEA and EM-800 on the development of DMBA-induced mammary carcinoma in the rat, thus suggesting the potential benefits of such a combination for the prevention of breast cancer in women while preserving or even increasing bone mass and maintaining a favorable lipid profile."[L131]

FEMALE HORMONE REPLACEMENT (OVER THE COUNTER)

Are people stuck with expensive, prescription-only estrogenic substances? Absolutely not! *Over the counter* ovarian and other glandular extracts offer the osteoporotic patient a good alternative to pharmaceutical estrogens. These glandulars do not purport to have been proven through methods acceptable to the FDA or AMA. However, millions of doses have been successfully taken by natural-medicine-inclined patients. Should the AMA and FDA, and other such alphabet concoctions be the only seal of approval to be respected? Consider how they have already struck out with Thalidomide, Phen-Phen, and others.

HOW DO I KNOW THAT MY HORMONES ARE LOW, HIGH, OR OK?

In our office we had a "rule of thumb" (more like a "rule of finger"), to determine hormonal status, a finger, introduced into the vagina, should normally feel a slight sensation of moisture, similar of that inside the lower lip. Not too wet, not too dry. Anything less indicated to us a need for hormone supplementation with raw ovary. How much ovary pills did we recommend to take? Enough to cause the vagina to be lightly lubri-cated. Swollen breasts or a drippy vagina (even spotting of blood) indi-cated one had taken too much. Women took 1 or more pills a day, and often went on 21 days on, 7 days off cycles, if they still had a uterus. Women who had undergone hysterectomies were taking them all year long.

GLANDULARS (PROTOMORPHOGENS)

As stated on page 244, a glandular is a piece of gland tissue or organ taken from beef (bovine glandular) or pork (porcine glandular) that supplies sev-eral active principles:
■ Biologically active hormones
■ Enzymes, vitamins
■ Hormone precursors
■ Minerals
■ Natural lipid factors
■ Soluble proteins

Scientific research has demonstrated that glandulars have tissue specific activity and exert significant biological effects in humans; thus bovine liver tissue has a biological effect on human liver, porcine pancreas tissue has a biological effect on human pancreas, and so forth. Glandulars offer a diversity of hormones and hormone related substances in a natural, non-toxic quantity for therapeutic, rejuvenative and preventive health care."[U121] Glandulars are frequently available in freeze-dried tablets, taken from uncontaminated cattle from New Zealand. Many of my patients have suc-cessfully used them for many years, with remarkable improvement in strength, well being and skeletal comfort. Vaginal dryness, which I asso-ciate with bone loss, is well corrected with the ovarian extracts. Lubrication when using the female glandulars is a good measure of tissue rejuvenation.

The most common glandulars used in our practice were:
■ *Raw orchic* or *raw male* (an extract of testicle and prostate, often has minerals and vitamins added—we avoided mixed glandulars)
■ *Raw ovary* or *raw female* (an extract of ovary and uterus, often has minerals and vitamins added—we avoided mixed glandulars)
■ *Raw pituitary* (an extract or freeze dried pituitary—we avoided mixed glandulars)

■ **Raw thyroid** (an extract or freeze dried thyroid—we avoided mixed glandulars)

HUMAN GROWTH HORMONE (HGH), REPLACEMENT AND AGING

Genetics, nutrition, environmental quality, spiritual life, all of these affect our aging. These processes control and are controlled by the release of certain substances produced in the body, the **hormones**.

According to state of the art research, only possible in the last decades, the condition commonly called **aging** is mediated primarily by the exhaustion and decrease in production of **HUMAN GROWTH HORMONE (HGH)**. This substance occurs naturally in the body under conditions of good health. It is produced in a small gland at the base of the brain, the **pituitary gland**. The blood levels of this substance, when tested by laboratory methods, are highest in childhood and youth, when the body develops and gains height. After that, these levels begin to wane, until at age 40 or so, they decrease very rapidly. It is because of this cycle that people can maintain weight, skin and muscle tone for 3 or 4 decades, regenerate body cells, recuperate from stress and injury. After the production decreases, they start aging at an accelerated pace: muscles atrophy, bones become less resistant, skin less vibrant and healthy, sexy muscles yield to unhealthy middle age spread.

Many of the age-related changes in body composition resemble those associated with growth hormone deficiency, and growth hormone secretion decreases with normal human ageing. With the availability of **recombinant human growth hormone (rhGH)**, it is now possible to test the metabolic and structural effects of growth hormone administration to adults. Administration of rhGH to healthy elderly people acutely promotes nitrogen retention and activates bone remodeling [sic]. Chronic administration may increase lean mass in men, but appears to give less impressive results in women. Changes in bone remodeling [sic] are not accompanied by dramatic increases in bone mass. Thus, it is not likely that daily administration of rhGH as a **single agent** will prove to be an effective means for regaining deficits in bone, but it may be possible to incorporate rhGH into a **multi-agent** [various drugs] strategy. In healthy older humans growth hormone can be given without obvious adverse effects on cardiovascular risk factors.[M021]

FUNCTIONS OF HGH

- Improve lean body mass
- Improve bone regeneration in osteoporosis
- Reduce body fat
- Regenerate the nervous system in conditions such as Alzheimers, Parkinsons and Multiple Sclerosis (MS), improving memory and function
- Thicken and strengthen skin and bones, reversing osteoporosis

TREATMENT WITH HGH

"Until recently, the use of growth hormone (GH) has been confined to the treatment of GH-deficient children. The advent of GH produced by recombinant DNA technology has increased the availability of GH. The increased availability of GH has made possible studies of the physiology and the possible therapeutic role of this hormone and its mediator [a substance that participates in activation by this hormone] *insulin-like growth factor*. One area where GH may play a therapeutic role is in the treatment of osteoporosis.[R111]

Today, commercially available human growth hormone is obtained by the technique of *genetic engineering*, producing a laboratory generated substance known or *recombinant*. This, when administered to growth hormone deficient individuals, following a proper protocol regularity, will improve lean body mass, reduce body fat, thicken and strengthen skin and bones. It has even been found to regenerate the nervous system in conditions such as *Alzheimers*, *Parkinsons* and *Multiple Sclerosis* (*MS*).

IS THERE ANY DANGER IN TAKING THIS TREATMENT?

Some of these substances may not be used when a person has prostatic or testicular cancer, and must be used cautiously when prostatic enlargement exists. These hormones are manufactured in the same way as insulin, vaccines and other biologic products made by recombinant or genetic engineering technology, so they have the same risks as these other substances.

SIDE EFFECTS WITH LOW DOSE HGH REPLACEMENT

The dose of recombinant HGH used in each individual is an important consideration in the therapy of aging, bones, a form of acquired HGH-deficiency. Pharmacological doses of HGH, which are too large, are often associated with clinical signs of HGH excess, including:

■ Carpal tunnel
■ Fluid retention
■ Hypertension
■ Joint pains (slight)

In our own experience, treatment with smaller, physiological doses, accompanied by intravenous vitamins and amino acids (chelation therapy) does not usually provoke such symptoms. Multiple studies support the conclusion that low dose HGH replacement is associated with minimal side-effects. It is already apparent that even these small doses, unassociated with symptoms of HGH excess, may be enough to achieve desired metabolic results.[L072]

BONE DENSITY AND HGH

Both growth hormone excess and deficiency lead to changes in the incidence of osteoarthritis. HGH has dramatic healing effects on the connective tissue, muscle, and the skeletal system. It rejuvenates and strengthens fragile, ulcerated skin, fractured bones that do not heal, and muscle strength. [M062]

> **HGH ADMINISTRATION MAY ACT TO REVERSE THE OSTEOPENIA PRESENT IN THE GH-DEFICIENT PATIENT**

The potential role of GH in the maintenance of the skeleton has recently been investigated. GH is known to:

■ Increase *thymidine* (amino acid) *incorporation* (addition)—in the test tube, at least, an indication of cellular activity
■ Increase significantly bone *Gla-protein*, a sensitive indicator of osteoblast function
■ Increases of 5% and 4% in spinal and cortical bone density over 12 months of therapy
■ Reverse the osteopenia (bone thinning) present in the GH-deficient patient
■ Stimulate osteoblast proliferation
■ Stimulate systemic and local production of *Insulin Like Growth Factor I*—a bone *mitogen* (a substance that invites cell division)

Positive, although variable changes in bone density have been demonstrated with administration of HGH. In a recent study intending to evaluate its effect on aging bones, using the sensitive bone mass measuring techniques of *quantitative tomography* and *single photon absorptiometry*, significant increases of 5% and 4% were demonstrated in spinal and cortical bone density over 12 months of therapy in GH-deficient adults. It thus appears that GH administration may act to reverse the bone loss present in the GH-deficient patient.

In a Swiss study of *insulin-like growth factor I* (*IGF-I*) which is dependent on HGH, it has been shown that this substance stimulates growth and maturation of cultured osteoblast-like cells and induces longitudinal bone growth in IGF-I-deficient rats, even if treated with a corticosteroid—which usually destroys bone.[B170]

"Decreased osteoblastic activity seems to be of major importance in the pathogenesis [develop- ment] of postmenopausal and senile osteoporosis[,] and several lines of evidence suggest that GH may become useful in treatment of osteoporosis. GH stimulates osteoblastic proliferation [multiplication] and differentiation [maturation] *in vitro* [in the test dish] and increases production of Insulin-like Growth Factor-I and II (IGF-I and IGF-II) which both have profound stimulatory effects on osteoblasts and are important local regulators of bone remodeling. GH affects several other osteotropic [bone up-building] hormones *in vivo* [in the live organism] and increases bone turnover while the effect on bone mass is less pronounced and depends on the skeletal compartment [part of the skeleton]."[B209]

"Growth hormone (GH) and insulin-like growth factors (IGFs) play a central role in skeletal growth and bone remodeling." In the test dish, both substances build tissue and protein; "... patients with *acromegaly* [a pathologic enlargement of the skeleton, extremities and jaws usually related to excesses of growth hormone] exhibit increased bone mass. Recent in vivo studies have demonstrated profound activation of bone remodeling that lasted for months after a single 1-week dose of GH or IGF-I."[E048]

HE SAID, SHE SAID: MORE OPINIONS ABOUT GROWTH HORMONE

We read that "Recently the cause of aging has been discovered by medical researchers. It has turned out to be quite simple. In an experiment at North

Dakota State University mice were treated by injections of either growth hormone or saline twice a week. After 6 months all of the mice with the saline injections were dead, but more than 90% of the growth hormone animals were alive. And so with little fanfare the major cause of age associated mortality was discovered. Experiments with aged humans have confirmed that the administration of growth hormone brings about signs of rejuvenation such as reduction of adipose tissue, as well as increases in **growth hormone-insulin-like growth factor 1**, muscle mass, bone density and skin thickness."[S131] [emphasis added] The next step is now for us to go ahead and discover why growth hormone secretion is suppressed with increasing age.

According to the marvelous tool known as the world wide web, we can see the opinion of various researchers in this field:[B230]

Daniel Rudman, M.D., writing in the "New England Journal of Medicine", tells us of the remarkable rejuvenating effects of HGH: "The effects of six months of human growth hormone on lean body mass and **adipose**-tissue [sic] were equivalent in magnitude to the changes incurred during 10-20 years of aging." [emphasis added]

From the V.A. Medical Center and Department of Medicine, Stanford University Medical Center, in a "Study of GH Therapy in the Elderly" (March 1992), the conclusion is that "It is possible that chronic physiologic GH and/or IGF-1 replacement therapy might reverse (or prevent) some of these 'inevitable' sequels of aging".

"Replacement therapy with Growth Hormone has shown beneficial/normalizing effect on...cardiac and renal function, thyroid hormone metabolism, bone metabolism, sweat secretion, total and regional fuel metabolism and psychological well-being."[J031]

Dr. Anthony Karpos, M.D. adds: "We really have something here which may be able to reverse some of the problems associated with aging."

Drs. Ramias, Shamos, and Schiller of St. Joseph Hospital Medical Center in Phoenix, AZ, found HGH to be a potent **anabolic** [protein building] agent: "Daily Administration of human growth hormone in the first week after trauma would enhance the metabolic status, resulting in reduced morbidity [illness] and earlier discharge from hospital."[R001] [emphasis added]

Dr. Jake Powrie, M.D. and Dr. Andrew Weissberger, St. Thomas Hospital, London, England, are of the opinion that "All adults with growth hormone deficiency should now be considered for growth hormone replacement therapy." (1995)

Dr. Rosen, M.D. and Dr. G. Johannsson, M.D. of University Hospital, Goteborg, Sweden, state in the journal "Hormone Research", 1995, that "There is no evidence suggestion that Growth Hormone Replacement Therapy causes any unfavorable long term side effects."

A TV program in England, Too Big Too Soon, broadcast on 20 February 1995, produced by Adam Bulmore, October Films, covered the saga of HGH, and among the points covered, they addressed that many people are interested and have benefitted from HGH therapy. At a presentation, the NARRATOR and producer, SEAN BARRETT, started by saying: "A new era of medicine has dawned. Bacteria, modified with human genes, produce huge quantities of biological drugs, perfect copies of human hormones. Synthetic human growth hormone is one of the first of this new generation of mass-produced genetic products. Using this potentially unlimited supply, scientists are quickly unravelling the role growth hormone plays in regulating our bodies from cradle to grave."

Without advising for or against usage in sports, it is interesting to hear what athletes had to say about the remarkable improvements they received from injections of HGH, Sportsman TIM BRUNER, said: "I don't lie about what I do, and the reason I don't lie is because I'm not ashamed of it, because basically every sport takes the drugs. The best way I could probably describe it is: steroids are like using regular gas, and growth hormone is closer to using super unleaded. It's a big difference." He added: "I went to Philadelphia for a contest and they contested ten lifts. Seven of them I'd never tried before, and in all ten events I set a record. Looking back after the fact, that's the only thing that could explain it, because I could not do some of those lifts even now." He added that top athletes - probably all of them used this enhancer, and that one could not compare a normal athlete who was just taking vitamins with a person that was taking enhancements, (of which HGH is the best).

HOWARD TURNEY, a Texas businessman, has invested his personal fortune in the selling of human growth hormone through a chain of private clinics called El Dorado. In January of 1991, he had palsy in his right hand, a gut "out to here", as he said, was on downhill skid...

The narrator says that "human growth hormone will have changed the face of the earth, because it will make people who are older and wise, who ordinarily would have retired or died, still be functional, still help increase the quality of life that we have in the world. I think it is the most important thing that's happened in 100 years, in 200 years - certainly from my standpoint the most important thing that happened in my life, in my whole lifetime. "

An El Dorado [a clinic devoted to HGH therapy] client stated that it was like [his] bones feel stronger, and you can feel a change going on inside—it's a strength inside, and [he does not] know if it's because [he has] never felt it, or what, but it's wonderful."

ANABOLIC EFFECTS OF HGH

Growth hormone, as well as DHEA and testosterone, are clearly anabolic hormones: they build tissue. As with increased age, our bodies break down tissue faster than we can repair them (*catabolism*), HGH tends to reverse the catabolic state.

One of HGH's most dramatic effects is on the connective tissue, muscle, and healing potential of the skeletal system. Fragile skin with ulcers, fractured bones that do not heal, and profound gains in muscle strength have been noted.

The potential role of HGH in the maintenance of the skeleton is its ability to make and repair these tissues. HGH stimulates osteoblast (bone) and fibroblast (supporting tissue) proliferation.[A040] In a recent study using the sensitive techniques of quantitative tomography and single photon absorptiometry, significant increases of 5% and 4% were demonstrated in spinal and cortical bone density over 12 months of therapy in HGH-deficient adults.[0010] It thus appears that HGH administration may act to improve skeletal repair of not only bone and skin but all organs as well.

MID-NINETIES HYPE:
A NOTE ABOUT "NATURAL PROGESTERONE"

Several sales organizations and books have popularized creams containing a semi-synthetic product derived from the estrogenic substance *diosgenin* from the Mexican yam (*dioscorea*), incorrectly dubbed "natural progesterone", are spreading information that is often not backed by appropriate research, and their literature is not annotated. I am not here to judge their information without having seen the proper data, but from my present experience, I would certainly not endorse this product as a proper treatment for osteoporosis, nor can I endorse the alleged scientific backing. I feel that everybody's products and books should stand on their own merits.

WHAT THE CATERPILLAR CALLS "THE END",
GOD CALLS A BUTTERFLY

Osteoporosis does not have to be the end of the line, but rather a beginning. Individuals who have never watched the quality of their food, their supplements, their habits, or heard about chelation therapy and growth hormone, now have a good reason to trade their couches for an exercise machine, and their drugs for supplements. New and stronger bone can replace the weakened ones, and they can at the same time improve their circulation, their spirit, their sex life.

SUPPORTIVE MEASURES

There are many actions a woman can take to prevent damage to her bones, joints, muscles, skin and hair after menopause, other than, or in addition to the HRT. Healthy lifestyle habits can slow down the aging process, revitalizing bones and tissues, helping them remain healthy and at peak function. The consensus is that some of these beneficial measures are:

Regular weight bearing exercise: walking or weight training, at least thirty minutes per day. Exercise stimulates the release of HGH (*somatotropin* or human growth hormone). This helps keep bones strong and intact and promotes good blood circulation.

Yoga or other stretching exercises: to keep your joints and muscles limber and flexible.

Stopping harmful practices: If you smoke, or if you drink to excess, QUIT!

Getting plenty of sunshine: It is my personal opinion (not necessarily supported by conventional wisdom or political correctness) not to believe the tales of science that badmouth life and health giving sunshine. Cancer of the skin and wrinkling from burning is vastly genetic (scottish-irish, welsh and german) and otherwise due to unbridled, irrational exposure, roasting instead of tanning. Protection from free radical damage through proper antioxidants and nutrition, good quality protein and supplementation of PABA (a B vitamin deficient in those genetic groups previously mentioned) is the safest method of protection against the free radical damage caused by solar radiation. Avoiding the acquisition of oncogenes, the cancer causing particles that exist in many products, especially genetically engineered biologic pharmaceuticals and vaccines, is paramount.

Drinking clean or purified water in quantities appropriate to the diet and exercise level. It is irrational, in my opinion, to recommend the intake of the same amounts of water for everybody, diluting excessively digestive juices and overburdening electrolyte sparing functions in the kidney. Tap water should be kept at a minimum, the more one drinks, the more pollutants one absorbs. One good way to measure appropriate water intake is by monitoring the color of urine, which should be straw, but people who take lots of vitamin or mineral supplements, even some medications often have much denser urine, and still do just fine. Water purifying systems should only be used if they are of excellent quality, in three stages, adding no harmful minerals to the water. Softened water is a no-no as a beverage, for cooking, and even for any prolonged showering or bathing. *Think of the ABCD of intelligent water intake, which should be*:
    Appropriate water for
    Bathing
    Cooking
    Drinking

Eliminating fluoride: putting appropriate four-stage filters to drinking, cooking and bathing water.

Avoiding cosmetics you don't absolutely need, because almost all of them contain substances that cause free radical damage. You will be surprised that it is quite easy to live without soaps, deodorants, toothpastes, creams and lotions. It is imperative to remember that skin is the largest absorptive organ of the body. Vanishing creams don't vanish, they soak in and go into your blood. Most are based on petroleum products, and you might as well take a bath in kerosene!

SKIN IS THE LARGEST ABSORPTIVE ORGAN OF THE BODY

Taking good care of your hair, using natural products if possible. Add color, fullness, shine. Avoid perms, if possible, all those chemicals cause further tissue damage if you are sensitive.

Consider electrolysis, plastic surgery, laser therapies, dental cosmetics. You repaint your walls and refinish your furniture, why should your body not deserve the same care? Looking great makes you feel good and active

THE ORIENTAL WAYS

Oriental medicine may not be for everybody, but it is enlightening to understand that there are other ways to look at illness and health, not only ours. That is why I will explore certain concepts in Chinese medicine, if only briefly. I am not either affirming or denying that the statements that follow are unquestionably correct, only offering them for information.[Y010]

According to Chinese medicine, there are five **Yin** organs which are considered the most important for our health and longevity...all of these five organs are mutually interrelated..." These organs are

- Heart
- Kidneys
- Liver
- Lungs
- Spleen

"Whenever any of these five organs is not functioning properly, sickness or even death can occur. Whenever there is a problem with one, the others are always involved too."

Chinese believe in the existence of "vital energy" or **Qi**. Qi deficiency, they say, is responsible for many problems. Low Qi can be caused by emotional depression and sadness, which can lead the Qi inward and make the body Yin. This deprives the outer body of Qi. When this happens, you will generally feel cold. If the problem persists for a long time, the muscles and tendons will be affected by the lack of Qi, and the joints will be weakened. Qi deficiency can have other causes, such as the weather. For example, your body's Qi is more deficient in the winter. Qi deficiency can also be caused by working for prolonged periods in a damp area, or by exposing your joints to the cold.

Some forms of disease are caused by defective genes, either acquired during life or inherited from one's parents. According to Chinese medicine, "the genes are considered the essence of your being. This essence is responsible for the production of hormones, from which Qi is generated. When this Qi is led to the brain, the spirit is raised. When all of these conversion processes are functioning normally, the immune system is strong and sickness is less likely."

Injuries, even if not serious may have significant results, the Qi imbalance can cause problems such as arthritis. When you are old, the Qi level in your body is low. Since your system is being deprived of the required amount of Qi, it starts to degenerate. One may learn how to slow down the aging process by building up the Qi in the body.

Stress includes both mental tension and physical tension, which are related and cannot be separated. Constant mental and physical tension increases pressure on joints. For example, some people are very tense and grind their teeth in their sleep, which can cause arthritis in the jaw. A lot of body tension is caused by the emotional disturbance which is related to your mental reaction to stressful events, an will decrease blood flow and nutrition of tissues, which may result in worsened osteoporosis.

Western medicine has found that the same treatment will not work equally well on all patients. Therefore, however alien and new to our way of thinking, I do not automatically brush off some of the treatment methods I discuss. After all, Western medicine is only in its infancy, and it may come to understand and accept these alternative remedies.

DIET

People who are experienced in Qigong have always considered food to be a significant influence on the condition of the Qi in the body. For this reason, diet is one of the main concerns of Chinese medicine. There is a well known saying: "You are what you eat." It is well known that improper diet is one of the main causes of acute episodes of gouty arthritis. The Chinese have found many different herbs that can ease the pain and reduce the swelling of arthritis. It has recently been discovered that protein, calories, and fats can reduce the inflammation of arthritis. Certain fish oils may interfere with the process of inflammation and therefore reduce the symptoms of rheumatoid arthritis.[U081][U091] Many individuals with osteoporosis also are sufferers of arthritis, and need all the help they can get.

CHANGE OF RESIDENCE

Since the Qi in your environment can affect the Qi in your body, arthritis sufferers should give serious consideration to this method. If the climate where you live is too damp or too cold, it may be affecting your arthritis. It has recently been discovered that the Qi in our bodies can be significantly affected by the electromagnetic fields generated by modern technology, and therefore cause some forms of cancer. For example, people who live near high tension power lines tend to get leukemias more often than those who do not. Perhaps similar environmental effects on arthritis will be found.

CHANGE OF LIFESTYLE:

Your lifestyle affects how the Qi circulates in your body. If you frequently feel ill, especially mentally, you might need to change your lifestyle. How you think and how you coordinate the Qi pattern in your body with the natural Qi is very important for your health. Whenever your Qi circulation is against the "Dao" (nature), you will be sick. You may find that walking for an hour or doing Qigong exercises every morning improves your Qi circulation.

CLOTHING

What you wear also affects the Qi in your body. In the winter you must stay warm, and especially protect your joints. Joints that are left unprotected can loose Qi very quickly.

It has been discovered that many man-made fibers can adversely affect the Qi distribution and circulation in the body. For example, polyester is known to cause Qi stagnation, and to prevent the body's Qi from exchanging with the environmental Qi. You may have noticed that clothing made of polyester can accumulate a considerable charge of static electricity in the winter. This builds up an electromagnetic field and affects the Qi circulation in your body.

SEXUAL ACTIVITY

Do you remember the admonition of the sixties: "Make love, not war!" Nothing more natural or healthy. There are many wonderful ways of improving the condition of body aches and pains. For example, it is reported that sexual activity can stimulate the adrenal glands to produce more corticosteroid, a hormone that reduces joint inflammation and pain. It is believed that sexual activity may also trigger the release of endorphins, a naturally occurring painkilling substance.[U080]

ACUPUNCTURE

Acupuncture is a method of encouraging the body to promote natural healing and to improve functioning. This is done by inserting needles and applying heat or electrical stimulation at very precise acupuncture points.

The classical Chinese explanation is that *channels of energy* run in regular patterns through the body and over its surface. These "channels", called *meridians*, are like currents flowing through the body, but are not always identical to the paths of blood flow and nerves. An obstruction in the movement of these energy rivers would act as a dam that backs up the flow in one part of the body and restricts it in others. Any obstruction and blockages or deficiencies of energy, blood and nervous pulses would eventually lead to disease.

Within this paradigm, it is asserted that the meridians can be influenced by *needling* the acupuncture points: the acupuncture needles unblock the obstruction at the dams, and reestablish the regular flow through the medians. Acupuncture treatments can therefore help the body's internal organs to correct imbalances in their digestion, absorption, and energy production activities, and in the circulation of their energy through the meridians.

Modern science explains the functions of acupuncture in 2 major ways:

Needling the acupuncture points stimulates the nervous system to release chemicals in the muscles, spinal cord, and brain. These chemicals will either change the experience of pain, or they will trigger the release of other chemicals and hormones which influence the body's own internal regulating system.

In traditional Chinese medicine *YIN* represents "-" (negative) and *YANG* represents "+" (positive). The main principle of Chinese medicine is to keep the YIN and YANG balance or bring YIN and YANG back to balance. YIN/YANG balance is the healthy state of the body. Modern science reveals that the very basic unit of the body is cell. Cells' movement follow the movement of electrons. The electrons inside cells act according to its own regular patterns. We call all these electrons in the living body bioelectrons.

Energy flow in the meridians is the direct or indirect transportation of bioelectrons. Meridians are the pathways where bioelectons move more frequently than other parts of the body. When positive and negative charges in the bioelectronic movements are not balanced, the cells would act abnormally — this is YIN and YANG imbalance. In Chinese medicine it is defined as "disease". It is a beginning stage of the physiological cells electrons movement. Only radical change of cell electron movement is admitted by Western medicine as "disease".

All the external factors, such as mechanical, physical, chemical, biological and internal factors such as mental, hereditary, constitutional can cause and force the body's bioelectrical movement into imbalances which would lead to disease.

BIOELECTRICAL MOVEMENT IMBALANCES HAVE VARIOUS CAUSES:

EXTERNAL	INTERNAL
mechanical	mental
physical	hereditary
chemical	constitutional
biological	

Acupuncture can force the bioelectrons to resume their normal and regular movement patterns, and YIN/YANG balance. The more acupuncture treatments the patient have, the longer the normal movement pattern of the bioelectrons can remain, until finally the electrons inside cells would not follow the abnormal movement pattern any more. Only at this point the problem can be deemed as solved and treated completely.[S100]

MORE ABOUT ACUPUNCTURE

Various cells including nerve cells (*neurons*), *embrionic* [from the unborn being] muscle cells (*myoblasts*) and embryonic connective tissue cells (*fibroblasts*) are sensitive to electric fields of physiological strength.[E049] Somite (embryonic body segment) fibroblasts move forward the negative (-) pole AT a very low voltage.[M110] Calcium flow is essential to acupuncture, results can be altered by using calcium channel blockers and calcium binders (chelators).[C131] In most cases, there is enhanced cell growth toward cathode (-) and reduced cell growth toward anode (+) in small, continuous, pulsed or focal electric fields.[M080 N100] Some fast growing tissues, particularly tumors, are electrically negative in polarity. If a current from positive pole is applied over a certain tumor, its growth can show significant retardation or even regression.[B060] This is consistent with the fact that the fluorescent dye *rhodamine* 123, which has a delocalized positive charge, binds preferentially to some cancer cells and inhibits the cell growth. [E140] [C060] [emphasis added]

Changes in limbs of frogs, for instance, can be preceded by a change in electric activity at the growth or organizing center several days before growth begins.

The distribution of organizing centers, acupuncture points and singular points in electric fields are closely related to the shape of the organism. For example, the ear lobe, which has no major nerves or blood vessels but has the most complex surface morphology, also has the highest density of acupuncture points. Many organizing centers are at the extreme points of curvature on body surface, i.e. the locally most convex or concave points.

A principle in electroacupuncture therapy is that positive pulse stimulation of a point sedates its corresponding function while negative pulse stimulation tonifies the function.[K081] This is analogous to the fact that cell growth is enhanced toward cathode and reduced toward anode in a pulsed electric field, in consistence with the model that the mechanism underlying acupuncture is similar to that of growth control.

Research on acupuncture, particularly the **endorphin** (internal morphine and opiate-like pain killers) effect of acupuncture analgesia and its blockage by **naloxone**, a drug which counteracts morphine and opiates, clearly shows that some effect of acupuncture is mediated through the nervous system.[P069] [emphasis added]

Satisfactory therapeutic effects were achieved in 116 cases with prolapse of lumbar intervertebral disc treated with non-surgical therapy. A very interesting discussion of traditional Chinese approaches can be obtained from the internet, at Non-Surgical Therapy For Prolapse of Lumbar Intervertebral Disc.[H090]

Not only do people with disc disease get treated with standard surgery, but they can receive a replacement disc (kinematic disc prosthesis model (SB Charite); this is considered "the best disc replacement compromise, and is the basis of the evolution of the prosthetic concept at the dawning of the year 2000. Clinical results of a homogeneous series of 105 cases with a mean follow-up of 51 months show 79% of the patients had an excellent result and 87% returned to work. Radiologically, these results correlated with restoration of a well balanced lordosis and with segmental mobility." But failure can occur if the patient also suffers from "posterior *facet* [small joints on the spine] arthritis, osteoporosis, structural deformities, and secondary facet pain."[L060]

WHAT IS CRANIAL ELECTROTHERAPY STIMULATION?
Cranial Electrotherapy Stimulation (*CES*) is the application of low-level pulsed electrical currents (usually less than 1 milliampere) applied to the head for medical and/or psychological purposes. There is now over 20 years of medical experience with CES in America. Presently, its use requires a prescription by a licensed health practitioner in the U.S. It is available without a prescription throughout the rest of the world.

Cranial electrotherapy stimulation has also been known by many other names:
- *Alpha sleep*
- *Electroanalgesia*
- *Electronarcosis*
- *Electrosleep* (the original name)
- *Neuroelectric therapy* (*NET*)
- *Transcranial electrotherapy* (*TCET*)

Cranial electrotherapy stimulation was first called electrosleep because it was thought to induce sleep. Most of the initial research was done in Russia. American human experiments were performed at the University of Texas Medical School in San Antonio, the University of Mississippi Student Counseling Center and the University of Wisconsin Medical School.

It has many indications, *chronic pain* being one of the most important ones.

"Cranial electrotherapy stimulation devices are generally similar in size and appearance to standard transcutaneous electrical nerve stimulators (TENS), but produce very different wave-forms. Standard milliampere-current TENS devices must never be applied transcranially. CES electrodes can be placed **bitemporally**, bilaterally in the hollow behind the ears just anterior to the mastoid processes, or clipped to the earlobes. This depends on the device being used.... No adverse effects or contraindications have been found from the use of CES, either in the U.S. or in other parts of the world. As with all electrical devices, caution is advised during pregnancy and for patients with a demand-type pacemaker. In addition, it is recommended that patients not operate complex machinery or drive automobiles during and shortly after a CES treatment."

Since we know that pain is a complex process involving the brain, it makes sense to add CES to the treatment of most pain patients. In fact, in many cases it is all that is needed to produce significant long-term pain relief. Cranial electrotherapy stimulation is believed to stimulate the production of **endorphins** (internally produced morphine). It probably also affects certain nerve centers: the **hypothalamus** causing changes in the hypothalamic neurohormonal regulatory mechanisms and the **reticular formation** of the brain stem.

"Immediately after a CES treatment, patients usually report feeling more relaxed. Some people feel somewhat inebriated for the first few minutes. This is a pleasant and very comfortable sensation. After several minutes to hours, the light-headed feelings usually disappear, the relaxed state remains and a profound sense of alertness is achieved. This relaxed/alert state will usually remain for an average of 12 to 72 hours after the first few treatments and then becomes cumulative from a series of treatments.

"Most patients relate feeling more relaxed, less distressed, while their minds remain alert and even more focused on mental tasks. They generally sleep better and report improved concentration along with heightened states of general well-being."[U092]

The manufacturers recommend not to confuse this device with *EMR* (*electro-magnetic radiation*) producing devices!

WHAT IS T.E.N.S.?

Transcutaneous Electrical Nerve Stimulation (T.E.N.S.) has been used for many years in the symptomatic relief and management of chronic, intractable pain, with great success. It has also been a tool in the management of post surgical and post-traumatic acute pain conditions.

"T.E.N.S. relieves pain by sending small, electrical impulses through electrodes placed on the skin to underlying nerve fibers. These fibers carry sensations such as touch, warmth, pressure and pain. T.E.N.S. can replace pain impressions from these fibers with a massage like sensation."

"Traditionally, drugs have been the primary means of controlling pain because they are simple, effective and in most cases, safe. However, there are many patients who are less tolerant of drugs and they may experience potentially harmful side effects, such as constipation, dizziness, nausea or depressed respiration[;] and there may also be the risk of addiction.

"T.E.N.S. is a safe, non invasive, drug-free medically proven method of pain management. T.E.N.S. may relieve pain from the following conditions:"[U092]

- Arthritis
- Back pain
- Carpal tunnel
- Fibromylagia
- Muscle tension or pain
- RSI

Osteoporosis often combines back and muscle tension pain.

SPINAL CORD STIMULATION (SCS)

Spinal cord stimulation (*SCS*) is an often very successful modality for the treatment of patients with low back and leg pain, some of which may be due to osteoporosis, osteoporotic fractures and nerve root problems. Pain relief will occur in up to 66% of patients, and they may each have up to a 75% improvement.[M140]

MASSAGE

Massage is a traditional therapy which consists in the kneading, rubbing, rolling and pressing of tissues done manually or with appropriate equipment. It is often done to alleviate the back pain associated to osteoporosis with, or without lumbar disc problems. The movement is often from above downward along both sides of the spinal column to relax the lumbar muscles. Massage and traction can:

- Eliminate the adhesive inflammation of the soft tissue surrounding the *nerve root* (the beginning part of the nerve where it comes out of the spine)
- Enlarge the *intervertebral space* (the gap between the vertebrae)
- Enlarge the *dural* capsule (the fibrous membranes around the spine and brain) and intervertebral foramen, thus a negative pressure is produced in the intervertebral space, that facilitates the replacement of intervertebral disc
- Lay a foundation for further manipulation
- Mechanically replace a prolapsed intervertebral disc to its original position
- Relax the spastic lumbar muscles
- Stretch the posterior longitudinal ligament and transverse ligament of the *fibrous ring* (a band that holds discs in place) to correct the lateral bending and posterior protruding abnormalities of the vertebral column

In some cases with short disease course, where severe symptoms make the general maneuver intolerable, specially qualified therapists believe that the manipulation can be performed under *extradural* anesthesia (a form of spinal anesthesia), or lumbar anesthesia. The lumbar muscular spasm should be fully relaxed, and the intervertebral space enlarged, so as to facilitate replacement of the prolapsed intervertebral disc, loose the nerve root adhesion, change the relation between the nerve root and prolapsed disc, restore the normal dynamic balance of vertebral column, and relieve or eliminate the clinical symptoms. However, violently forceful maneuvers which may induce medically caused (*iatrogenic*) injury should be avoided.

Massage is commonly contraindicated for certain types of patients, but opinions on this subjects often differ:
- Senile patients
- Patients with cardiovascular diseases
- Patients with central prolapse of the disc
- Patients with significant bony proliferation or calcification of the prolapse
- Patients who have a prolonged disease course and have been treated many times without satisfactory therapeutic results and with frequent recurrences.

A dear, wonderful chiropractor I know, who often, and very rapidly got me out of spasms and postural problems, uses verbal coaxing to entice my body to adjust itself. He talks to the body... — "Tell her to stretch, to balance itself" — ...And it works! He is using a form of *ideokinetic* imagery and flexibility. Ideokinetic imagery is a postural development technique that involves using movement images to gain subcortical control over the spinal musculature. If you add sit-ups so as to combine this with abdominal strength training, it is a wonderful method for improving the spinal angles of lordosis and kyphosis and reducing low back pain.

Experimental investigations prove the effectiveness of these treatments for low back pain. Findings indicated that ideokinetic imagery had a positive effect on the spinal column and low back pain. Spinal angles improve significantly, there often is complete cessation of low back pain. Ideokinetic imagery is an inexpensive and noninvasive technique to improve poor posture and alignment.

PROTECTIVE MEASURES AGAINST FALLING
"Assuming that a large proportion of osteoporotic fractures are a consequence of traumatic falls, and are not spontaneous due to osseous weakness, preventive measures in elderly people are best directed to...."[G030]
- Avoid over-treating hypertension (danger of *orthostatic hypotension*, a sudden drop in blood pressure when changing from a lying or recumbent, to an upright position)

- Avoid unnecessary *hypnotics* and *tranquilizers* (pills to make you calm and sleepy, which can cause dizziness and/or confusion)
- Correct visual impairments
- Counteract muscular weakness (exercise strengthens muscles, improves circulation, has a positive effect on agility and reflexes)
- Guard against unnecessary obstacles in the home (clutter is very dangerous, causing falls or slips. Beware of throw rugs!)
- Improve agility (makes getting around easier)

PREVENTING FALLS

Strategies to prevent falls are important in elderly patients who may fall frequently for a variety of reasons, such as from the effects of drugs. Specific environmental interventions can minimize home hazards that increase the chances of falling. The maintenance of a good level of physical activity during the earlier part of life is associated with better balance and less falls at an old age.

Osteoporotic patients with fractures or breaks should recognize the benefits of rapid return to function and avoidance of prolonged immobilization.

"Although falls are a major factor in the occurrence of femoral neck fractures, fall types and frequency have not been studied in detail. A few case-reports have demonstrated that *bone insufficiency* can lead to *femoral neck fracture* and that some falls occur as a result of acute pain *preceding* the fracture...femoral neck fractures due to bone insufficiency have ranged from 3% to 24%." [emphasis added] [M070]

Do people actually fall from a standing position as they break their hip? Some do, but these falls often have some early warnings:
- 5.9% experienced acute pain before the fall
- 9.8% reported trivial trauma before the break
- 15.7 reported no trauma before the break
- 45.5% had hip pain during the weeks preceding the fracture, more often than not only in the hip that was subsequently fractured

Spontaneous fracture (no fall) was preceded by the following symptoms in the hip:
- Gradually worsening pain
- Pain during the preceding weeks

- Pain in the inguinal or *crural* area
- Recent onset of pain, less than 3 months

The most important step in dealing with fractures in osteoporotic patients, is to prevent injuries.

PREVENTION OF OSTEOPOROSIS

From a financial point of view, osteoporosis is a medical, social and economical problem in developed countries. Prevention of the harm caused by bone loss remains the only realistic approach to effect a reduction in the burden related to this disorder. Primary prevention of osteoporosis is based on efforts to reach a maximal peak bone mass at the end of the growth period and, subsequently, at the time of menopause.[R030] [emphasis added]

In comparing several of the available options, researchers in Belgium considered that a systematic screening of asymptomatic post-menopausal women followed by the induction of hormonal replacement therapy in high risk subjects appears to be an interesting cost/benefit strategy in terms of reasonable attribution of health resources. They reached this decision after comparing this approach to the other well known treatments, such as nasal administration of calcitonin and bisphosphonates, and *experimental estrogen receptor modulators*, not on the market yet.

The likelihood of developing osteoporosis can be reduced by improving one's lifestyle:

- Adequate nutrient intake
- Appropriate physical activity
- Estrogen replacement in postmenopausal women
- Limiting alcohol and cigarette consumption
- Plenty of sunshine
- Weight-bearing exercises, such as walking or playing tennis

Many of these issues have generated major research efforts and considerable controversy. *Establishment* medicine feels that despite our vast body of knowledge, there is great need for additional research on understanding the biology of human bone, defining individuals at special risk, and developing safe, effective, low-cost strategies for fracture prevention.

Alternative medicine, not shackled by big money constraints, such as patentability of products and corporate wars, on the other hand, looks at those who are having problems in the present, confident that the techniques it uses are effective and appropriate in "the here and now", and can solve problems *today*, not at an uncertain future date.

CALCIUM AND ESTROGENS:
THE (ALMOST) WINNING COMBINATION

Ultimately a combination of calcium and estrogens appears to be the winning formula.

In a Japanese study performed at the Osaka University, post-menopausal and elderly women were treated either with calcium (lactate), by itself, or with calcium and *estriol*. The test was continued for 10 months. At the end, when *before* and *after* measurements of bone density in the lumbar vertebrae of the test subjects were compared with each other, there was no doubt that only the group receiving the additional estrogens did well. Half of the calcium...[only] groups actually lost bone mass![N080] [emphasis added] The alternatives, as seen by this author, do not disagree, they simply offer easy to obtain plant or ovary derived estrogens which are ubiquitous in nature, and available to the public.

**ONLY CALCIUM ACCOMPANIED BY ESTROGENS
INCREASES BONE MASS**

HGH (HUMAN GROWTH HORMONE) THE SUPREME APPROACH

At a time when it is almost impossible to secure growth hormone for the treatment of severe growth hormone deficiency, it is premature to consider the administration of this substance as a routine preventative. However, we can envision times when this may be a reality, and for those fortunate to be able to defy the restrictions and discrimination of insurance companies, the therapies are available in selected centers outside the US.

ULTIMATE PREVENTION OF OSTEOPOROSIS (SUMMING UP)

DO NOT
- Eat packaged, artificial, processed and devitalized foods
- Smoke or use tobacco products

- Drink alcoholic beverages excepting sparingly
- Drink coffee excepting sparingly
- Drink sodas, excepting sparingly
- Take medications, if you can correct problems nutritionally and naturally
- Become a couch potato
- Let yourself run low on estrogen for many years before correcting the deficiency
- Miss out on sunshine

DO

- Drink alcohol only in moderation
- Drink caffeine only in moderation
- Avoid tobacco
- Keep a positive calcium intake all of your life
- Consider HRT and discuss it with your doctor if you are going to use prescription medication
- Do demand supporting information about any endorsements of extraneous stuff such as progesterone, etc.

WHAT WAS MY PREVENTION PROGRAM WHEN I WAS IN PRACTICE?

All people are different, having individualized metabolisms and chemistries, lifestyles and activity levels. No fixed rules are possible. However, certain basics work for almost anybody. I used to recommend:

ENVIRONMENT:

Should be kept clean and cheerful, avoiding any unnecessary chemicals, dust, allergens, particles, bacteria, etc. Abundant light and plenty sunshine, unbridled by sun screening products (unless the patient is of Scottish-Irish-German-Welsh descent, and has a congenital deficiency of PABA in his/her skin. Avoidance of "electrically contaminated" rooms: minimizing fuse-boxes, equipment, even clock radios and wiring in and around the area where the person lives. In polluted inner cities live in high-rise buildings, "far from the madding crowd". In suburbia, avoid highly transited spots. Watch open fireplaces (gas or wood), they soil the air if not well vented. If allergic, avoid carpeting, waxes, polishes, preferable use a water-filtered vacuum cleaner (the advantages are well worth the investment)*.

NUTRITION IN GENERAL:
What were my recommendations when I was in practice?

FIRST: READ LABELS!
Avoid additives, even if those additives are commercially used vitamins and minerals. Beware of "enriched" foods. Original, quality foods do not need any enriching. Some products out there actually have no additives, excepting potential contaminants acquired during their growing period.

A varied diet with clean water, good quality protein, abundant fruits, vegetables, grains and animal products.

Water should generally be purified, few waters are reliable. Purifiers should be three stage devices, less stages produce filtered waters of unreliable quality.

Fruits should be whole fruits. Juices, which compress the sugar, water and vitamins of several fruits into one glass, are hidden sources of excess calories, and should be considered a treat, not a beverage.

Vegetables must be eaten in balance with proteinaceous food. Excess fiber can cause worsening of osteoporosis. Green vegetables and products high in fiber, such as whole grains, may deplete minerals. Juices may be appropriate in deficiency states, or as a cleansing device, but may be too concentrated for many. Some juices, such as carrot, have as much sugar as certain fruits.

Sugar, sweets, dry fruit, only sparingly: excesses affect calcium metabolism adversely.

Dairy products should preferably be non-pasteurized, non-homogenized. One must realize that milk is contaminated with environmental pollutants, vitamin D, synthetic growth hormone, all of which may both help and hurt the osteoporotic patient, depending on dosage. One glass of milk a day appears to be a must for a healthy bone structure, particularly if coffee or tea are drunk.

Meats should be quality, lean, preferably from non-hormonized, un-drugged, un-vaccinated cattle. All fat should be trimmed off. In baked meats, cook them slowly, so that fat melts and is removed. Meat should never be ground meat that has oxidized. If you must grind it, select a clean, non fat piece such as sirloin, and grind it before use.

Be sure to add soy products, especially fermented soy products to your diet.

BEWARE OF HIDDEN TOXINS IN COSMETICS: when in doubt, do not use. Lotions and soaps should *never* contain mineral oils. Remember that rubbing alcohol is also toxic. Beware of anti-wrinkle creams. Do not use progressive hair colorings.

SUPPLEMENTS

Secure a good supply of vitamins and minerals. Remember that there are natural ovary preparations, and that if your estrogen is low you must replace it, either from soy, ovary or even prescription, if you do not have a choice.

Some of these supplements may be on your "to buy" list. Principally, vitamin C, multi-vitamins, raw glandulars (ovary, testicle—male—and/or thyroid). The amounts you may want to use are your decision, or by recommendation of your health practitioner.

A 25.000 (<u>not</u> beta-carotene)	EPA (marine lipids) (prevents clotting)
ACIDOPHILUS	GARLIC PILLS
B2	GENISTEIN
B3-NIACIN 250 TIMED RELEASE	GLUTAMINE
B5-PANTOTHENIC ACID 500 MG.	LECITHIN
B6-PYRIDOXINE 100	LITHIUM CHELATED
BORON	MOLYBDENUM
B12 sublingual	MULTIMINERALS IN
	MEGADOSE
B COMPLEX 100	POTASSIUM 99
C POWDER 5000 MG/CC	RAW FEMALE
C 1000 TABLETS	RAW MALE
	(ORCHIC AND PROSTATIC)

CALCIUM & MAGNESIUM
   GLUCONATE
CARNITINE
CHROMIUM 500
Co-Q-10
DHEA
DLPA 750
E 400
ENZYMATIC DIGESTANT

RAW THYMUS
RAW THYROID
SAW PALMETTO HERB
SELENIUM
SHARK CARTILAGE
TRACE ELEMENTS
VITAMIN D
ZINC

Seek help with physical and electric medicine: chiropractors, acupuncturists, energy machines, etc.

Sleep soundly, exercise regularly.
Remember, Love! God Loves You!

GLOSSARY

1,25-dihydroxylcholecalciferol: a form of vitamin D

1,25 dihydroxy-vitamin D: Rocaltrol®

16 alpha-hydroxyestrone: 16 alpha-OHE1, breakdown product of estrogen

16 alpha-OHE1: breakdown product of estrogen

17-beta-estradiol: a form of estrogen

25-hydroxycholecalciferol: a form of vitamin D

7-dehydrocholesterol: a form of cholesterol

acacia: a tree which supplies a gum used in pharmaceuticals

acetaminophen: generic Tylenol

acetylcholine: a neuro-transmitter

acetylsalicylic acid: aspirin

acid: a molecule, such as battery or stomach acid, which contains the chemical group COOH, and turns the litmus paper to the lower pHs

acidophilus bacteria: friendly bacteria of the colon

ACTH: adreno-cortico-tropic hormone, a pituitary hormone which induces the formation of adrenal hormones

activated ergo-calciferol: D2, the major synthetic form of provitamin D

active principle: the specific drug in a medicine product

acupuncture: a method of natural healing by inserting needles and applying heat or electrical stimulation at very precise acupuncture points

acupuncture points: specific locations on the body that are centers of electric energy

acutane, retin-a: an acne medication which was taken off the market because of its side effects

adaptogen: substance which helps the body adapt to stress

ADFR: a complex system of several drugs to attempt to treat osteoporosis

adrenal hormones: hormonal secretions of the adrenal glands above the kidney: cortisone, adrenalin, etc.

ageusia: inability to taste

agranulocytosis: deficiency of neutrophils, a type of white blood cell

albumin: a part of the body proteins

aldehyde: dehydrogenated alcohol, any of various highly reactive compounds characterized by the group CHO

alendronate, alendronate sodium: a non-hormonal drug for osteoporotic bone

alkali: turns litmus paper to higher numbers, substances which neutralize acids, such as baking soda

alkaline phosphatase: an enzyme related to bone metabolism

Alkphase-B®: a monoclonal antibody test for measuring bone alkaline phosphatase

Allium sativum L. single clove variety: garlic

alloy: a metal combination

allyl: isopropyl

Alopecia: baldness, hair loss

Alpha-methyl-proline: a methylated amino acid

alpha-tocopherol: a form of vitamin E

alpha 1-blockers: drugs that are relatively contraindicated in elderly patients with hypertension

ALT: a common liver function test.

alternative: applied to medicine, non-drug, non invasive orientation

aluminum: a metal that is very abundant and light aluminum hydrochloride: product used to keep moisture out of packaged goods; an antiperspirant

AMA: American Medical Association

amalgam fillings: dental silver fillings, the most important source of mercury exposure in the general population

amino-acids: chemicals containing an amino and an acid group, components of proteins

aminoglycosides: certain antibiotics

anabolic: protein building

anabolism: protein buildup

anaphylaxis: severe allergic reaction

androgens: male hormones

androstenedione: a male type hormone of the adrenals

angiogenesis: formation of new blood vessels

anhydrous: dehydrated

anion: an ion which is negatively charged, which has gained one or more electrons

anosmia: inability to smell

methionine: a sulphur containing amino acid

acetaldehyde: a toxin resulting from the metabolism of alcohol in drinkers and cigarette smokers

antacid: a medication to reduce stomach acid

antibodies: substances generated in the body in response to an antigen anticonvulsant: medication which controls seizures

antigen: can induce the production of a binding chemical which can fit the antigen as a key fits a lock

antioxidants: substances which fight against biologic rusting

antipyresis: fever control through action on the mid-brain heat-regulating center

antiresorptive Therapy: treatment against bone destruction

6-Glucose-monophosphte-dehydrogenase or 6-gmpd: an enzyme that may exist in anomalous forms (isoenzymes)

Arginine: amino acid

arrhythmia: irregular heart rhythm

arsenic: environmental toxin

artificial fluoridation: addition of fluoride to public water supply

ASA: Acetyl-Salycilic-Acid, aspirin

ascorbates: vitamin C salts

ascorbic acid: a water soluble vitamin that has anti-oxidant activity

aspartates: salts of aspartic acid

asthma: lung disease with narrowing of bronchial tubes and wheezing

barium chloride,"barii chloridum", BaCl2.2H2O: a barium salt

barium sulphate BaSO4: insoluble salt, and used for body imaging

barium sulphide BaS: barium salt, was used as a hair remover

baroreceptor: pressure receptor

BB, bb, or Bb: names of different types of VDRs

beclomethasone: a substance frequently contained in inhaled corticosteroids

beta-blockers: a family of cardiovascular medicines

beta carotene: a pro-vitamin A

beta endorphin: a naturally occurring chemical which resembles opiates, which induces a sense of well-being, released by the pituitary into the brain

betadine: iodine containing antiseptic

BGH: Recombinant Bovine Growth Hormoner—a genetically engineered drug

BHA (butylated hydroxyanisole): synthetic antioxidant

BHT (butylated hydoxytoluene): synthetic antioxidant

bilateral oophorectomy: removal of both ovaries

bile: secretion from the gall-bladder

bio-available: absorbable into the body

bioavailability: the percentage at which the body can soak up a substance

biochemical markers: chemicals which indicate a certain biologic process has taken place, and can be tested in the lab

bioflavonoids: companion substances to vitamin C

biotin: a water-soluble vitamin and member of the B-complex family.

bismuth: mineral

bisphosphonates (Fosamax® alendronate): osteoporosis drugs

bithionol: antiparasitic drug

bone alkaline phosphatase: an enzyme found on the surface of osteoblasts

Bone Paste, Norian SRS®Skeletal Repair System: a kind of bone glue or fixer

boron: mineral

bradycardia: slow heart rate

brittle bone disease: osteoporosis
bronchospasm: narrowing of bronchial tubes
BST-Recombinant Bovine Somatotropine: a genetically engineered substance that causes growth and fattening of animals
buffered: a solution, chemically arranged to always remain at a proper pH
bullous rash: rash with blistering
butylated hydoxytoluene (BHT): synthetic antioxidant
butylated hydroxyanisole (BHA): synthetic antioxidant
cadmium: bluish-white metallic element
caffeine: alkaloid from coffee and other plants
calciferol: a form of vitamin D
calcimar: a non-hormonal drug to treat osteoporosis
calcitonin: a hormone secreted by the thyroid gland in mammals, by the ultimobranchial gland of birds and fish
calcitonin-salmon: a fish hormone used to treat osteoporosis
calcitriol: 1,25(OH)2-vitamin D3, natural vitamin D
calcium ascorbate: a buffered, less acidic form of vitamin C
calcium carbonate: an inorganic form of calcium
calcium lactate: a chelated calcium
cancer induction: "sowing the seed", introducing the cancer gene or oncogene
cancer promotion: activating the "expression" of the cancer gene
carbonates: salts of carbonic acid
carboxy: a chemical group, carbon monoxide
carcinogenesis: cancer causation
carcinogenicity: Ability to cause cancer
carcinogens: cancer-causing substances
cardiovascular failure: weak heart
carnauba wax: filler for pharmaceutical products
carotenoid: precursors of vitamin A
propyl gallate: synthetic antioxidant
castration: removal of the ovaries or testicles
catabolism: protein breakdown
catalase: red blood cell enzyme that breaks down hydrogen peroxide
cation: an ion with a positive electrical charge, which has lost one or more electrons
cells: each one of the small units of which tissues are built
cellulose: substance used to make paper and filler of medications and tablets
centrally acting blood pressure agents: blood pressure medicines such as reserpine, methyldopa and clonidine
cerebrospinal: elating to the brain and spine
chelates: molecules of an amino acid binding to a metal
chelation therapy: cleansing of toxins and plaque through an amino acid
chemotherapeutic agents: cancer treatment which stop cell growth
chloasma: brown spots on the face, upper lip, mid line of abdomen, more noticeable in people with darker skin pigment
chlorofluorocarbon: propellant
chloroform: anesthetic
chlorophyll: the green pigment of plants
chloruresis: the elimination of chloride through urine
cholecalciferol: vitamin D3, found in animals, mainly in fish liver oils
choline: a substance which is a precursor of acetylcholine, a
neurotransmitter
chondrocytes: cells which form cartilage
chorea: St. Vitus's Dance
chromium picolinate: an insulin-sensitizing chelate of chromium and picolinic acid, a nutrient
dehydroepiandrosterone-sulfate: DHEA, anabolic hormone
cimetidine: acid suppressor

citrate: salts of citric acid and minerals
citric acid: acid contained in fruits
clear cell vaginal cancer: a type of cancer
clitoromegaly: enlarged clitoris
clonidine: an medication
co-enzyme Q: an enzyme which helps regulate the rhythm of the heart
cobalt: a mineral
coenzyme: a factor which assists the action of an enzyme
collagen: a gelatinous, gristle type substance, that derives its name from the Latin colla, glue
collagen type I: the major protein of bone matrix
colloidal minerals: a system of liquid and minerals in which the particles are of a size intermediate between a solution and a suspension
colostrum: the first secretion of the mother's breasts after giving birth
complete protein: proteins in which all essential amino-acids are present complex carbohydrates: starches, dextrines and maltoses
compton scattering: bone density study
computerized axial tomography: CAT scan, which can measure bone density in the spine
congestive heart failure: weakness of the heart causing the backing up of fluid
conjugated equine estrogen: estrogens from mares' urine
conjugated estrogens: pharmaceutical hormones
conjunctivitis: pink eye
conjunctivitis sicca: pink eye
connective tissue matrix: support or holding protein matter
copper: mineral
cortical bone: smooth and uniform bone, which forms the external envelope of the skeleton
cortisone: orticosteroid drug
coumarin: blood thinner
cresol: antiseptic, a constituent of lemon flavoring
carnitine: an amino acid, normal component of animal protein
croscarmellose Sodium: additive to some medications
cross-linking: a braiding arrangement of the collagen fibers in bone
cross-links: braids or arrangements of the collagen fibers in bone
cortical bone: Compact surface bone, which appears smooth and uniform, it forms the external envelope of the skeleton
crural: inguinal
cushing's syndrome: a condition where the adrenal glands overproduce cortisone
cyanide: poison
cyclophosphamide: pesticide
Cycrin® 2.5mg: medroxyprogesterone
cysteine: sulphur containing amino-acid
cytochrome oxidase: enzyme
cytochrome P-450: multi-function oxidase, helps detoxify petroleum distillates and other toxins
cytotoxin: toxic to cells at large D-alpha-tocopheryl succinate could completely improve the situation. Vitamin E can protect
D&C Red 2825 mg: industrial color D&C Red No. 27aluminum lake, dibasic calcium phosphate, FD&C Blue No. 1 aluminum lake, lactose anhydrous, magnesium
D&C Red No. 27aluminum lake: industrial color
D&C Yellow 10: industrial color D2 or activated ergo-calciferol, is the major synthetic form of provitamin D
D3: or cholecalciferol: "natural" vitamin D, is found in animals, mainly in fish liver oils
daidzein: soybean milk isoflavones
degraded: broken down chemically
delatestryl: Testosterone Enanthate Injection
deoxypyridinoline: bone chemical, derivative of lysine
depo-provera: a hormonal contraceptive found to cause innumerable side effects
DES: during pregnancy have an increased risk of clear cell vaginal cancer later in life

DHEA: dehydro-epi-androsterone
diaphysis: the shaft part of the bone
dibasic calcium phosphate: Salt of Calcium
Didronel®: a bisphosphonate drug
differentiation: in a cell, becoming more mature and less invasive
digestive enzymes: substances that help the digestive process
digitalis: a heart drug
dilantin: an anti-epileptic drug
Dimethyl Amino Ethanol (DMAE): is a nutritional supplement
DMAE: a nutritional supplement that supports the old wives' tale that fish is a great brain food.
direct antacids: unite directly with free acid in the stomach
diuretics: fluid medicines
delatestryl: Testosterone Enanthate Injection
endogenous: internally produced DNA the genetic material in the cell nucleus
dual-energy x-ray absorptiometry (DXA): bone density scanning machine dual photon densitometer, which measures the spine or hip bone
dural: relating to the fibrous membranes around the spine and brain
DXA: bone density scanning machine
Dyspnea: shortness of breath, difficulty breathing
ectopic calcification: abnormal locations of calcium deposits
eczema: weepy rash
edema: fluid retention, swelling
elastin: a chief component of elastic tissue
Electro Immuno Absorbency: a genetically engineered antibody test using electric currents
electron transport chains oxidases: NADPH, amino acids,
electrophoresis: a process that separates chemicals by running an electric current through a solution
ELISA: Electro Immuno Absorbency, a genetically engineered antibody test
ellagic acid: inhibits cytochrome p450-mediated activation of NMBA
endemic: prevalent most of the time
endogenous: internally produced
endometriosis: disease characterized by the proliferation of womb-lining cells in other tissues and organs, also known as chocolate cysts endorphin: internally produced morphine.
enterolactone:
ENZYMES: activators of chemical processes, without being part of the chemical process themselves
epiphyseal chondrocytes: cartilage forming cells from the heads of long bones epiphyseal growth plates: areas between the end of the shaft and the neck of the heads of the bones
epistaxis: nosebleed
equol: flavonoid
estrogen: hormone produced predominantly in the first half of the menstrual cycle
Erythema multiforme: rash of varied appearances
Erythema nodosum: rash that creates bumps under the skin
essential amino acids: they are not manufactured by the human body, and must be provided by food intake). They are eight in the adult, in children as many as ten of the amino-acids may qualify as essential.
establishment: the conventional wisdom in medicine
establishment medicine: AMA (American Medical Association) type medicine, focused on surgery and drugs
Estrace®: pharmaceutical estrogen
Estrace®: Estradiol Vaginal Cream: Usp, 0.01% is used in the treatment of vulval and vaginal atrophy in menopausal women with or without osteoporosis.
estradiol 2- hydroxylation: chemical process affecting estrogen estradiol form of estrogen
estradiol valerate: horse derived estrogen
estradiol valerate: form of estrogen
estriol: form of estrogen
estrogen-responsive tissues: tissues that react when stimulated by estrogen
estrogen 2-hydroxylase: enzyme which acts upon estrogen
estrogen is a female hormone that is primarily produced during the first half of the menstrual cycle

estrone: form of estrogen
ethanol: alcohol ethinyl estradiol: form of estrogen
ethyl acetate: a compound naturally found in many fruits, such as apples, peaches, and pears. It is used in a process to absorb the caffeine in decaffeinated coffee
Ethylene-diamino-tetraacetic acid (EDTA): a synthetic amino acid that scavenges — chelates undesirable minerals
ethylene vinyl acetate copolymers EVAC: plastic substance
exfoliative dermatitis: peeling condition of skin
F-344: Fischer 344, strain of laboratory rat
fatty acids are:
FD&C Blue 1: an industrial color
FD&C Blue No. 1: aluminum lake: an industrial color
FD&C Blue No. 1: an industrial color
FD&C Red 4025 mg: an industrial color
FD&C Yellow 6: an industrial color
FD&C Yellow No. 5: tartrazine, an industrial color
FD&C Yellow No. 5: an industrial color
Feng Shui: pronounced 'phong schway', part of an ancient Chinese philosophy of nature
FIA: a substance used in virology, the main component of which is mineral oil
fibrillar collagen: linear strands of collagen
fibroids: connective tissue tumors of the uterus
Fischer 344: strain of laboratory rat
folic acid: one of the B vitamin familial hyperlipidemia. Bone of the B-complex vitamins, follicle stimulating hormone (FSH)
follicular phase: first two weeks of the menstrual cycle
Fosamax®: a non-hormonal drug for osteoporotic bone
fracture: a break through the bone
free radical molecule: molecules which react destructively with others, causing the oxidizing of fats —lipid peroxidation —in cell membranes
free radicals: atoms or molecules which react destructively with others, causing the oxidizing of fats —lipid peroxidation —in cell membranes
Freund's incomplete adjuvant oil: a substance used in virology, the main component of which is mineral oil fructose, fruit sugar
adenosine triphosphate (ATP): energy substance
kinase enzymes: certain activating enzymes
tyrosine-phospho-kinase: certain activating enzymes
furosemide: a diuretic, also known as Lasix
GABA: gamma-amino-butiric-acid, a polyunsaturated fatty acid
gallium: a metal, liquid at room temperature
gastrin: a hormone which stimulates gastric acid secretion gastritis
genes: particles of genetic information
genistein: hormone like substance present in soy and other plant products
germanium: element glandular or Protomorphogen is a derivative of glandular tissue, usually freeze dried
globulin: part of the body proteins glucocorticoids such as cortisone, prednisone
gluconates: a salt with gluconic acid
glutamine: amino acid
glutathion-reductase: GS, an antioxidant
glycerophosphates: molecules conteining glycerol and phosphorus
glycol: a family of chemicals of which the best known is poly-ethylene-glycol, or PEG., common antifreeze
gonadotropin: a hormone that stimulates ovaries and testicles
GPT a common liver function test.
graft-versus-host interactions: reaction against a foreign tissue
growth hormone: HGH
GS: glutathion-reductase
hair analysis: a simple and inexpensive way to tell whether the person has been exposed.
halogens: literally "salt formers", chlorine, fluorine, bromine and iodine are halogens
healing bands: areas of over-hardened bone

hematemesis: vomiting blood
hematuria: urinating blood
heme: blood pigment
hemoglobin: red pigment of red blood cells
hemolysis: dissolution of red blood cells
hemoptysis: coughing up blood
hemorrhagic eruption: rash accompanied by bleeding
herpes viruses: chicken-pox, small-pox, herpes simplex and zoster, Epstein Barr or chronic fatigue viruses
hesperidin: bioflavonoid
hexachlorophene: Phisohex, a surgical skin cleanser
HGH: human growth hormone
hip protector: device to protect the hips of the elderly
hirsutism: increase of body hair
histamine: a substance produced in an allergic reaction which causes redness, swelling and itching
histidine: amino acid
histomorphometry: an invasive analysis, usually performed on a bone biopsy
holistic: in medicine, referring to the total person
homogenized milk: processed to minimize the size of the fat globules
hormone replacement therapy: the use of hormones for therapeutic purposes after menopause or surgery
HRT: the use of hormones for therapeutic purposes after menopause or surgery
human growth hormone: HGH
hydrochlorothiazide: a diuretic
hydrogen peroxide H2O2: peroxide, oxidized water
hydroxyapatite: the predominant structural form of calcium in human bone tissue
Hydroxypropyl Methylcellulose: a filler for pharmaceuticals
hyper-reninaemia: excess rennin, a kidney hormone
hypercalcemia: increased blood calcium
hypercalcuria: excessive urinary calcium
hyperkeratosis: calluses and hard skin
hyperparathyroidism: excessive production of the parathyroid hormone
hyperprolactinemia: a condition in which the pituitary gland, located in the skull directly above the nose, and under the brain, overproduces the milk releasing hormone prolactin)
hypertension: high blood pressure
hypocoagulability: decreased clotting ability of the blood
hypoglycemia: condition characterized by low blood sugar
hypogonadism: low glandular performance
hypokinesia: decreased mobility
hyponatremia: decreased serum sodium
hypothalamic: related to the mid-brain area
hypothalamus: mid-brain
iatrogenic: medically caused
IBD: irritable bowel disease, gastrointestinal inflammation, diarrhea, pain
ibuprofen: a non-steroidal analgesic or NSAID
IDDM: insulin dependent diabetes mellitus
iliac crest: the prominent part of the hip
immugen: a brand of immune globulins from whey
immunoglobulins or Ig: certain proteins active in the immune process
in vitro: literally, "in glass", in the test tube or dish
incomplete protein: essential amino-acids are not all present
inert ingredients: all ingredients other than the main drug; they constitute the filler, the bulk of the pill, and its color
inflammatory bowel disease: IBD, gastrointestinal inflammation, diarrhea, pain
ingesting: Taking food or drink into your body
insulin-like growth factors: a hormonal substance related to youth and tissue repair, IGF
insulin dependent diabetes mellitus: diabetes which must be treated with insulin, IDDM
insulin: pancreatic hormone

interferon: anti-viral
interleukin-6 related illnesses: immunologic disorders
interstitial nephritis: form of kidney disease
intervertebral foramen: small opening between two vertebral apophyses (appendages)
intervertebral space: the gap between the vertebrae
intranasally: given as a nasal spray
iodine: mineral
ion: an atom or group of atoms which has lost or gained one or more orbiting electrons, becoming able to conduct electricity
ipriflavone: acts predominantly as an inhibitor of bone resorption.
iron: mineral
ischaemia: lack of oxygen supply due to circulatory inefficiency
isoenzymes: similar enzymes
isopropyl to "denature" it: that is why it is not burdened by high alcohol taxes. It is uncertain to me whether Itai-Itai disease, literally "it hurts, it hurts", severe cadmium poisoning
intravascular hemolysis: disintegration of red blood cells inside blood vessels),
IUs: international units
juxtaglomerular apparatus hyperplasia: kidney damage
kaempferol: flavonoid
Kaffee Veredlvngs Werk: European Water Process to decaffeinate, using methylene chloride in a process similar to the Swiss water process.
kaliuresis: urinating too much potassium
keratinization: the full maturation of epithelial or surface cells
ketoprofen: another member of the NSAIDS, also known as Orudis
KI: potassium iodide, a toxic substance frequently added to table salt
KVW: European Water Process to decaffeinate, using methylene chloride in a process similar to the Swiss water process.
kyphosis: hunched back, curving from back to front
L-thyroxine: thyroid substance
lactates: derivatives of lactic acid
lactose: milk sugar
lactose intolerance: condition of mal-digestion and allergy to the milk sugar lactose
laryngeal edema: swelling of the wind-pipe
Lasix: fluid pill, furosemide
lactose reduced milk: milk with less milk sugar
lead: a mineral, toxic to humans
lecithin: substance abundant in brain and egg yolk, clears fat out of the blood vessels
licorice: used in candy and as herbal remedy
lignan: botanical compound in bark
linoleic acid: unsaturated fatty acid - flax oil
linoleic (LN) acid: unsaturated fatty acid - flax oil
linolenic (LNA) acids: unsaturated fatty acid - flax oil
lipid peroxidation: oxidizing in fats
lipogranuloma: small nodules in fat
lithium: a mineral
lithium carbonate: allegedly as a therapeutic agent for the treatment of bipolar or manic-depressive disorders. Despite much evidence of its worthlessness
litmus paper: treated paper which changes colors depending whether a substance is acid or alkaline
looser zones: woven, thickened areas of bone
lordosis: swayback
lumbar: low back
lumbar disc problems: a narrowing or damage to the gelatinous discs that are located between each two vertebrae
lymphoma: tumor of the lymph glands
lysine: an amino acid necessary to bone chemicals pyridinoline and deoxypyridinoline
macrominerals: iron, copper, calcium, etc.
macrominerals: minerals necessary in large amounts

magnesium: mineral, an important enzymatic activator.
magnesium stearate: magnesium salt
matrix: the soft, pliable, proteinaceous bone structure bed
mask of pregnancy: brown spots on the face, upper lip, mid line of abdomen, more noticeable in people with darker skin pigment
medullary cavity: central space in the shaft of the bone
medullary interstitial cell hyperplasia: kidney damage
medullary bone: trabecular or cancellous, in small beehive cells, built in small scales and tubules
melasma: mask of pregnancy, brown spots on the face, upper lip, mid line of abdomen, more noticeable in people with darker skin pigment
melena: tarry stools, usually due to blood in them
menadione: vitamin K3
menaphthone: vitamin K3
menaquinone: form of vitamin K
menarche: first menstrual period
Mercurochrome, Merthiolate: red antiseptic, containing the toxin mercury. mercury is a substance which is highly toxic to animals and humans. Even very low levels may suppress necessary selenium function. Mercury can be responsible for arthritic and neurologic symptoms, which may add to, or mimic, osteoporotic pains and disabilities.
meridians: channels of energy in Acupuncture
mesenteric lymph node histiocytosis: inflammation in the glands in the abdominal cavity
mestranol: horse estrogen
metabolic bone disease: bone disorder caused by various imbalances
metalloenzymes: enzymes bound to a metal atom
metaphysis: shaft of the long bones
metastatic calcification: calcium deposits in soft tissues
metastatic disease: scattering of cancer throughout the body
methemoglobin: blood pigment that has been modified to where it can no longer carry oxygen
methionine: sulphur containing amino-acid
methrotrexate: may cause changes in the elimination leading to elevated serum levels and increased toxicity.
methyl methacrylate monomer: in cosmetic nail products
methylene chloride: chemical used in both direct and indirect decaffeination methods
methylparaben: additive
miacalcin: a non-hormonal drug for osteoporotic bone
microfractures: small breaks in the structural tiny scales that make up the bone
microvascular complications: damage to tiny blood vessels
milk-alkali syndrome: condition caused by the intake of too much milk and antacid
milligram (mgr.): One thousandth of a gram
mineral hydrocarbon MHC: white oils and waxes
mineral oil: petroleum product
mineralization: deposit of calcium salts into the matrix
minerals: elements of the soil, also contained in foods
miso: soy product
mitral valve: heart valve
modulators: modifiers of a process
molybdenum: trace element
monoclonal antibody: antibodies derived from a group of daughter cells which originate from one mother cell
mRNA: messenger RNA, a measure of genetic function for osteocalcin, a bone-specific marker
multiple myeloma: a usually fatal bone marrow cancer which destroys the bone itself
mutations: genetic changes
Myalgia: muscle pain
myoglobin: a protein which is found only in muscle tissue
myopia: nearsightedness
myxedematous: suffering from hypothyroid swelling
N-acetyl-cysteine (NAC): a commercial cysteine and anti-toxic factor. N-methyl-N-nitro-N-nitrosoguanidine MNNG, N-nitroso-N-ethylurea,

N-telopeptides: proteinaceous ends of cross-linked collagen regions in bone N-telopeptides of bone collagen

naphthalene: the chemical in mothballs

naproxen sodium: a non-steroidal analgesic or NSAID

naturally decaffeinated: no specific "natural process" exists

necrosis: cell and tissue death in the living body

neoplasms: malignant tumors

nephrolithiasis: kidney stones

nephrotic syndrome: chronic kidney disease

neuro-transmitter: substance which permits neurologic conduction

neuroleptics: tranquilizers

neurons: nerve cells

neurotoxin: toxin affecting the nervous system in particular

neutron activation: bone density study

nickel: is NIDDM

nigari: a compound found naturally in ocean water

nitrates: chemical compounds

NMBA: esophageal-specific carcinogen

NNK: a potent environmental carcinogen generated during tobacco processing and smoking. The carcinogenic response to tobacco smoking is modulated by nutritional factors.

non-collagen proteins: proteins that are not gristle-like

non-insulin dependent diabetes mellitus: diabetes type II, manageable by diet

non-essential: manufactured in the human body

nonovulatory cycle: monthly period where no ovulation took place

Norian SRS®Skeletal Repair System: a really bionic medicine, is a new substance for mending bone made of calcium and phosphoric acid.

NSAIDS: Non steroidal antiinflammatories

nuclear estrogen receptor: a DNA-binding protein which is found in estrogen-responsive tissues

nucleic acids: components of DNA and RNA

nulliparity: not having had any babies

O2*: superoxide oxygen radical

ocular neuritis: inflammation of the nerve of the eye

off-label indication: a mode of use of a drug that has not been specifically approved by the FDA, but has been approved for other conditions

oncogenes: cancer genes, abnormal genetic particles which cause cancer

onycholysis: separation of the nails

oophorectomy: ovarian resection

orotates: salts of orotic acid, an amino acid

orthostatic hypotension: a sudden drop in blood pressure when changing from a lying or recumbent, to an upright position

Orudis: ketoprofen another member of the NSAIDS.

Oruvail: long acting, prescription strength of Orudis

osseous metaplasia: soft tissue turns into bony tissue in the insertions of muscles and tendons

Osteogenic: bone building

ostein: bone protein, which is rich in collagen

osteoblasts: cells that form bone

osteocalcin: non-collagen bone protein

osteochondrosis: development of hardened tissue in muscle insertions

osteoclasts: cells that digest the surface of old bone

osteoclasts cells that aid the reabsorption or breakdown of already existing bone

osteoid matrix: the proteinaceous basis of the bone

osteomalacia: poor mineralization of bone and the inability of the bones to handle stress

osteopenia: thinning of bones

osteophytes: outgrowth of bony material

osteopontin: mRNA concentrations increased

osteoporosis: bone weakening due to malformation of bone matrix

Osteomark®: the NTx Test

ovarian follicle: where the egg cell forms.

oxides: compound containing oxygen oxydases, which may add an electron to an oxygen molecule. For example, paba: para-amino-benzoic-acid

Paget's disease of the bone: accelerated, inappropriate bone formation

palpitation: perceptible heart beat

Panax Ginseng, also called Asian, Chinese or Korean Ginseng. The second is Panax Ginseng: the "stress herb"

Panax Quinquefolius: American Ginseng

pantothenic acid: vitamin B5

papilloma: genital wart

paraffin waxes: a family of petroleum derivatives that are unctuous to touch

paraplegia: paralysis

parathyroid glands: located on both sides of the thyroid

parathyroid hormone: hormone of the parathyroid gland

parathyroid hormone by the parathyroid glands: located on both sides of the thyroid

paresthesia: false feelings due to neurologic or chemical disorders, such as "pins and needles"

pathological fractures: fractures due to preexisting illness, not accidents peak bone mass

PEG: poly-ethylene-glycol, antifreeze PEITC

penetrative resorption: dissolving bone mass deeply into the bone

peptic ulcer: stomach ulcer

percutaneous penetration: entry via the skin

periodic table of Mendelejeff: an organizational charting of chemical elements

periosteum: membrane which surrounds bone

peripheral vascular disease: poor circulation

petrolatum: Vaseline

pharyngitis: sore throat

phenacetin: analgesic, similar to acetaminophen

phenytoin: Dilantin, an anti-epileptic drug

phosphatase: enzyme which affects the metabolism of phosphorus

phosphate: compound, containing phosphorus

photodensitometry: bone density study

photolysis: the chemical breakdown of a substance, induced by light

photosensitivity: sensitivity to light

phylloquinone: vitamin K1

phytate: compound of mineral and phytic acid

phytic acid: substance contained in plants and grains, which can bind minerals in the digestive tract, making them unabsorbable

phyto-estrogens: plant-derived estrogens

pituitary gonadotropin: hormones of the pituitary which stimulate the ovaries or testicles

pituitary gland: located in the skull directly above the nose, and under the brain

platelets: small bodies in the blood which promote clotting

pokeweed: a plant

pokeweed mitogen: a plant product from the pokeweed plant, that stimulates white blood cells, and the immune process

policythemia: an abnormal increase of the number of red blood cells

poly-ethylene-glycol: antifreeze

Polysorbate 20: a detergent often found in cosmetics

porphyria: a disorder of the metabolism of porphyrins, derivatives of hemoglobin

porphyrins: derivatives of hemoglobin

Posilac®: bovine growth hormone

post-partum mastitis: inflammatory condition of the breasts after giving birth

potassium: mineral, part of the "electrolytes" of the body

potassium iodide: KI, a toxic substance frequently added to table salt

potassium nitroprusside: a precursor of cyanide, often added to table salt

povidone-iodine: iodine containing molecule, a surgical antiseptic. Toxin.

povidone: iodine containing molecule, a surgical antiseptic. Toxin.

PPITC: like the isothiocyanates, ellagic acid

PPM: Parts per million.

prasterone: DHEA pre-ovulatory or nonovulatory cycles, and in these, estrogen alone is the primary determinant

precholecalciferol: precursor of a vitamin D

prednisone: corticosteroid drug

Prempro®: A brand of combination estrogen-progesterone

preovulatory cycle: period before ovulation

primary hyperparathyroidism: insufficient production of parathyroid hormone

primary ovarian failure: improper ovulation of unknown cause

pro-vitamin D: precursor of vitamin D

probenecid: chemical

progesterone: hormone predominantly of the second half of the menstrual cycle, and pregnancy

progestogen: hormone of the progesterone family

prolactin: milk releasing hormone

Propylene Glycol: antifreeze

Propylparaben: chemical used in making cosmetics

prostaglandin: hormones related to inflammation and blood pressure

protein: substance formed from smaller building blocks called amino-acids, primary component of muscle (meat), milk, cheese, eggs, etc.

proteoglycans: molecules that contain proteins and sugars

pruritus: itch

pseudoarthrosis: false joint

psoriasis: skin disease with disorderly, misaligned growth of skin cells and layers

PTH: parathyroid hormone

purpura: condition characterized by bruising

purpuric rash: rash with bruising

pyridines: commonly used chemicals, are also less toxic to subjects well supplied with methionine

pyridinoline: bone chemical, derivative of lysine

pyridoxal: form of vitamin B6

pyridoxamine: form of vitamin B6

pyridoxine: a water soluble nutrient

pyridoxine: form of vitamin B6

Pyrilinks: Tests for pyridinoline and deoxypiridinoline

Qi: vital energy

quadriplegia: paralysis of all four extremities

quercetin: flavonoid

quinones: a certain family of drugs

quintile: one fifth

RA: rheumatoid arthritis

rad: a unit of radiation

radiogrammetry: bone study for the measurement of cortical thickness

radiographic absorptiometry: bone density scanning by X-Ray

ranitidine: an antacid - Zantac

raw male or raw orchic: an extract of freeze dried testicle and prostate, often has minerals and vitamins added

raw ovary or raw female: an extract of freeze dried ovary and uterus, often has minerals and vitamins added

raw pituitary: an extract or freeze dried pituitary

raw thyroid: an extract or freeze dried thyroid

RDA: recommended dietary allowance

Recombinant Bovine Growth Hormone: BGH a genetically engineered drug

red No 40: industrial color

redox cycling: oxidation and reduction

reduced glutathion: an antioxidant

renal failure: malfunctioning of the kidneys

renal tubular blockade: impaired kidney function

resorption cavities: newly digested areas of the bone, where bone matter has been redissolved

retinal hemorrhage: bleeding into the retina of the eye

retinaldehyde: vitamin A-like drug

retinal pigmentation: granules of colored materials deposited in the retina of the eye

Reyes syndrome: a rare bleeding disorder that occurs when aspirin is used in some immunosuppressed children suffering from chicken pox rheumatoid arthritis or RA: inflammatory connective tissue disease, deforming joints, with pain and other degenerative and autoimmune reactions

rhinitis: a cold

Rickets: bone malformation due to vitamin D deficiency in children

Risedronate: bisphosphonate

RNA: the genetic material in the cell's body

Rocaltrol®: 1,25 dihydroxy-vitamin D

retinoic acid acutane: retin-a

rubbing alcohol: grain alcohol "denatured" by the additive isopropyl

rutin: bioflavonoid

salicylates: forms of salicylic acid or aspirin

salt sensitivity: condition marked by a rise in blood pressure after salt consumption is increased, or a fall in high blood pressure after consumption is cut

saponin glycosides: 4-ring steroid-like chemicals with attached sugar molecules that make a foam when shaken in water

sarcoidosis: pulmonary disease

scurvy: severe deficiency of vitamin C

secondary hyperparathyroidis: a condition which involves a disorderly production of parathyroid hormone, due to another disorder, such as malnutrition

secondary osteoporosis: osteoporosis due to some previous disease or medication

selenium: is a member of the powerful serotonin — a brain neurotransmitter that controls our moods, appetite, sleep
patterns, and sensitivity to pain

serum: clear part of blood

sex hormone-binding globulin: a protein that attaches to sex hormones

SHBG: sex hormone-binding globulin

Short-term: Lasting 14 days or less.

sialic acid: a substance which increases when cancer occurs, and is connected to its ability to spread

sialil-transferase: enzyme related to sialic acid

silicon Dioxide: an "inert" ingredients in pills

simethicone: detergent or surfactant

simple carbohydrate: glucose, sucrose, fructose

spinal cord stimulation SCS: electric treatment for spinal pain

singh Index of femoral trabecular pattern: bone density study

single and dual energy computed tomography: bone density study

single and dual photon absorptiometry: bone density study

single photon densitometer: device which measures the density of the forearm

skin patches: fabric or plastic skin dressings which carry a medication

sodium: element, electrolyte

sodium arsenite: toxic arsenic salt

sodium Benzoate: preservative

sodium fluoride: rat poison, also used as an additive to drinking water

sodium Lauryl Sulfate: an "inert" ingredients in pills

sodium salicylate: an aspirin-like substance

sodium Starch Glycolate: an "inert" ingredients in pills

soluble: Dissolves well in liquid.

solution: the particles are small enough to dissolve completely,

sorbitan Monolaurate: ingredient used as a filler in medications

soy flour: made from roasted soybeans that have been ground into a fine powder

soy milk: is the rich, creamy product of whole soybeans

soy protein: proteins from soy

spermatogenesis: production of sperm

spondylosis: spurs and bridging between spinal vertebrae

squamous cell dysplasia of the cervix: anomaly of the mucous membrane of the mouth of the womb

stannuous fluoride: combination of the toxic substances fluoride and tin, used in making toothpaste

starch: polisaccharide, complex carbohydrate in substances such as potatoes, rice, etc.

stearic acid: an "inert" ingredients in pills

steroids: chemical group which comprises many hormones

strontium: mineral

sucrose: table sugar

supercritical Carbon Dioxide: decaffeination by carbon dioxide at a high temperature and pressure.

superoxide anion: highly reactive oxidant

superoxide dismutase: antioxidant

superoxide oxygen radical: O2*-.

suspension: particles in a liquid, which form a sediment and the mix has to be shaken up

Swiss Water Process: decaffeination process

T4-T8: trunk vertebrae 4-8

tachycardia: fast heart beat

Tagamet: cimetidine, acid suppressor

talc: the mineral in talcum powder

Tamoxifen: cancer drug

tannin: substance found in tea and other products, can chelate metals

tartrazine: an industrial coloring agent which can cause asthmatic attacks

tempeh: pronounced 'tem-pay' a traditional Indonesian food, a chunky, tender cake of soybeans

teratogenesis: induction of malformations

testosterone: male hormone

tetany: muscle spasms

tetracycline: an antibiotic

textured soy protein, TSP or TVP: a registered trademark of the Archer Daniels Midland Company, a nutritious extender in a variety of food products

thiazide: diuretic, fluid or water pill

thoracic: related to the trunk of the body

Thrombocytopenia: decrease in the number of platelets

thymus: a gland in the anterior neck intimately related with the immune process

thyrotoxicosis: thyroid gland overproduces hormone

tin: a metal which is toxic to the body

titanium dioxide: a whitening agent frequently used as a "filler" (inert ingredient) in tablets and pills

tobacco: a plant used to make cigarettes, cigars, etc.

tofu: soybean curd

trabecular bone: medullary bone

Trace elements: zinc, chromium, etc.

trace elements: small amounts

Transcutaneous Electrical Nerve Stimulation (T.E.N.S.): electrotherapy

transdermal: through the skin, usually the application of a medicated patch to the naked skin

transient ischemic attacks: TIA's or small strokes:

TIA's: transient ischemic attacks or small strokes: triglycerides are used in a direct contact method of decaffeination.

Trihalomethanes: anesthetic, carcinogenic chemicals caused by halogens such as chlorine and fluorine added to water supplies containing organic matter

Trypsin inhibitor: TI, an enzyme blocker

TI: Trypsin inhibitor, an enzyme blocker

TSH: thyroid function test which measures a pituitary hormone which induces thyroid hormone production in the thyroid gland

Tylenol: acetaminophen

type I collagen: connective tissue proteins, a specific form of gristle

type II collagen - RCII: connective tissue proteins, a specific form of gristle

tyrosine: is a basic building block of the all-important thyroid hormones, and of skin pigments.

ultrasound: bone density scanning by special sound frequencies, something like a "sonar"

under-carboxylation: decreased binding of the chemical group carboxy

urethane, URE: a genotoxin, causing mutations

urinary N-telopeptide crosslinks: derivatives from bone protein

urticaria: allergic rash, with welts

uterine fibroids: benign tumors of the womb

vaginal adenosis: glands in vagina

vaseline: petrolatum, an ointment

vasodilation: enlargement of blood vessels

VDR gene: vitamin D receptor gene

vegetarianism: nutrition favoring non-animal-source foods

ventricular arrhythmia: irregular heart beat originating in the ventricles (a certain chamber of the heart)

vertebrae: backbones

vertigo: dizziness, loss of balance

vinyl chloride: a chemical used as a growth factor, and also to make pharmaceutical patches

virilism: development of male characteristics in a female

virilization: the development of male traits

vitamin A: carotenoids

vitamin B1: thiamine

vitamin B2: riboflavin

vitamin B3: niacin

vitamin B5: pantothenic acid

vitamin B6: also called pyridoxine, a water soluble nutrient

vitamin C: ascorbic acid, a water soluble vitamin

vitamin D: calciferol, a generic name for several fat-soluble vitamin variants, related to each other, all of which are sterols, cholesterol-like substances

vitamin D receptor: site on cells that attaches to vitamin D

vitamin K1: phylloquinone, from food sources

vitamin K2: menaquinone, formed by bacteria in the intestines

vitamin K3: menaphthone, or menadione, which is synthetic

warfarin: anticoagulant, blood thinner, Coumadin

water number: the percentage of water in a food product

wholistic: holistic, in medicine, referring to the total person

x-ray: a method of examining the structure of the body by using rays which penetrate through tissue

xanthine: caffeine, teine

xanthine oxidase: a strong former of free radicals

XO: xanthine oxidase

Yang: in Chinese philosophy, the male principle

YIN: in Chinese philosophy, the female principle

Zantac: ranitidine, an antacid

zinc stearate: a salt of zinc

zirconium complexes: minerals in underarm deodorants and cosmetics

REFERENCES

A010 Abate G; Taormina F; Brillante C; Fraccalaglio L, Cattedra di Geriatria, Universita degli Studi G. D'Annunzio, Chieti, "The effects of the carbocalcitonin + arginine-lysine-lactose, combination in senile involutional osteoporosis", MINERVA MED. 1994 May;85(5):253-9, NLM CIT. ID: 94301501,

A020 Abbott L., Nadler J., Rude R.K., Department of Endocrinology, LAC+USC Medical Center 90033, "Magnesium deficiency in alcoholism: possible contribution to Osteoporosis and cardiovascular disease in alcoholics", ALCOHOL. CLIN. EXP. RES. 1994 Oct;18(5):1076-82, NLM CIT. ID: 95150250

A021 ACOG Technical Bulletin 166. Reproduced with permission of the publisher; copyright 1992. American College of Obstetricians and Gynecologists. "Hormone Replacement Therapy" Washington, DC: American College of Obstetricians and Gynecologists; 1992.

A022 AQUIRE Database, ERL-Duluth, U.S. EPA. http://mail.odsnet.com/TRIFacts/207.html

A030 Adlercreutz C.H., Goldin B.R, Gorbach S.L., Hockerstedt K.A., Watanabe S., Hamalainen E.K., Markkanen M.H., Makela T.H., Wahala K.T., Department of Clinical Chemistry, Helsinki University Central Hospital, Finland. "Soybean phytoestrogen intake and cancer risk", NUTR 1995 Jul;125(7):1960

A030 Alfrey, Allen C., MD. (1995) "Toxicity of detrimental metal ions - Aluminum" (Guy Berthon, editor), Handbook of Metal-Ligand Interactions Biological Fluids - BIOINORGANIC MEDICINE, Volume 2, Marcel Dekker, Inc., New York, pages 735 - 748.

A040 Amato G, Carella C, Fazio S et al. "Body Composition, Bone Metabolism, and Heart Structure and Function in Growth Hormone (GH)-Deficient Adults Before and After GH Replacement Therapy at Low Doses" JOURNAL OF CLINICAL ENDOCRINOLOGY AND METABOLISM 1993; 77:1671 -1676.

A050 Amoroso E.C., Perry J.S., PHILOS. TRANS. R. SOC. LOND. B. BIOL. SCI., "The existence during gestation of an immunological buffer zone at the interface between maternal and foetal tissues", 1975 Jul 17;271(912):343-61, NLM CIT. ID: 75218061,

A060 Anderson F.H., Francis R.M., Faulkner K., Musculoskeletal Unit, Freeman Hospital, Newcastle upon Tyne, UK, "Androgen supplementation in eugonadal men with osteoporosis-effects of 6 months of treatment on bone mineral density and cardiovascular risk factors", BONE 1996 Feb;18(2):171-7, NLM ID: 96430061,

A070 Angus, R. M. and Eisman, J. A., "Osteoporosis: the Role of calcium intake and Supplementation" MEDICAL JOURNAL OF AUSTRALIA, June 20th 1988, Vol. 148, N° 12, pp. 630—633

A080 Angus, R. M.,Eisman, J. A., MEDICAL JOURNAL OF AUSTRALIA, June 20th 1988, Volume 148, Number 12, Pages 630—633

A081 Aroonsakul, C., Personal communication

A090 ASIDY-A. BINGHAM-S. SETCHELL-K.,"Biological Effects of Isoflavones in Young Women", BRITISH JOURNAL OF NUTRITION, 1995, OCT, V74, N4, P587-601. ISSN0007-1145.

A100 Ayres S/; Tang M/; Subbiah MT., Department of Internal Medicine, University of Cincinnati Medical Center, OH 45267-0540, USA, "Estradiol-17beta as an antioxidant: some distinct features when compared with common fat-soluble antioxidants" J. LAB. CLIN. MED. 1996 Oct; 128(4):367-75, 344-5, NLM CIT. ID: 96430803

B008 Bailey A.J., Wotton S.F., Sims T.J., Thompson P.W., Department of Veterinary Medicine, University of Bristol, Langford, UK, "Biochemical Changes in the Collagen of human osteoporotic bone matrix", CONNECT. TISSUE. RES. 1993;29(2):119-32, NLM CIT. ID: 94007802,

B009 Baird D.D., Umbach D.M., Lansdell L., Hughes C.L., Setchell K.D., Weinberg C.R., Haney A.F., Wilcox A.J., Mclachlan J.A., National Institute of Environmental Health Sciences, Research Triangle Park, North Carolina 27709, USA, "Dietary intervention study to assess estrogenicity of dietary soy among postmenopausal women", J. CLIN. ENDOCRINOL. METAB. 1995 May, 80(5):1685-90, NLM CIT. ID: 95263734,

B010 Banerjee A.K., Lane P.J., Meichen F.W., "Osteoporosis and Vitamin C", AGE AGEING 1978 Feb;7(1):16-8, NLM CIT. ID: 78141843

B020 Barregard L., Lindstedt G., Schütz A & Sallsten G., "Endocrine Function in mercury exposed chloralkali workers" OCC. ENVIRON. MED. 51:536-540 (1994)

B030 Barrett-Connor E., Chang J.C., Edelstein S.L., Department of Family and Preventive Medicine, University of California, San Diego 92093-0607, "Coffee-associated osteoporosis offset by daily milk consumption. The Rancho Bernardo Study", JAMA 1994 Jan 26;271(4):280-3, NLM CIT. ID: 94125501

B040 Bartsioka et al., "Lead Poisoning and dental caries in the Broken Hill Hominid" J. HUM. EVOL. (1993), 24(3):243-249.

B141 Bates, B., "Estrogen Use High Among Postmenopausal Docs", FAMILY PRACTICE NEWS, Southern California Bureau, October 15, 1997, p. 9

B050 Bauer D.C., Orwoll E.S., Fox K.M., Vogt T.M., Lane N.E., Hochberg M.C., Stone K., Nevitt M.C., Division of General Internal Medicine, University of California, San Francisco, USA, "Aspirin and NSAID Use in older women: effect on bone mineral density and fracture risk. Study of Osteoporotic Fractures Research Group", J. BONE. MINER. RES. 1996 Jan;11(1):29-35,, NLM CIT. ID: 96366517,

B051 Baylink, D.J. et al., "Treating postmenopausal Osteoporosis", FAM. PRACT. RECERT., Vol. 19, No. 9(SUPPL), Sept. 1997

B060 Becker RO, Marino AA. Electromagnetism and life. Albany: State Univ. of New York, 1982.

B070 Beiraghi S., Atkins S., Rosen S., Wilson S., Odom J., Beck M., "Effect of calcium lactate in erosion and S. mutans in rats when added to Coca-Cola", PEDIATR. DENT. 1989 Dec;11(4):312-5, NLM CIT. ID: 90310753

B071 Bellati U., Liberati M., Clinica Ostetrica e Ginecologica, Universita degli Studi, G. D'Annunzi, Cheti, "Experience Regarding the use of Arginine-Lysine-lactose treatment in menopausal osteoporosis", MINERVA MED 1994 Jun;85 (6):327-32, NLM ID. 94366544,

B072 Bellows C.G., Aubin J.E., Heersche J.N., MRC Group in Periodontal Physiology, Faculty of Dentistry, University of Toronto, Ontario, Canada,"Differential Effects of fluoride during initiation and progression of Mineralization of Osteoid nodules formed in vitro", J. BONE MINE. RES. 1993 Nov;8(11):1357-63, NLM CIT. ID: 94091183

B080 Benagiano G; Fraser I.,"The Depo-Provera Debate. Commentary on the Article 'Depo-Provera, a critical analysis'", CONTRACEPTION 1981 Nov;24(5):493-528, NLM CIT. ID: 82094376,

B090 Benagiano G; Fraser I.,"The Depo-Provera Debate. Commentary on the Article 'Depo-Provera, a critical analysis'", CONTRACEPTION 1981 Nov;24(5):493-528, NLM CIT. ID: 82094376,

B100 Bengtsson BA. The Consequences of Growth Hormone Deficiency in Adults. ACTA ENDO- CRINOLOGICA 1993;128 (Suppl 2):2-5.

B110 Bengtsson BA, Eden S, Lonn L et al. "Treatment of Adults with Growth Hormone (GH) Deficiency with Recombinant Human GH" JOURNAL OF CLINICAL ENDOCRINOLOGY AND METABOLISM 1993;76;309- 317.

B120 Bercovitz et al., "Tooth type as an indicator of exposure to lead of adults and children" ARCH. ORAL BIOL. (1990) 35(11):895-898.

B130 Berlin K., Gerhardsson L., Borjesson J,. Lindh E., Lundstrom N., Schutz A., Skerfving S., Edling C., "Lead intoxication caused by skeletal disease", Scand J. Work Environ. Health. 1995 Aug. 21 (4): 296-300 []

B140 Bernal S.D, Lampidis T.J, Summerhayes I.L, Chen L.B., "Rhodamine 123 selectively reduces clonal growth of carcinoma cells in vitro, SCIENCE 1982;218: 1117.

B141 BIBLE, THE, Leviticus 7:23

B150 Bigler J.M., Abetel G., Krieg MA., Wimpfheimer C., Burnand B., Thiebaud D., Burckhardt P., Department de medecine interne, CHUV, Lausanne, "Importance of the clinical profile in the post-menopausal osteoporosis screening by Densitometry", SCHWEIZ. MED. WOCHENSCHR. 1996 Aug 6;126(31-32):1347-51, NLM CIT. ID: 96364185

B160 Bigler J.M., Abetel G., Krieg MA., Wimpfheimer C., Burnand B., Thiebaud D., Burckhardt P., Department de medecine interne, CHUV, Lausanne, "Importance of the clinical profile in the post-menopausal osteoporosis screening by Densitometry", SCHWEIZ. MED. WOCHENSCHR. 1996 Aug 6;126(31-32):1347-51, NLM CIT. ID: 96364185

B170 Binz K., Schmid C., Bouillon R., Froesch ER., Jurgensen K., Hunziker E.B., Department of Medicine, University Hospital, Zurich, Switzerland, "Interactions of insulin-like growth factor I with dexamethasone on trabecular bone density and mineral metabolism in rats", EUR. J. ENDOCRINOL. 1994 Apr;130(4):387-93, NLM CIT. ID: 94214651,

B171 Black M.M; Leis H.P. Jr., Kwon S., "The breast cancer controversy. A natural experiment", JAMA 1977 Mar 7;237(10):970-1, NLM CIT. ID 77097375

B172 Blumenthal N.C., Cosma V., Skyler D., LeGeros J., Walters M., Department of Bioengineering, Hospital for Joint Diseases Orthopaedic Institute, New York, New York 10003, USA, "The Effect of Cadmium on the Formation and Properties of Hydroxyapatite in Vitro and its Relation to cadmium toxicity in the skeletal system", CALCIF. TISSUE. INT. 1995 Apr;56(4):316-22, NLM CIT. ID: 95285389,

B180 Bo-Linn G.W., Davis G.R., Buddrus D.J., Morawski S.G., Santa Ana C., Fordtran J.S., "An Evaluation of the Importance of gastric acid secretion in the Absorption of dietary calcium", J. CLIN. INVEST. 1984 Mar.,73(3):640-7, NLM CIT. ID: 84162593,

B181 Bowser, Andrew, "Povidone-Iodine May Suppress Thyroid Function", FAMILY PRAC-TICE NEWS, Nov. 15, 1997

B182 Bradford, L., Chem. 1, Fall 96. WWW http://crystal.biol.csufresno.edu:8080/projects/31.html

B190 Bravo G., Gauthier P., Roy PM., Payette H., Gaulin P., Harvey M., Peloquin L., Dubois M.F., Department of Community Health Sciences, University of Sherbrooke, Canada, "Impact of a 12-month exercise program on the physical and psychological health of osteopenic women", J. AM. GERIATR. SOC.1996 Jul;44(7):756-62, NLM ID. 96268240,

B200 Breant V., Aulagner G., Laffont-Mevel A., Lafaure A., Fusselier M., Pharmacologie Clinique Pediatrique, Hopital Debrousse, Lyon, "Contamination of ternary mixtures of parenteral nutrition by barium" ANN. PHARM. FR. 1993;51(6):273-82, NLM CIT. ID: 94205934

B209 Brixen K., Kassem M., Eriksen E..F., Nielsen H.K., Flyvbjerg A., Mosekilde L, Department of Endocrinology and Metabolism, Aarhus University Hospital, Denmark, "Growth Hormone (GH) and adult bone remodeling: the potential use of GH in Treatment of Osteoporosis", J. PEDIATR. ENDOCRINOL. 1993 Jan-Mar;6(1):65-71, NLM CIT. ID: 93386294,

B210 Bruce., M.R., PhD. "Aluminum: a neurotoxic product of acid rain", Accounts of Chemical Research, 1994:27;204-210.

B220 Buglass, Dan. "Is school milk Safe to Drink? THE SCOTSMAN. 1/25/96;" p32.

B230 Bulmore, Adam, Producer, October Films "Too Big Too Soon", A TV program in England, broadcast on 20 February 1995

C010 Capo M.A., Sevil M.B., Lopez M.E., Frejo M.T., Department of Toxicology, School of Veterinary Medicine, Universidad Complutense de Madrid, Spain, "Ethylene glycol action on Neurons and its cholinomimetic effects", J. ENVIRON. PATHOL. TOXICOL. ONCOL. 1993 Jul-Sep;12(3):155-9, NLM CIT. ID: 94246557,

C020 Carroll D., Jadad A., King V., Wiffen P., and others, "Single-dose, randomized, double-blind, double-dummy cross- over comparison of Extradural and i.v. Clonidine in chronic pain", Oxford Regional Pain Relief Unit, Churchill Hospital, BR. J. ANAESTH. 1993 Nov;71(5):665-9, Unique Identifier: MEDLINE 94072311

C030 Carroll, Robert Todd , (Reproduced from "The Skeptic's Dictionary", a book published on the www, authorized for reproduction by its author, . Minor editing added).

C040 Chaitow, L., N.D., D.O.©1990

C050Chalkley S.M., Chisholm DJ., Department of Endocrinology, St Vincent's Hospital, Darlinghurst, NSW.,"Cushing's Syndrome from an inhaled gluco-corticoid [published erratum appears in MED. J. AUST. 1994 Jul 18;161(2):176] [see comments] MED. J. AUST. 1994 May 16;160(10):611, 614-5, NLM ID. 94232029 COMMENT: MED. J. AUST. 1995 Mar 20;162(6):333,

C060 Chen LB. Fluorescent labeling of mitochondria. Methods Cell Biol 1989; 29: 103-120,

C070 Chinese Pain Center, "How Does Acupuncture Work?"

C080 Chonan O., Takahashi ., Kado S., Nagata Y., Kimura H., Uchida K., Watanuki M., Yakult Central Institute for Microbiological Research, Kunitachi, Japan, "Effects of calcium gluconate on the Utilization of Magnesium and the Nephrocalcinosis in rats fed excess dietary phosphorus and calcium", J. NUTR. SCI.VITAMINOL. (TOKYO) 1996 Aug., 42(4):313-23, NLM CIT. ID, 97062894,

C081 Choudhury A.R., Das T., Sharma A., Talukder G., Centre for Advanced Study in Cell and Chromosome Research, Department of Botany, University of Calcutta, India,"Inhibition of clastogenic effects of arsenic through continued oral administration of garlic extract in Mce in Vivo", MUTAT.RES.1997 Aug 14;392(3):237-42, NLM CIT. ID: 97438248,

C090 Clinical Center Office of Clinical Reports & Inquiries, Building 10B"Medicine for the Layman Arthritis," , Room 1C255, Bethesda, Maryland, 20892CMA Webspinners

C100 CMAJ August 15, 1996 (vol 155, no 4), INTERNATIONAL DIGEST , CMA Webspinners

C110 Conn H.O., Poynard T., "Corticosteroids and peptic ulcer: meta-analysis of adverse events during steroid therapy", Yale University School of Medicine, West Haven, Connecticut, J. INTERN. MED. 1994 Dec;236(6):619-32, NLM CIT. ID: 95081753, COMMENT: J. INTERN. MED. 1994 Dec, 236(6):599-601, ACP J Club 1995 May-Jun, 122(3):81

C120 Constantinou A., Huberman E.: Department of Surgical Oncology, College of Medicine,University of Illinois at Chicago 60612. (Proc. Soc. Exp. Biol. Med. 1995 Jan., 208(1):109-15)

C130 Consumer vinegar test for determining calcium disintegration", Mason N.A., Patel J.D., Dressman J.B., Shimp L.A., College of Pharmacy, University of Michigan, Ann Arbor 48109-1065., AM. J. HOSP. PHARM. 1992 Sep., 49(9):2218-22, NLM CIT. ID,92397896,

C131 Cooper MS, Schliwa M. Transmembrane Ca2+ Fluxes in the Forward and reversed galvanotaxis of fish epidermal cells", PROG. CLIN. BIOL. RES. 1986; 210: 311-318.

C140 Cranton, Elmer M. and Frackelton, James P., This is a greatly oversimplified explanation of what actually occurs. For those of you with a decided interest in the scientific technicalities, you can send for the manuscript entitled FREE RADICAL PATHOLOGY IN AGE-ASSOCIATED DISEASES: TREATMENT WITH EDTA, NUTRITION AND ANTIOXIDANTS by Doctors Elmer M. Cranton and James P. Frackelton. For a fuller explanation of the many issues involved, written in popular form for the general public, you might enjoy reading BYPASSING BYPASS by Dr. Elmer M. Cranton and Arline Brecher. Both publications, as well as others, are available from the American College of Advancement in Medicine, 23121

Verdugo Drive Suite 204, Laguna Hills CA 92653, (714) 583-7666. Telephone before ordering to find out costs, or you may purchase them from our office or in the bookstore. A new book, FORTY SOMETHING FOREVER, by Arlene Brecher, is a wonderful addition to many already great publications.

C141 Crawford, R.D., "Proposed Role for a Combination of citric acid and ascorbic acid in the Production of dietary iron overload: a fundamental cause of Disease", Department of Chemistry and Biochemistry, Loyola Marymount, University, Los Angeles, California 90045, USA, BIOCHEM. MOL MED. 1995 Feb., 54(1):1-11, NLM CIT. ID: 96002217

C141 Cuesta A., Revilla M., Villa LF., Hernandez ER., Rico H., Department of Medicine, Alcala de Henares University, Madrid, Spain, "Total and regional bone mineral content in Spanish professional ballet dancers", CALCIF.TISSUE.INT, Mar;58(3):150-4, NLM CIT. ID: 97005258,

C150 Cuneo RC, Salomon F, Wiles CM et al. "Growth Hormone Treatment in Growth Hormone Deficient Adults. II. Effects on Exercise Performance" JOURNAL OF APPLIED PHYSIOLOGY 1991;70:

C160 CYBER-DIET: http://www.CyberDiet.com/foodfact/vitmins/vitcnew.html

D010 Dalen, Hallberg and Lamke: "Bone Mass in obese subjects"

D020 Daniell H.W., "Post-menopausal tooth loss. Contributions to Edentulism by Osteoporosis and cigarette smoking", ARCH. INTERN. MED. 1983 Sep;143(9):1678-82, NLM CIT. ID: 83307717

D021 Daugherty, Jane. "Should milk drinkers be Alerted to Use of Hormone?" THE DETROIT NEWS. 11/20/95; page unknown.

D022 De Cree C; Lewin R; Barros A., Department of Applied and Experimental Reproductive Endocrinology, Institute for Gyneco-Endocrinological Research, Leuven, Belgium, "Hypoestrogenemia and Rhabdomyelysis (Myoglobinuria) in the female judoist: a new worrying phenomenon?", J. CLIN. ENDOCRINOL. METAB. 1995 Dec;80(12):3639-46, NLM CIT. ID: 96094410,

D 023 Dean D.D., Schwartz Z., Bonewald L., Muniz OE., Morales S., Gomez R., Brooks B.P., Qiao M., Howell D.S., Boyan B.D., Department of Orthopaedics, University of Texas Health Science Center at San Antonio 78284-7774, "Matrix vesicles produced by osteoblast-like cells in culture become significantly enriched in proteoglycan-degrading metalloproteinases after addition of beta-glycerophosphate and ascorbic acid" Calcif. Tissue. Int. 1994 May; 54(5) :399- 408, NLM CIT. ID: 94340467, ABSTRACT

D030 Dekker, 1988: 526-55.

D031 Del Favero C., Rossini G., Tufarulo L., Ciancio ML., Sopransi M., Martegani A., Borghi C., Campi R., Fugazzola C., Ospedale Valduce, Como, "Mammography changes associated with hormone replacement therapy in post-menopausal patients", RADIOL. MED. (Torino) 1997 Mar; 93(3):210-3, NLM CIT. ID, 97324839,

D040 Dequeker, J., Goris, P. and Uytterhoeven, R., "Osteoarthritis and Osteoporosis, anthropometric study" JOURNAL OF THE AMERICAN MEDICAL ASSOCIATION, March 18th, 1983, Vol. 249, № 11, pp. 1448—1451

D050 Developmental Biology. New York: Plenum, 1985;2:112-6.

D051 Dhir H., Roy A.K., Sharma A., Department of Botany, University of Calcutta, India, "Relative Efficiency of Phyllanthus emblica fruit extract and ascorbic acid in modifying lead and aluminium-induced sister-chromatid exchanges in mouse bone marrow." ENVIRON. MOL. MUTAGEN. 1993;21(3):229-36, NLM CIT. ID: 93215622

D060 Diaz M., Cooper C., Kanis J., Felsenberg D., ARC Epidemiology Research Unit, Manchester University, UK., European Vertebral Osteoporosis Study Group, O'Neill T.W., Silman A.J., Naves"Influence of Hormonal and Reproductive Factors on the Risk of vertebral deformity in European Women" OSTEOPOROS. INT. 1997;7(1):72-8, NLM CIT. ID: 97226944

[]

D070 Diddle A.W., Smith I..Q.,"Post-menopausal Osteoporosis: the Role of Estrogens, SOUTH. MED. J. 1984 Jul;77(7):868-74, NLM CIT. ID: 84250353

D080 Douillet C., Bost M., Accominotti A., Borson-Chazot F., Ciavatti M., National Institute of Health and Medical Research, Unit 331, Bron, France, "In Vitro and in vivo effects of Selenium and Selenium with Vitamin E

D090 Dubin N., "Effect of different mammographic radiation exposures on predicted benefits of screening for breast cancer", STAT. MED. 1982 Jan-Mar;1(1):15-24, NLM CIT. ID 84044013

E000 Eastell R; Vieira NE; Yergey AL; Wahner HW; Silverstein MN; Kumar R; Riggs BL., Endocrine Research Unit, Mayo Clinic, Rochester, Minnesota 55905, "Pernicious Anaemia as a risk factor for Osteoporosis", CLIN. SCI. (COLCH.) 1992 Jun;82(6):681-5, NLM CIT. ID: 92323865,

E001 EatRight Cyberdiiet, 1996, 1996http://www.CyberDiet.com/foodfact/vitmins/vitmins.html

E010 Edelson, S. B. M.D., F.A.A.F.P., F.A.A.E.M. • Environmental and Preventive Health Center of Atlanta, 3833 Roswell Road, Suite 110 • Atlanta, GA 30342 • (404) 841-0088 • FAX: (404) 841-6416, The Chelation Phenomenon: A Natural Biochemical Process. Home Page (http://www.EnvPrevHealthCtrAtl.com)

E011 Edelson, Stephen B. M.D., F.A.A.F.P., F.A.A.E.M.© 1995 http://www.ephca.com/dmso.htm

E020 Effect of dietary fat on fluoride absorption and tissue fluoride retention in rats. McGown E.L; Kolstad D.L; Suttie J.W., J. NUTR., 106: 4, 1976 Apr, 575-9, Abstract

E021 El-Nahas S.M., Mattar F.E., Mohamed A.A., Cell Biology, National Research Centre, Dokki, Cairo, Egypt, "Radioprotective Effect of Vitamins C and E", MUTAT. RES. 1993 Feb;301(2):143-7, NLM CIT. ID: 93116777, ABSTRACT

E022 Ene-Obong H.N., Department of Home Science and Nutrition, University of Nigeria, Nigeria."Content of Antinutrients and in vitro protein digestibility of the African yambean, pigeon and Cowpea", PLANT FOODS HUM. NUTR. 1995 Oct., 48(3):225-33, NLM CIT. ID: 96430303

E030 Ensrud KE., Black DM., Harris F., Ettinger B., Cummings S.R., Department of Medicine, VA Medical Center, Minneapolis, MN 55417, USA, "Correlates of kyphosis in older women. The Fracture Intervention Trial Research Group", J. AM. GERIATR. SOC. 1997 Jun;45(6):682-7, NLM ID. 97324555,

E040 Ensrud KE., Black DM., Harris F., Ettinger B., Cummings S.R., Department of Medicine, VA Medical Center, Minneapolis, MN 55417, USA, "Correlates of kyphosis in older women. The Fracture Intervention Trial Research Group", J. AM. GERIATR. SOC. 1997 Jun;45(6):682-7, NLM ID. 97324555, RACT

E041 Enterline P.E; Day R; Marsh G.M., Department of Biostatistics, Graduate School of Public Health, University of Pittsburgh, PA 15261, USA, "Cancers Related to Exposure to Arsenic at a copper smelter", OCCUP. ENVIRON MED.1995 Jan;52(1):28-32, NLM CIT. ID: 95211219,

B049 Erhardt J.G., Lim S.S., Bode J.C., Bode C., "Department of Nutrition Physiology at Hohenheim University, Stuttgart, Germany, "A diet rich in fat and Poor in dietary fiber increases the in vitro formation of reactive oxygen species in human feces" J. NUTR. 1997 May;127(5):706-9, NLM CIT. ID: 97307648,

E048 Eriksen E.F., Kassem M., Brixen K., Aarhus Bone and Mineral Research Group, AarhusAmtssygehus, Denmark, "Growth Hormone and insulin-like growth factors as anabolic therapies for osteoporosis", HORM. RES. 1993;40(1-3):95-8, NLM CIT. ID: 94131408,

E049 Erickson CA. "Morphogenesis of the neural crest", In: Browder LW, editors. DEVELOPMENTAL BIOLOGY. New York: Plenum, 1985;2:528.

E050 Ershler W.B., Sun W.H., Binkley N., Gravenstein S., Volk M.J., Kamoske G., Klopp R.G., Roecker E.B., Daynes R.A., Weindruch R., Department of Medicine, University of Wisconsin-

Madison, "Interleukin-6 and aging: blood levels and mononuclear cell production increase with advancing age and in vitro production is Modifiable by dietary restriction", LYMPHOKINE CYTOKINE RES. 1993 Aug;12(4):225-30, NLM CIT. ID: 94032765,

E060 Ershler W.B., Sun W.H., Binkley N., Gravenstein S., Volk M.J., Kamoske G., Klopp R.G., Roecker E.B., Daynes R.A., Weindruch R., Department of Medicine, University of Wisconsin-Madison, "Interleukin-6 and aging: blood levels and mononuclear cell production increase with advancing age and in vitro production is Modifiable by dietary restriction", LYMPHOKINE CYTOKINE RES. 1993 Aug;12(4):225-30, NLM CIT. ID: 94032765,

E070 Evans W.J., "Exercise, Nutrition and Aging", Human Physiology Laboratory, U.S. Department of Agriculture, Human Nutrition Research Center on Aging, Tufts University, Boston, MA 02111, J. NUTR. 1992 Mar., 122(3 Suppl):796-801, NLM CIT. ID: 92177081

F010 Feng W., Marshall R., Lewis-Barned N.J., Goulding A.,"Low follicular oestrogen levels in New Zealand women consuming high fibre diets: a risk factor for osteopenia? [see comments], Department of Human Nutrition, Otago School of Medicine, University of Otago, Dunedin", N. Z. MED. J. 1993 Oct 13;106(965):419-22, NLM CIT. ID: 94020576, COMMENT: N. Z. MED. J. 1993 Nov 24;106(968):510,

F020 Ferris BD; Klenerman L; Dodds RA; Bitensky L; Chayen J., Department of Orthopaedics, Northwick Park Hospital, Harrow, Middlesex, "Altered Organization of non-collagenous bone matrix in Osteoporosis", UK, BONE 1987;8(5):285-8, NLM CIT. ID: 88107195,

F030 Finkenstedt G., Skrabal F., Gasser RW., Braunsteiner H., Lactose absorption, milk consumption, and fasting blood glucose concentrations in women with idiopathic osteoporosis", BR. MED. J. (Clin Res Ed) 1986 Jan 18;292(6514):161-2, NLM CIT. ID: 86105025,

F040 Fitzpatrick, Phil. "More on Monsanto". PEACE AND JUSTICE NEWS. April 1997; p.8.

F041 Fleming K.H., Heimbach J,T., TAS, Flour Mill, Washington, DC 20007, "Consumption of Calcium in the U.S.: food sources and intake levels" J. NUTR. 1994 Aug., 124(8 Suppl):1426S-1430S, NLM CIT. ID: 94343028,

F050 Flieger, K., "Aspirin: A New Look at an Old Drug" in the January-February 1994 FDA CONSUMER"

F060 Forst T., Pfutzner A., Kann P., Schehler B., Lobmann R., Schafer H., Andreas J., Bockisch A., Beyer J., Department of Endocrinology and Internal Medicine, University Hospital Mainz, Germany, "Peripheral osteopenia in adult patients with insulin-dependent diabetes mellitus", DIABET MED. 1995 Oct., 12(10):874-9, NLM CIT. ID: 96114547

F070 Fotsis T., Department of Oncology and Immunology, Children's University Hospital, Ruprecht- Karls-Universitat, Heidelberg, Federal Republic of Germany, "Genistein, a dietary-derived inhibitor of in vitro angiogenesis", PROC NATL ACAD.SCI. USA 1993 Apr 1, 1990(7):2690-4)

F080 Fotsis T., Pepper M., Adlercreutz H., Hase T., Montesano R., Schweigerer L., Department of Oncology and Immunology, Children's University Hospital, Ruprecht-Karls Universitat, Heidelberg, Germany, J. NUTR. 1995 Mar., 125(3 Suppl):790S-797S

F081 Franceschi R.T., Iyer B.S., Cui Y., Department of Periodontics, Prevention, and Geriatrics, University of Michigan School of Dentistry and Biological Chemistry, University of Michigan School of Medicine, Ann Arbor, "Effects of ascorbic acid on collagen matrix formation and osteoblast differentiation in murine MC3T3-E1 cells.", J. BONE MINER. RES. 1994 Jun;9(6):843-54, NLM CIT. ID: 94360783, ABSTRACT

F090 Frank et al., "Comparison of lead levels in human permanent teeth from Strasbourg, Mexico City, Mexico, and rural zones of Alsace, France" J. DENT. RES. (1990), 69(1):90-93.

F091 Friedman A.J., Ravnikar V.A., Barbieri R.L., "Serum steroid hormone profiles in post-menopausal smokers and Nonsmokers", FERTIL. STERIL. 1987 Mar;47(3):398-401, NLM CIT. ID: 87162565,

F100 Friend D.R., Catz P., Heller J., Okagaki M., Controlled Release and Biomedical Polymers Department, SRI International, Menlo Park, California 94025, "Transdermal delivery of levonorgestrel. V. Preparation of devices and evaluation in vitro", PHARM. RES. 1989 Nov;6(11):938-44, NLM CIT. ID: 90083000, ABSTRACTDaugherty, Jane. "Should milk drinkers be Alerted to Use of Hormone?" THE DETROIT NEWS. 11/20/95; page unknown.

G010 Galley H.F., Thornton J., Howdle P.D., Walker B.E., Webster NR., Clinical Oxidant Research Group, St James's University Hospital, Leeds, UK, "Combination oral antioxidant supplementation reduces blood pressure" CLIN. SCI. (Colch) 1997 Apr;92(4):361-5, NLM CIT. ID: 97319131,

G020 Garg A., Bonanome A., Grundy S.M., Unger R.H., Breslau N.A., Pak C.Y., Department of Internal Medicine, University of Texas Southwestern Medical Center, Dallas, "Effects of dietary carbohydrates on Metabolism of Calcium and other Minerals in normal subjects and Patients with noninsulin-dependent diabetes mellitus", J. CLIN. ENDOCRINOL. METAB. 1990 Apr;70(4):1007-13, NLM CIT. ID: 90203124,

G021 Gavaler J.S., Rosenblum E.R., Deal S.R., Bowie B.T., Women's Health Research Program, Oklahoma Medical Research Foundation, Oklahoma City 73104, "The phytoestrogen congeners of alcoholic beverages: current status", PROC. SOC. EXP. BIOL. MED. 1995 Jan., 208(1):98-102, NLM CIT. ID: 95199384,

G030 Gerber N.J., Department of Rheumatology, University Hospital, Berne, Switzerland, "Prophylaxis of falls and Treatment of Fractures", BAILLIERES. CLIN. RHEUMATOL. 1993 Oct;7(3):561-71, NLM CIT. ID: 94123364,

G040 Gertz B.J., Holland S.D., Kline W.F., Matuszewski B.K., Freeman A., Quan H., Lasseter K.C., Mucklow J.C., Porras A.G., Merck Research Laboratories, Rahway, NJ 07065-0914, USA, "Studies of the oral bioavailability of Alendronate" CLIN. PHARMACOL. THER. 1995 Sep;58(3):288-98, NLM CIT. ID: 96003609

G050 Ghatak A., Brar M.J., Agarwal A., Goel N., Rastogi A.K., Vaish A.K., Sircar A.R., Chandra M., Division of Clinical and Experimental Medicine, Central Drug Research Institute, Lucknow, India, "Oxy free radical system in heart failure and therapeutic role of oral vitamin E", INT. J. CARDIOL. 1996 Dec 6;57(2):119-27, NLM CIT. ID: 97165502,

G060 Gold D.T., Department of Psychiatry, Duke University Medical Center, Durham, NC 27710, USA, "The clinical impact of vertebral fractures: quality of life in women with osteoporosis", BONE 1996 Mar;18(3 Suppl):185S-189S, NLM ID. 96261800,

G070 Gold D.T., Department of Psychiatry, Duke University Medical Center, Durham, NC 27710, USA, "The clinical impact of vertebral fractures: quality of life in women with osteoporosis", BONE 1996 Mar;18(3 Suppl):185S-189S, NLM ID. 96261800,

G071 Goldman, E.L., "ERT Shows No Risk in Breast Ca Survivors", FAMILY PRACTICE NEWS, New York Bureau, October 15, 1997, p. 9

G080 Gordan G.S.,"Dead wrong—estrogens, osteoporosis cancer and public policy" J. MED., 1980; 11 (2-3) :203-22, NLM CIT. ID: 81008271,

G081 Gosiewska A., Wilson S., Kwon D., Peterkofsky B., Laboratory of Biochemistry, National Cancer Institute, Bethesda, Maryland 20892, "Evidence for an in vivo role of insulin-like growth factor-binding protein-1 and -2 as inhibitors of collagen gene expression in vitamin C-deficient and fasted guinea pigs", ENDOCRINOLOGY 1994 Mar;134(3):1329-39, NLM CIT. ID: 94164037, ABSTRACT

G082 Goyer R.A., "Toxic and essential metal interactions", ANNU. REV. NUTR. 1997;17:37-50, NLM CIT. ID: 97382927,

G083 Grauer A., Reinel H.H., Lunghall S., Lindh E., Ziegler R., Raue F., Department of Internal Medicine 1, Endocrinology and Metabolism, University of Heidelberg, Germany,"Formation of neutralizing antibodies after treatment with human calcitonin", AM. J. MED. 1993 Oct;95(4):439-42, NLM CIT. ID: 94027124,

G090 Greendale G.A., Barrett-Connor E., Edelstein S., Ingles S., Haile R., Division of General Internal Medicine, UCLA School of Medicine, "Dietary sodium and bone mineral density: results of a 16-year follow-up study", J. AM. GERIATR. SOC. 1994 Oct, 42(10):1050-5, NLM CIT. ID: 95015554

G091 Greenhills Ginseng Limited, Copyright ©1997 http://www.ginseng.ca/gi02002.htm

G100 Greger J.L., Krzykowski C.E., Khazen R.R., Krashoc C.L., "Mineral utilization by rats fed various commercially available calcium supplements or milk" J. NUTR. 1987 Apr., 117(4):717-24, NLM CIT. ID, 87225292,

G110 Greger J.L., Krashoc C.L., Department of Nutritional Sciences, University of Wisconsin, Madison, "Effects of a Variety of calcium sources on mineral metabolism in anemic rats" DRUG. NUTR. INTERACT. 1988., 5(4):387-94, NLM CIT. ID, 89196240,

G120 Grisso J.A., Kelsey J.L., O'Brien L.A., Miles C.G., Sidney S., Maislin G., LaPann K., Moritz D., Peters B., Center for Clinical Epidemiology and Biostatistics, School of Medicine, University of Pennsylvania, Philadelphia 19104-6021,"Risk Factors for hip fracture in men. Hip Fracture Study Group" USA, AM. J. EPIDEMIOL. 1997 May 1., 145(9):786-93, NLM CIT. ID: 97288230,

G130 Gudmand-Hoyer E., Division of Gastroenterology, Gentofte University Hospital, University of Copenhagen, Hellerup, Denmark, "The clinical significance of disaccharide maldigestion" AM. J. CLIN. NUTR. 1994 Mar;59(3 Suppl):735S-741S, NLM CIT. ID: 94160931

G140 Gur E., Waner T., Barushka-Eizik O., Oron U., Life Science Research Israel, Ness Ziona, "Effect of Cadmium on Bone Repair in young rats", J. TOXICOL. ENVIRON. HEALTH. 1995 Jul;45(3):249-60, NLM CIT. ID: 95333209,

H009 Haas, Elson M., M.D. STAYING HEALTHY WITH NUTRITION, ©

H010 Haller E., "Eating Disorders. A Review and Update, Langley Porter Psychiatric Institute, University of California, San Francisco, School of Medicine 94143, WEST. J. MED. 1992 Dec;157(6):658-62, NLM CIT. ID: 93118296

H020 Haller E., "Eating Disorders. A Review and Update, Langley Porter Psychiatric Institute, University of California, San Francisco, School of Medicine 94143, WEST. J. MED. 1992 Dec;157(6):658-62, NLM CIT. ID: 93118296

H030 Hamamoto, H. et al. (1993) BIO/TECHNOLOGY 11, 930-932

H040 Hansen M., Florescu A., Stoltenberg M., Podenphant J., Pedersen-Zbinden B., Horslev-Petersen K., Hyldstrup L., Lorenzen I., Department of Rheumatology, Hvidovre Hospital, University of Copenhagen, Denmark, "Bone loss in rheumatoid arthritis. Influence of disease activity, duration of the disease, functional capacity, and corticosteroid treatment" Scand J. RHEUMATOL 1996;25(6):367-76, NLM CIT. ID: 97149663 []

H050 Hansen C, Werner E, Erbes HJ, Larrat V, Kaltwasser JP, "Intestinal calcium absorption from different calcium preparations: influence of Anion and Solubility", OSTEOPOROS. INT. 1996; 6(5): 386-93

H060 Hasegawa K., Homma T., Uchiyama S., Takahashi H.E.,Department of Orthopaedic Surgery, Niigata University School of Medicine, Ichiban-cho, Japan, "Osteosynthesis without instrumentation for vertebral pseudarthrosis in the osteoporotic spine", J. BONE JOINT SURG. BR. 1997 May;79(3):452-6, NLM ID. 97324159,

H070 Heiserman, David L. Exploring Chemical Elements and their Compounds. USA: TAB Books, 1992.

H071 Hermel M.B., Murdock M.G.,"Microdose Mammography", CANCER 1976 Nov;38(5):1947- 51, NLM CIT. ID 77046868

H072 Herzberg M., Lusky A., Blonder J., Frenkel Y., Institute of Clinical Biochemistry, Chaim Sheba Medical Center, Tel Hashomer, Israel, "The Effect of Estrogen replacement therapy on Zinc in Serum and Urine", OBSTET. GYNECOL. 1996 Jun;87(6):1035-40, NLM CIT. ID: 96240588,

H080 Heshan, W., Department of Medical Service,#C Training Bureau of the State Sports Committee, Beijing 10006, THE JOURNAL OF TRADITIONAL CHINESE MEDICINE

H090 Heshan,Wang, Department of Medical Service,#C Training Bureau of the State Sports, Committee, Beijing 10006, "Non-Surgical Therapy For Prolapse of Lumbar Intervertebral Disc", Appearing originally in THE JOURNAL OF TRADITIONAL CHINESE MEDICINE

H100 Hinder, R. A., Stein, J. H. , "Oxygen-Derived Free Radicals", ARCH. SURG. 1991; 126:104-105

H110 Hofbauer L.C., Heufelder A.E., Medizinischen Klinik, Klinikums Innenstadt der Ludwig-Maximilians- Universitat Munchen, Deutschland, "Pathogenesis of post-transplantation osteopathy", WIEN. MED. WOCHENSCHR. 1996;146(12):253-7, NLM CIT. ID: 96399764

H111 Hojima Y; Behta B; Romanic A.M; Prockop D.J., Department of Biochemistry and Molecular Biology, Jefferson Medical College, Thomas Jefferson University, Philadelphia, Pennsylvania, MATRIX. BIOL. "Cadmium ions inhibit procollagen C-proteinase and cupric ions inhibit procollagen N-proteinase",1994 Mar;14(2):113-20, NLM CIT. ID: 94340209,

H120 Holick M.F.,"Noncalcemic Actions of 1,25-Dihydroxyvitamin D3 and clinical applications" Department of Medicine, Boston University Medical Center, MA 02118, USA, BONE 1995 Aug;17(2 Suppl):107S-111S, NLM CIT. ID: 96019100

H130 Holick M.F., Department of Medicine, Boston University Medical Center, MA 02118,"Environmental Factors that Influence the cutaneous production of vitamin D" AM. J. CLIN. NUTR. 1995 Mar;61(3 Suppl):638S-645S, NLM CIT. ID: 95185438

H139 Hopper J.L., Seeman E., Faculty of Medicine Epidemiology Unit, University of Melbourne, Carlton, Australia,"The bone density of female twins discordant for tobacco use [see comments] N. ENGL. J. MED. 1994 Feb 10;330(6):387-92, NLM CIT. ID: 94111742, COMMENT: N. ENGL. J. MED. 1994 Feb 10;330(6):430-1

H140 Horn-Ross P.L; Barnes S; Kirk M; Coward L; Parsonnet J; Hiatt R.A., Northern California Cancer Center, Union City 94587, USA, "Urinary phytoestrogen levels in young women from a multiethnic population", CANCER EPIDEMIOL. BIOMARKERS PREV. 1997 May;6(5):339-45, NLM CIT. ID: 97294009,

H141 Hughes, E.F., "Alternative Medicine: What Works, and What Do You Tell Your Patients", FAM. PRACT. NEWS., Vol 19, No. 11, Nov. 1997, pp 63-86

H150 Hultman P., Johansson U., Turley S. J., Lindh U., Enestrom S. & Pollard K. M. "Adverse immunological effects and immunity Induced by dental amalgam and Alloy in Mice", FASEBJ 8:1183-1190 (1994) []

H160 Human Services, Public Health Service, National Institutes of Health.

H170 Hunt J.L., Sato R., Heck E.L., Baxter C.R.,"A critical evaluation of povidone-iodine absorption in thermally injured patients", J. TRAUMA 1980 Feb;20(2):127-9, NLM CIT. ID: 80117950,

H180 Hutchins A.M., Slavin J.L., Lampe J.W., Department of Food Science and Nutrition, University of Minnesota, St. Paul, USA, "Urinary isoflavonoid phytoestrogen and lignan excretion after Consumption of Fermented and unfermented soy products", J. AM. DIET. ASSOC. 1995 May., 95(5):545-51, NLM CIT. ID: 95238817,

I010 Isenbarger D.W., Chapin B.L., William Beaumont Army Medical Center, El Paso, Texas 79920-5001, USA,"Osteoporosis. Current pharmacologic options for prevention and treatment", POSTGRAD. MED. 1997 Jan;101(1):129-32, 136-7, 141-2, NLM ID. 97161437,

J010 Johansson C., Mellstrom D., Department of Geriatric Medicine, Vasa Hospital, University of Gothenburg, Sweden. "An earlier fracture as a risk factor for new fracture and its association with smoking and menopausal age in women", MATURITAS 1996 May;24(1-2):97-106, NLM CIT. ID: 96386703

J020 Johnston DG, Bengtsson BA. "Workshop Report: the Effects of Growth Hormone and Growth Hormone Deficiency on Lipids and the Cardiovascular System" ACTA ENDOCRINOLOGICA 1993;128 (Suppl 2): 69-70.

J030 Johnston J.D., Department of Chemical Pathology, United Medical School, Guy's Hospital, London, "Smokers have less dense bones and fewer teeth", J. R. SOC. HEALTH. 1994 Oct;114(5):265-9, NLM CIT. ID: 95147239

J031 Jorgensen, Christian, Copenhagen, Denmark, in EUROPEAN JOURNAL OF ENDOCRINOLOGY, 1994:

K010 Kanda T., Wada M., Kawamori R., Kubota M., Kamada T., Department of Internal Medicine, Osaka Prefectural General Hospital, "A study of osteopenia in elderly diabetic patients", NIPPON RONEN IGAKKAI ZASSHI 1995 Mar;32(3):183-9, NLM CIT. ID: 95319084

K011 Kanis J.A., Pitt F.A., Department of Human Metabolism, University of Sheffield, UK, "Epidemiology of Osteoporosis", BONE 1992;13 Suppl 1:S7-15, NLM CIT. ID 92256072, ABSTRACT

K020 Kannus P., Leppala J., Lehto M., Sievanen H., Heinonen A., Jarvinen M., UKK Institute for Health Promotion Research, Tampere, Finland, "A rotator cuff rupture produces permanent osteoporosis in the affected extremity, but not in those with whom shoulder function has returned to normal" J. BONE MINER. RES. 1995 Aug;10(8):1263-71, NLM ID. 96172230,

K030 Kannus P., Leppala J., Lehto M., Sievanen H., Heinonen A., Jarvinen M., UKK Institute for Health Promotion Research, Tampere, Finland, "A rotator cuff rupture produces permanent osteoporosis in the affected extremity, but not in those with whom shoulder function has returned to normal" J. BONE MINER. RES. 1995 Aug;10(8):1263-71, NLM ID. 96172230,

K040 Kapuscinski P., Talalaj M., Borowicz J., Marcinowska-Suchowierska E., Brzozowski R., Department of Internal Medicine, Postgraduate Medical Education Centre, Warsaw, Poland, "An analgesic effect of synthetic human calcitonin in patients with primary osteoporosis", MATER. MED. POL. 1996 Jul-Sep;28(3):83-6,NLM ID. 97310125,

K050 Kawai S., Mizushima Y., "Minimizing side effects of gluco-corticoid therapy", Institute of Medical Science, St. Marianna University School of Medicine, NIPPON RINSHO 1994 Mar;52(3):767-72, NLM CIT. ID: 94217309

K060 Keitel W., Rheumazentrum Magdeburg-Vogelsang, "Backache from the internal medicine-rheumatologic viewpoint", Z. ARZTL. FORTBILD. (JENA) 1997 Jan;90(8):671-6, NLM ID: 97213387,

K070 Keiver K., Herbert L., Weinberg J. Department of Anatomy, University of British Columbia, Vancouver, Canada, "Effect of maternal ethanol consumption on Maternal and fetal calcium metabolism", ALCOHOL. CLIN. EXP. RES. 1996 Oct;20(7):1305-12, NLM CIT. ID: 97060940

K080 Kelsey: [letter]. Lancet 1987;1:802.

K081 Khan P.K., Sinha S.P., Department of Zoology, Bhagalpur University, India, "Antimutagenic Efficacy of higher doses of Vitamin C", MUTAT. RES. 1993 Jan;298(3):157-61, NLM CIT. ID: 93116754, ABSTRACT

K090 Kincl F.A., Ciaccio L.A.,"Suppression of immune responses by Progesterone", Endocrinol Exp 1980 Mar;14(1):27-33, NLM CIT. ID: 80245816,

K091 Kleerekoper M., Nelson D.A., Peterson E.L., Wilson P.S., Jacobsen G., Longcope C., Department of Internal Medicine, Wayne State University, Detroit, Michigan 48201, "Body Composition and gonadal steroids in older white and black women [published erratum appears in J. CLIN. ENDOCRINO. METAB. 1995 May;80(5):1540]

K092 Knight D.C., Eden J.A., Royal Hospital for Women, New South Wales, Australia "A Review of the clinical effects of Phytoestrogens" OBSTET. GYNECOL 1996 May;87(5 Pt 2):897-904, NLM CIT. ID: 96200662

K100 Knox T.A., Kassarjian Z., Dawson-Hughes B., Golner B.B., Dallal G.E., Arora S., Russell R.M., US Department of Agriculture Human Nutrition Research Center on Aging, Tufts University, Boston, "Calcium absorption in elderly subjects on high- and low-fiber diets: effect of gastric acidity, AM. J. CLIN. NUTR. 1991 Jun;53(6):1480-6, NLM CIT. ID: 91241057,

K110 Kolega J. The cellular basis of epithelial morphogenesis. In: Browder LW, editors.

K120 Koloszar S., Gellen J., Kovacs L,"The value of plasma prolactin level determination in the diagnosis of postmenopausal osteoporosis", Szent-Gyorgyi Albert Orvostudomanyi Egyetem Szuleszeti es Nogyogyaszati Klinika, ORV. HETIL. 1997 Jan 12;138(2):71-3, NLM CIT. ID: 97176464

K130 Kwon D.J., Kim J.H., Chung K.W., Kim J.H., Lee J.W., Kim S.P., Lee H.Y., Department of Obstetrics and Gynecology, Catholic University Medical College, Uijeongbu Saint Mary's Hospital, Gyeonggi-do, Korea, "Bone mineral density of the spine using dual energy X-ray absorptiometry in patients with non-insulin-dependent diabetes mellitus", J. OBSTET. GYNAECOL. Res. 1996 Apr;22(2):157-62, NLM CIT. ID: 96280292

L000 Lark, S. M.   M.D.,"Osteoporosis & Other Physical Changes" excerpted from THE ESTROGEN DECISION SELF HELP BOOK, Celestial Arts, Berkeley

L010 LaBan M.M., Wilkins J.C., Sackeyfio A.H., Taylor R.S., Department of Physical Medicine and Rehabilitation, William Beaumont Hospital, Royal Oak, MI 48073, USA, "Osteoporotic stress fractures in anorexia nervosa: etiology, diagnosis, and review of four cases", ARCH. PHYS. MED. REHABIL. 1995 Sep;76(9):884-7, NLM ID. 95398555,

L020 Lacronique, J., "Primum non nocere: inhaled corticoids", REV. PNEUMOL.CLIN. 1996;52(2):137-43 []

L030 Lamartiniere C.A., Moore J., Holland M., Barnes S., Department of Pharmacology and Toxicology, University of Alabama at Birmingham 35294-0019, "Neonatal genistein chemoprevents mammary cancer", PROC SOC EXP. BIOL MED., 1995 Jan;208(1):120-3

L040 Laroche M; Lasne Y; Felez A; Moulinier L; Bon E; Cantagrel A; Leophonte P; Mazieres B., Service de Rhumatologie, CHU Rangueil Toulouse, "Osteocalcin and Smoking", REV. RHUM. ED. FR. 1994 Jun;61(6):433-6, NLM CIT. ID: 95135366

L050 Leb G; Warnkross H; Obermayer-Pietsch B, " Thyroid hormone excess and Osteoporosis", Acta Med. Austriaca 1994;21(2):65-7

L060 Lemaire J.P., Skalli W., Lavaste F., Templier A., Mendes F., Diop A., Sauty V., Laloux E., Centre d'Etude et de Chirurgie du Rachis, Point Medical, Dijon, France, "Intervertebral disc prosthesis. Results and prospects for the year 2000", CLIN.ORTHOP. 1997 Apr.,(337):64-76, NLM ID: 97283044,

L061 Leveille S.G., LaCroix A.Z., Koepsell T.D., Beresford S.A., Van Belle G., Buchner D.M., Center for Health Studies, Group Health Cooperative of Puget Sound, Seattle, Washington,USA., "Dietary Vitamin C and bone mineral density in postmenopausal women in Washington State, USA.", J. EPIDEMIOL. COMMUNITY. HEALTH 1997 Oct;51(5):479-85, NLM CIT. ID: 98086592, ABSTRACT

L070 Levy J.R., Murray E., Manolagas S., Olefsky J.M., "Demonstration of insulin receptors and modulation of alkaline phosphatase activity by Iinsulin in rat osteoblastic cells", ENDOCRINOLOGY 1986 Oct;119(4):1786-92, NLM CIT. ID: 87004333,

L071 Lewis S.J., Heaton K.. UK, "Lower serum oestrogen concentrations associated with faster intestinal transit", BR. J. CANCER. 1997;76(3):395-400, NLM CIT. ID: 97394492, ABSTRACT

L072 Lichten, Edward M., M.D., P.C.,29355 Northwestern Hwy, Suite 120, Southfield, Michigan 48034, phone 1(248)358-3433, Correspondence by E-mail to: usdoctor@usdoctor.com, fax: 1 (248) 358-2513 "Will growth hormone prove to be the first 'anti-aging' medication?"

L080 Lim S.K., Won Y.J., Lee J.H., Kwon S.H., Lee E.J., Kim K.R., Lee H.C., Huh K.B., Chung B.C., Department of Internal Medicine, Yonsei University College of Medicine, Seoul, Korea, "Altered hydroxylation of estrogen in Patients with postmenopausal osteopenia" J. CLIN. ENDOCRINOL.METAB. 1997 Apr, 82(4):1001-6, NLM CIT. ID: 97255217 []

L090 Lips P., Agnusdei D., Caulin F., Cooper C., Johnell O., Kanis J., Liberman U., Minne H., Reeve J., Reginster J.Y., de Vernejoul MC., Wiklund I., Department of Endocrinology, Free University Hospital, Amsterdam, The Netherlands,"The development of a European questionnaire for quality of life in patients with vertebral osteoporosis", SCAND. J. RHEUMATOL. SUPPL. 1996;103:84-5., discussion 86-8, NLM ID. 96272923 (abstract present)

L100 Lips P., Cooper C., Agnusdei D., Caulin F., Egger P., Johnell O., Kanis J.A., Liberman U., Minne H., Reeve J., Reginster J.Y., de Vernejoul M.C., Wiklund I., Department of Endocrinology, Academisch Ziekenhuis Vrije Universiteit, Amsterdam, The Netherlands, "Quality of Life as outcome in the treatment of osteoporosis: the development of a questionnaire for quality of life by the European Foundation for Osteoporosis", OSTEOPOROS INT.1997;7(1):36-8, NLM ID., 97226937,

L110 Lips P., Agnusdei D., Caulin F., Cooper C., Johnell O., Kanis J., Liberman U., Minne H., Reeve J., Reginster J.Y., de Vernejoul MC., Wiklund I., Department of Endocrinology, Free University Hospital, Amsterdam, The Netherlands,"The development of a European questionnaire for quality of life in patients with vertebral osteoporosis", SCAND. J. RHEUMATOL. SUPPL. 1996;103:84-5., discussion 86-8, NLM ID. 96272923 (abstract present)

L120 Lips, P., Graafmans, W.C., Ooms M.E., Bezemer, D., Bouter, L.M,. "Vitamin D Supplementation and fracture incidence in elderly persons" ANN. INTERN. MED. 1996; 124: 400-6.

L130 Lubec G; Labudova O; Seebach D; Beck A; Hoeger H; Hermon M; Weninger M, "Alphamethyl-proline restores normal levels of bone collagen Type I synthesis in ovariectomized rats", Life. Sci. 1995;57(24):2245-52 []

L131 Luo S., Sourla A., Labrie C., Belanger A., Labrie F., Medical Research Council Group in Molecular Endocrinology, CHUL Research Center and Laval University, Quebec, Canada, "Combined Effects of Dehydroepiandrosterone and EM-800 on bone mass, serum lipids, and the Development of dimethylbenz(A)anthracene-induced mammary carcinoma in the Rat", ENDOCRINOLOGY 1997 Oct;138(10):4435-44 NLM CIT. ID: 97462734

L140 Lux G., Hagel J., Backer P., Backer G., Vogl R.., Ruppin H.,. Domschke S.., Domschke W.., Acupuncture inhibits vagal gastric acid secretion stimulated by sham feeding in healthy subjects. GUT 1994;35:1026-9.

L150 Lyles K.W., Gold D.T., Shipp K.M., Pieper C.F., Martinez S., Mulhausen P.L., Aging Center, Duke University Medical Center, Durham, NC 27710, "Association of osteoporotic vertebral compression fractures with impaired functional status" AM. J. MED. 1993 Jun;94(6):595-601, NLM CIT. ID: 93282434,

M010 Mahmoodian F., Gosiewska A., Peterkofsky B., Laboratory of Biochemistry, National Cancer Institute, Bethesda, Maryland 20892-4255, USA, "Regulation and Properties of bone alkaline phosphatase during vitamin C deficiency in guinea pigs", ARCH. BIOCHEM. BIOPHYS. 1996 Dec 1;336(1):86-96, NLM CIT. ID: 97108717

M020 Makita K., Department of Obstetrics and Gynecology, School of Medicine, Keio University, Tokyo, "Correlation of bone mineral density with lumbago and vertebral fracture in climacteric women", NIPPON SANKA FUJINKA GAKKAI ZASSHI 1995 Jan;47(1):55-62, NLM ID. 95146868,

M021 Marcus R., Holloway L., Butterfield G., Department of Medicine, Stanford University Aging Study Unit, VA Medical Center, Palo Alto, CA 94304, "Clinical Uses of growth hormone in older people", J. REPROD. FERTIL. SUPPL. 1993;46:115-8, NLM CIT. ID: 93301884,

M030 Markham RB., White A., Goldstein A.L., "Selective immunosuppressive activity of steroids in mice inoculated with the Moloney Sarcoma Virus (38503)", PROC. SOC. EXP. BIOL. MED. 1975 Jan;148(1):190-3, NLM CIT. ID: 75158429,

M040 Markham RB., White A., Goldstein A.L., "Selective immunosuppressive activity of steroids in mice inoculated with the Moloney Sarcoma Virus (38503)", PROC. SOC. EXP. BIOL. MED. 1975 Jan;148(1):190-3, NLM CIT. ID: 75158429,

M050 Marsh G, Beams HW. Electrical control of morphogenesis in regenerating Dugesia tigrina. J

M051 Maskarinec G., Wilkens L., Meng L., Cancer Research Center of Hawaii, Honolulu 96813, USA, "Mammography Screening and the Increase in breast cancer incidence in Hawaii", CANCER EPIDEMIOL. BIOMARKERS. PREV. 1997 Mar;6(3):201-8, NLM CIT. ID 97227166, ABSTRACT

M052 Mason N.A., Patel J.D., Dressman J.B., Shimp L.A., College of Pharmacy, University of Michigan, Ann Arbor 48109-1065, "Consumer vinegar test for determining calcium disintegration", AM. J. HOSP. PHARM. 1992 Sep., 49(9):2218-22, NLM CIT. ID,92397896,

M060 Massey, L.K. "Acute Effects of dietary caffeine and Sucrose on urinary mineral excretion in healthy adolescents" NUTR. RES. 8(9): 1988, contributed to the www by Noel Peterson, N.D., American Association of Naturopathic Physicians

M061 Matsen, F. III MD Chairman, Department of Orthopaedics, University of Washington, Seattle, USA From the www.

M062 Matteucci BM, "Metabolic and endocrine disease and Arthritis", CURR.OPIN.RHEUMATOl 1995 Jul;7(4):356-8

M070 Maugars Y., Dubois F., Berthelot J.M., Dubois C., Prost A., Rheumatology Department, Nantes Teaching Hospital, France, "Pain Due to bone insufficiency as a symptom heralding femoral neck fracture", Rev. Rhum. Engl. Ed. 1996 Jan;63(1):30-5, NLM ID. 97076703,

M071 McCaffery, P.,BS, Victoria University of Wellington, New Zealand, 1981, PhD, Otago University, New Zealand, 1987, Current appointments: Assistant Scientist, Division of Developmental Neurosciences, Shriver Center Instructor in Psychiatry, Harvard Medical School (www)

M080 McCaig C.D., "Spinal neurite regeneration and regrowth in vitro depend on the polarity of an applied electric field", DEVELOPMENT 1987;100: 31-41.

M090 McCarty M.F.,"Anabolic Effects of Insulin on Bone Suggest a Role for chromium picolinate in preservation of bone density", MED. HYPOTHESES. 1995 Sep, 45(3):241-6, NLM CIT. ID: 96130665

M100 McGauley GA, Cuneo RC, Salomon F et al. Psychological Well-Being Before and After Growth Hormone Treatment in Adults with Growth Hormone Deficiency. Hormone Research 1990;33 (suppl. 4):52-54.

M110 McGinnis ME, Vanable JW Jr. Voltage gradients in newt limb stumps. Prog Clin Biol ResCooper MS, Schliwa M. Transmembrane Ca2+ fluxes in the forward and reversed

M011 McGown E.L, Kolstad D.L, Suttie J.W., "Effect of dietary fat on fluoride absorption and tissue fluoride retention in rats" J. NUTR., 106: 4, 1976 Apr, 575-9, Abstract

M012 McGrady, Pat, "THE PERSECUTED DRUG: THE STORY OF DMSO", NEW REVISED EDITION, 1973, Charter Book, N.Y.,N.Y.

M120 Mechcatie, Elizabeth, Senior Writeer, "FDA Panel Gives Bone Ultrasound Device its Vote", FAMILY PRACTICE NEWS, 1997, Sept. 15, p. 6Isenbarger D.W., Chapin B.L., William Beaumont Army Medical Center, El Paso, Texas 79920-5001, USA, "Osteoporosis. Current pharmacologic options for prevention and treatment", POSTGRAD. MED. 1997 Jan;101(1):129-32, 136-7, 141-2, NLM ID. 97161437,

M130 Medical Economics, Physician's Desk Reference,

M140 Meglio M., Cioni B., Visocchi M., Tancredi A., Pentimalli L., Istituto di Neurochirurgia, Universita Cattolica, Roma, Italia, "Spinal cord stimulation in low back and leg pain", STEREOTACT. FUNCT. NEUROSURG. 1994;62(1-4):263-6, NLM ID. 95357556,

M150 Merck & Co., Osteoporosis -

M151 Messina, M., PhD, and Messina, V., MPH, RD, "The Simple Soybean and Your Health"

M152 Metz JA; Anderson JJ; Gallagher P.N. Jr., Department of Nutrition, School of Public Health, University of North Carolina at Chapel Hill 27599-7400, "Intakes of calcium, phosphorus, and Protein, and physical-activity level are Related to Radial bone mass in young adult women [see comments]" AM. J. CLIN. NUTR. 1993 Oct;58(4):537-42, NLM CIT. ID: 93392896 COMMENT: AM. J. CLIN. NUTR. 1994 Sep;60(3):455-6,

M160 Meyers A.M., Feldman C., Sonnekus M.I., Ninin D.T., Margolius L.P., Whalley N.A., Department of Medicine, Johannesburg Hospital, "Chronic laxative abusers with pseudo-idiopathic oedema and autonomous pseudo-Bartter's syndrome. A spectrum of metabolic madness, or new lights on an old disease?" S. AFR. MED. J. 1990 Dec 1;78(11):631-6, NLM CIT. ID: 91068129

M170 Michnovicz J.J., Galbraith R.A., Laboratories of Biochemical Endocrinology and Metabolism- Pharma- cology, Rockefeller University Hospital, New York, N.Y., "Cimetidine inhibits catechol estrogen metabolism in women" METABOLISM 1991 Feb;40(2):170-4, NLM CIT. ID: 91109575,

M180 Millard P.S., Rosen C.J., Johnson K.H., Eastern Maine Medical Center, Bangor, USA, "Osteoporotic vertebral fractures in post-menopausal women", AM.FAM.PHYSICIAN.1997 Mar;55(4):1315-22NLM ID. 97226082,

M190 Millard P.S., Rosen C.J., Johnson K.H., Eastern Maine Medical Center, Bangor, USA, "Osteoporotic vertebral fractures in postmenopausal women", AM.FAM.PHYSICIAN.1997 Mar;55(4):1315-22NLM ID. 97226082,

M200 Miller M.J., Lonardo E.C., Greer R.D., Bevan C., Edwards D.A., Smith J.H., Freeman J.J., Exxon Biomedical Sciences, Inc., East Millstone, New Jersey, "Variable Responses of Species and Strains to white mineral oils and paraffin waxes", 08875-2350, USA, REGUL. TOXICO.L PHARMACOL. 1996 Feb;23(1 Pt 1):55-68, NLM CIT. ID: 96207364

M210 Miller,Benjamin F., M.D., THE COMPLETE MEDICAL GUIDE, Simon and Schuster, New York,

M211 Mirkin, G., Home Page (http://www.wdn.com/mirkin)

M220 Monegal A., Navasa M., Guanabens N., Peris P., Pons F., Martinez de Osaba M.J., Rimola A., Rodes J., Munoz-Gomez J,. Service of Rheumatology, Hospital Clinic i Provincial, University of Barcelona, Spain."Osteoporosis and bone mineral metabolism disorders in cirrhotic patients referred for orthotopic liver transplantation", CALCIF. TISSUE. INT. 1997 Feb;60(2):148-54, NLM CIT. ID: 97178789

M221 Monsonego E., Baumbach W.R., Lavelin I., Gertler A., Hurwitz S., Pines M., Institute of Animal Science, Agricultural Research Organization, The Volcani Center, Bet Dagan, Israel, "Generation of growth hormone binding protein by avian growth plate chondrocytes is dependent on cell differentiation." Mol. Cell. Endocrinol. 1997 Nov 30;135(1):1-10, NLM CIT. ID: 98113980, ABSTRACT

M222 Montague, P. "Is BGH in Trouble?" PLANET ENN. 4/1/96 http://www.enm.com/feature/fe040196/ feature5.htm

M230 Monteleone G.P. Jr., Browning D.G., "Nutrition in women. Assessment and counseling", Prim. Care. 1997 Mar 24(1):37-51

M240 Monti E., Sinha B.K., "Antiproliferative Effect of Genistein and adriamycin against estrogen-dependent and independent human breast carcinoma cell lines", Institute of Pharmacology, University of Milan, Italy. ANTICANCER RES. 1994 May-Jun;14(3A):1221-6)

M250 Moran C.E., Sosa E.G., Martinez S.M., Geldern P., Messina D., Russo A., Boerr L., Bai J.C., Clinical Department, Hospital de Gastroenterologia Dr Carlos Bonorino Udaondo, Universidad del Salvador, Buenos Aires, Argentina, "Bone mineral density in Patients with pancreatic insufficiency and Steatorrhea", AM. J. GASTROENTEROL. 1997 May., 92(5):867-71, NLM CIT. ID: 97293150

M260 Mousavi Y., Department of Clinical Chemistry, University of Helsinki, Meilahti Hospital, Finland, "Genistein is an effective stimulator of sex hormone-binding globulin production in hepatocarcinoma human liver cancer cells and suppresses proliferation of these cells in Culture", STEROIDS 1993 Jul., 58(7):301-4

M270 Munoz-Torres M., Jodar E., Escobar-Jimenez F., Lopez-Ibarra PJ., Luna J.D., Endocrine Division (Catedra Medicina Interna I), University Hospital, Granada, Spain,"Bone mineral density measured by dual X-ray absorptiometry in Spanish patients with insulin-dependent diabetes mellitus: CALCIF. TISSUE. INT. 1996 May, 58(5):316-9, NLM CIT. ID: 96269817

M280 Mussener A., Klareskog L., Lorentzen J.C., Kleinau S., Department of Rheumatology, Karolinska Hospital, Stockholm, Sweden, "TNF-alpha dominates cytokine mRNA Expression in lymphoid tissues of rats developing collagen- and oil-induced arthritis", SCAND. .J IMMUNOL. 1995 Jul;42(1):128-34, NLM CIT. ID: 95357613

M290 Miyata T., Kawai R., Taketomi S., Sprague SM Department of Internal Medicine, Branch Hospital, Nagoya University School of Medicine, Japan, "Possible involvement of advanced glycation end-products in bone resorption" Nephrol. Dial. Transplant. 1996;11 Suppl 5:54-7 NLM CIT. ID: 97197248,

N010 Nakagawa R., Laboratory of Environmental Science, Faculty of Science, Chiba University, Japan, "Concentration of mercury in Hair of diseased people in Japan", Chemosphere 1995 Jan;30(1):135-40, NLM CIT. ID: 95179489,

N020 Nash J.F., Gettings S.D., Diembeck W., Chudowski M., Kraus A.L.,The Proctor & Gamble Co., Cincinnati, OH 45241, USA, "A toxicological review of topical exposure to white mineral oils", Food. Chem. Toxicol. 1996 Feb;34(2):213-25, NLM CIT. ID: 96197382

N030 National Institutes of Health, Office of Communications, "PREMATURE GRAYING MAY BE A SIGN OF BONE DISEASE", NIH HEALTHLINE—October/November 1994, (301) 496-1766, (301) 402-0395,Compuserve 74201-1057, NIH's National Center for Research Resources, by Clifford J. Rosen, M.D., at the Maine Center for Osteoporosis Research and Education, "PREMATURE GRAYING MAY BE A SIGN OF BONE DISEASE", JOURNAL OF CLINICALENDOCRINOLOGY AND METABOLISM (Vol. 79, No. 3, 1994)

N040 National Resource Center: osteoporosis and related bone

N041 Newman, Unknown, 1993)

N050 Nguyen T.V., Kelly P.J., Sambrook P.N., Gilbert C., Pocock N.A., Eisman J.A., Bone and Mineral Research, Garvan Institute of Medical Research, St. Vincent's Hospital, Sydney, New South Wales, Australia,"Lifestyle factors and bone density in the elderly: implications for osteoporosis prevention" J. BONE. MINER. RES. 1994 Sep;9(9):1339-46, NLM CIT. ID: 95117574

N060 NIH Healthline—October/November 1994

N070 NIH, Optimal Calcium Intake. NIH CONSENSUS STATEMENT 1994 June 6-8; 12(4):1-31

N071 NIH, National Institutes of Health, NATIONAL INSTITUTE ON AGING, U.S. Department of Health and Human Services, Public Health Service, 1991

N080 Nishibe A., Morimoto S., Hirota K., Yasuda O., Ikegami H., Yamamoto T., Fukuo K., Onishi T., Ogihara T., Department of Geriatric Medicine, Osaka University Medical School, Japan,"Effect of estriol and bone mineral density of lumbar vertebrae in elderly and postmenopausal women", NIPPON RONEN IGAKKAI ZASSHI 1996 May;33(5):353-9, NLM CIT. ID: 96344758 []

N090 Nishio K, Miura K, Ohira T, Heike Y, Saijo N: Pharmacology Division, National Cancer Center Research Institute, Tokyo, Japan, "Genistein, a tyrosine kinase inhibitor, decreased the Affinity of p56lck to Beta-Chain of interleukin-2 receptor in human natural killer (NK)-rich cells and decreased NK-mediated cytotoxicity"PROC SOC EXP. BIOL. MED. 1994 Nov;207(2):227-33

N091 Nordin B.E., Robertson A., Seamark R.F., Bridges A., Philcox J.C., Need A.G., Horowitz M., Morris H.A., Deam S., "The relation between calcium absorption, serum dehydroepiandrosterone, and vertebral mineral density in postmenopausal women, J. CLIN. ENDOCRINOL. METAB.1985 Apr;60(4):651-7, NLM CIT. ID: 85131612,

N100 Nuccitelli R. "The involvement of transcellular ion currents and electric fields in pattern formatio",. In: Malacinski GM, editor. PATTERN FORMATION. New York: Macmillan, 1984.

O010 O'Halloran DJ, Tsatsoulis A, Whitehouse RW et al. "Increased Bone Density after Recombinant Human Growth Hormone (GH) Therapy in Adults with Isolated GH Deficiency" JOURNAL OF CLINICAL ENDOCRINOLOGY AND METABOLISM 1993;76:1344-1348.

O020 O'Hara, D., "Osteoporosis", AMERICAN MEDICAL NEWS, 1997 Oct.6, p. 20-28

O030 Ogihara T., Hiwada K., Matsuoka H., Matsumoto M., Shimamoto K., Ouchi Y., Abe I., Fujishima M., Morimoto S., Nakahashi T., Mikami H., Kohara K., Takasaki M., Takizawa S., Kiyohara Y., Ibayashi S., Eto M., Ishimitsu T., Nakamura T., Masusa A., Takagawa Y., [Guidelines on treatment of hypertension in the elderly, 1995—a tentative plan for comprehensive research projects on aging and health— Members of the Research Group for "Guidelines on Treatment of Hypertension in the Elderly", Comprehensive Research Projects on Aging and Health, the Ministry of Health and Welfare of Japan] Department of Geriatric Medicine, Osaka University Medical School, NIPPON RONEN IGAKKAI ZASSHI 1996 Dec;33(12):945-75, NLM CIT. ID: 97212139,

O039 Okano T.,Department of Hygienic Sciences, Kobe Pharmaceutical University, (ed.) "Menopause: The Alternative Way. Facts and Fallacies of the Menopause Industry", AustralianWomen's Research Centre, Geelong, Victoria. pp. 62-80,"Effects of essential trace elements on bone turnover—in relation tothe osteoporosis, NIPPON RINSHO 1996 Jan;54(1):148-54, NLM CIT. ID: 96155324, :

O040 Oldenhave A., Jaszmann L.J., Everaerd W.T., Haspels A.A., Faculty of the Social Sciences, Department of Women Studies, Leiden University, The Netherlands, "Hysterectomized women with ovarian conservation report more severe climacteric complaints than do normal climacteric women of similar age" AM. J. OBSTET. GYNECOL. 1993 Mar;168(3 Pt 1):765-71, NLM CIT. ID: 93206994

O050 Okano, T., Department of Hygienic Sciences, Kobe Pharmaceutical University, "Effects of essential trace elements on bone turnover—in relation to the osteoporosis", NIPPON RINSHO 1996 Jan;54(1):148-54, NLM CIT. ID: 96155324,

P010 Pagliacci M.C., Smacchia M., Migliorati G., Grignani F., Riccardi C., Nicoletti I.: Istituto di Medicina Interna e Scienze Oncologiche e Dipartimento di Medicina Clinica, Patologia e Farmacologia, Universita di Perugia, Italy."Growth-inhibitory effects of the natural phyto-oestrogen genistein in MCF-7 human breast cancer cells" EUR. J. CANCER, 1994;30A(11):1675-82

P020 Paier G.S., College of Nursing, University of Arizona, Tucson, USA, "Specter of the crone: the experience of vertebral fracture", ANS ADV. NURS. SCI. 1996 Mar;18(3):27-36, NLM ID. 96230902,

P030 Papazian, R., "An FDA Guide to Nonprescription PainRelievers, From 1995 FDA CONSUMER

P040 Pashko L.L., Rovito R.J., Williams J.R., Sobel E.L., Schwartz A.G., "Dehydroepiandrosterone (DHEA) and 3 beta-methylandrost-5-en-17-one: Inhibitors of 7,12-dimethylbenz[a]anthracene (DMBA)-initiated and 12-O- tetradecanoylphorbol-13-acetate (TPA)-promoted skin papilloma formation in Mice", CARCINOGENESIS 1984 Apr;5(4):463-6, NLM CIT. ID: 84156946,

P050 Pavia C., Siiteri P.K., Perlman J.D., Stites D.P., "Suppression of murine allogeneic cell interactions by sex hormones" J. REPROD. IMMUNOL. 1979 Jan-Feb;1(1):33-8, NLM CIT. ID: 81027964, T

P051 PDR Electronic Library, Medical Economics, 1996

P052 Pekelharing H.L., Lemmens A.G., Beynen A.C., Department of Laboratory Animal Science, State University, Utrecht, The Netherlands, "Iron, Copper and zinc status in rats fed on diets containing various concentrations of Tin", BR. J. NUTR. 1994 Jan., 71(1):103-9, NLM CIT. ID: 94145962 []

P060 Persson I., Bergkvist L., Lindgren C., Yuen J., Department of Cancer Epidemiology, University Hospital, Uppsala, Sweden,"Hormone replacement therapy and major risk factors for reproductive cancers, osteoporosis, and cardiovascular diseases: evidence of Confounding by exposure characteristics", J. CLIN. EPIDEMIOL. 1997 May;50(5):611-8, NLM CIT. ID: 97324549,

P069 Philip W.J, Martin J.C, Richardson J.M, Reid D.M., Webster J., Douglas A.S., "Decreased Axial and periph.bone density in patients takinG long-term warfarin", QJM 1995 Sep;88 (9): 635-'40 []

P070 Porter R.W., Ralston S.H., University of Aberdeen, Department of Orthopaedics, Scotland, "Pharmacological management of back pain syndromes", DRUGS 1994 Aug;48(2):189-98, NLM ID. 95080013,

P080 Preisinger E., Alacamlioglu Y., Pils K., Bosina E., Metka M., Schneider B., Ernst E., Department of Physical Medicine and Rehabilitation, University of Vienna, Austria, "Exercise therapy for osteoporosis: results of a randomised controlled trial", BR. J. SPORTS. MED. 1996 Sep;30(3):209-12, NLM ID. 97044041, Preisinger E., Universitatsklinik fur Physikalische Medizin und Rehabilitation, Wien., "Physical Therapy in Osteoporosis", WIEN. MED. WOCHENSCHR. 1994;144(24):612-8, NLM ID. 95224981,

P081 Preisinger E., Universitatsklinik fur Physikalische Medizin und Rehabilitation, Wien., "Physical Therapy in Osteoporosis", WIEN. MED. WOCHENSCHR. 1994;144(24):612-8, NLM ID. 95224981,

P090 Public Health Service,Office of Disease Prevention and Health Promotion, Peer Review Status: Externally Reviewed, Chapter 46: Estrogen and Progestin,

R000 RA-11123-10023126. Eli Lilly

R001 Ramias, Shamos, and Schiller of St. Joseph Hospital Medical Center in Phoenix, AZ, May 1992, JOURNAL OF SURGERY, VOL 111, 495-502.

R010 Rao A.V., Sung M.K.: Department of Nutritional Sciences, University of Toronto, Ontario, Canada., J NUTR,1995 Mar, 125(3 Suppl):717S-724S

R011 Reddy B.V., Reddy P.R. School of Life Sciences, University of Hyderabad, India, "Effects of vanadyl sulphate on ornithine decarboxylase and progesterone levels in the Ovary of Rat", BIOCHEM. INT. 1989 Feb;18(2):467-74, NLM CIT. ID: 89351024

R020 Reference Guide for VITAMINS

R030 Reginster J.Y., Unite d'Exploration du Metabolisme Osseux et du Cartilage Articulaire, Universite de Liege, Belgique,"Evaluation of the preventive role of estro-progestogens and non-hormonal therapies in postmenopausal osteoporosis", J. GYNECOL. OBSTET. BIOL. REPROD. (Paris) 1996;25(7):677-83, NLM CIT. ID: 97124859 []

R031 Reginster J.Y., Unite d'Exploration du Metabolisme Osseux et du Cartilage ArticulaireUniversite de Liege, Belgium, "Miscellaneous and experimental agents", AM. J. MED. SCI. 1997 Jan;313(1):33-40, NLM CIT. ID: 97154446,

R040 Ribot et al.: "The effect of obesity on post-menopausal bone loss and the risk of osteoporosis"

R050 Ribot, Tremollieres and Pouilles "Risk factors for osteoporosis and associated fractures" :

R060 Ribot, C.,Tremollieres, F., Pouilles, J. M., Bonneu, M., Germain F. and Louvet, J. P. "Obesity and post- menopausal bone loss: the influence of Obesity on vertebral density and bone turnover in post-menopausal women", BONE, 1987, Vol. 8, N° 6, pp. 327—331

R070 Rikans L.E., Kosanke S.D., "Effect of Aging on liver glutathione levels and hepatocellular injury from carbon tetrachloride, allyl alcohol or galactosamine" DRUG CHEM. TOXICOL.1984;7(6):595-604, NLM CIT. ID: 85203531,

R080 Rock C.L.; Saxe G.A.; Ruffin M.T. 4th; August D.A.; Schottenfeld. D., Program in Human Nutrition, School of Public Health, University of Michigan, Ann Arbor 48109, USA,"Carotenoids, Vitamin A, and estrogen receptor status in breast cancer", NUTR. CANCER. 1996;25(3):281-96, NLM CIT. ID: 96367457

R090 Rojas L.X., McDowell L.R., Cousins R.J., Martin F.G., Wilkinson N.S., Johnson A.B., Velasquez J.B., Animal Science Department, University of Florida, Gainesville 32611, USA, "Interaction of different organic and inorganic zinc and copper sources fed to Rats" J. TRACE ELEM. MED. BIOL. 1996 Sep., 10(3):139-44, NLM CIT. ID: 97061526Crawford, R.D., "Proposed Role for a Combination of citric acid and ascorbic acid in the Production of dietary iron overload: a fundamental cause of Disease", Department of Chemistry and Biochemistry, Loyola Marymount, University, Los Angeles, California 90045, USA, BIOCHEM. MOL MED. 1995 Feb., 54(1):1-11, NLM CIT. ID: 96002217

R091 Ross Laboratories. Ross Flier about glutamine

R110 Rozhinskaia L.Ia., Marova E.I., Rassokhin B.M., Purtova G.S., Bukhman A.I., Oganov V.S., Rakhmanov A.S., Bakulin A.V., Rodionova S.S., Mishchenko B.P., "Osteopenic Syndrome in Liquidators of the aftereffects of the accident at the Chernobyl power plant", PROBL. ENDOKRINOL. (Mosk) 1994 Jul-Aug;40(4):24-7, NLM ID. 95062087,

R111 Rubin C.D., Department of Internal Medicine, University of Texas Southwestern Medical Center, Dallas 75235-8889, "Southwestern internal medicine conference: growth hormone—aging and Osteoporosis", AM. J. MED. SCI. 1993 Feb;305(2):120-9, NLM CIT. ID: 93151280,

R120 Rubin P., Therapeutic acupuncture: a selective review. South Med J 1977;70: 974-7.

R130 Rubin Y., Kessler-Icekson G., Navon G, School of Chemistry, Tel-Aviv University, Israel, "The Effect of Furosemide on Calcium ion concentration in myocardial cells." CELL CALCIUM 1995 Aug., 18(2):135-9, NLM CIT. ID: 96049302,

R140 Ryan PJ., Blake G., Herd R., Fogelman I., Department of Rheumatology, Guy's Hospital, London, United Kingdom, "A clinical profile of back pain and disability in patients with spinal osteoporosis", BONE 1994 Jan-Feb;15(1):27-30, NLM ID. 94296734,

S010 Sabo D.; Reiter A.; Pfeil J.; Gussbacher A.; Niethard F.U., "Modification of bone quality by extreme physical stress, "Bone density measurements in high-performance athletes using dual-energy x-ray absorptiometry", Z. Orthop. Ihre. Grenzgeb. 1996 Jan.-Feb.,134(1):1-6 []

S020 Salomon F, Cuneo RC, Hesp R et al. "The Effects of Treatment with Recombinant Human Growth Hormone on Body Composition and Metabolism in Adults with Growth Hormone Deficiency" NEW ENGLAND JOURNAL OF MEDICINE 1989;321:1797-1803.

S021 Sarma L; Kesavan PC, School of Life Sciences, Jawaharial Nehru University, New Delhi, India, "Protective Effects of Vitamins C and E against gamma-ray-induced chromosomal damage in mouse", INT. J. RADIAT. BIOL. 1993 Jun;63(6):759-64, NLM CIT. ID: 93301546

S030 Satoh K.; Sakagami H., Analysis Center, School of Pharmaceutical Sciences, Showa University, Tokyo, Japan, ANTICANCER RES 1996 Sep-Oct, 16(5A):2885-90, NLM CIT. ID, 97074976

S040 Schachter, M., M.D., P.A.,1996, "THE PREVENTION OF POST-MENOPAUSAL OSTEOPOROSIS"

S050 Schaller J.P; Milo G.E; Blakeslee J.R Jr; Olsen R.G; Yohn D.S., "Influence of glucocorticoid, estrogen, and androgen hormones o Transformation of human cells in Vitro by feline sarcoma virus" CANCER. RES. 1976 Jun;36(6):1980-7, NLM CIT. ID: 76186072,

S051 Shang, Charles, Boston University School of Medicine, Box 275, 80 E. Concord Street,Boston, MA 02118, Telephone: 617-825-5812 Email: cshang@acs.bu.edu

S060 Scher K.S., "Prevention of wound infection: the comparative effectiveness of topical and systemic cefazolin and povidone-iodine", AM. SURG. 1982 Jun;48(6):268-70, NLM CIT. ID: 82204490,

S070 Schneider H.P., Birkhauser M., "Does HRT Modify the Risk of gynecological cancers?" Int. J. FERTIL. MENOPAUSAL. STUD. 1995;40 Suppl. 1:40-53 []

S080 Schryver, H.F., DVM, D.L. Millis DVM, J. Williams DVM, and H.F. Hintz DVM., Metabolism of some essential minerals in ponies fed high levels of aluminum. CORNELL VET., 986:76;354-360.

S090 Shang C, Lou M, Wan S. Bioelectrochemical oscillations. Science Monthly [Chinese]

S100 Shang, Charles, "The Mechanism of Acupuncture", The Chinese Pain Center, 2219 S. Hacienda Blvd. Suite #203, Hacienda Heights, CA, USA, TEL: (818) 369 0078, (818) 330 8233

S110 Sherblom A.P., Smagula R.M., Moody C.E., Anderson G.W., "Immunosuppression, sialic acid, and sialyltransferase of bovine serum as a function of progesterone concentration", J. REPROD. FERTIL. 1985 Jul;74(2):509-17, NLM CIT. ID: 86011148,

S111 Shore R.E., Hempelmann L.H., Kowaluk E., Mansur P.S., Pasternack B.S., Albert R.E., Haughie G.E., "Breast Neoplasms in women treated with x-rays for acute postpartum mastitis", J. NATL. CANCER. INST. 1977 Sep;59(3):813-22, NLM CIT. ID 77252356

S120 Shvets V.N., Pankova A.S., "Effect of alpha-hydroxydimethyl-gamma-aminopropylidene bisphosphonate on the bone tissue of rats during hypokinesia", KOSM. BIOL. AVIAKOSM. MED. 1989 Jan-Feb;23(1):27-31, NLM CIT. ID: 89217722.,

S130 Siiteri PK., Febres F., Clemens LE., Chang RJ., Gondos B., Stites D., "Progesterone and Maintenance of pregnancy: is progesterone nature's immunosuppressant?", ANN. N. Y. ACAD. SCI. 1977 Mar 11;286:384-97, NLM CIT. ID: 79060686

S131 Douglas Skrecky, "The Cause Of Aging, North Dakota State University Experiment", LONGEVITY REPORT 33, p. 4.

S140 Sinaki M., Itoi E., Rogers J.W., Bergstralh E.J., Wahner H.W., Department of Physical Medicine and Rehabilitation, Mayo Clinic and Mayo Foundation, Rochester, Minnesota, USA, "Correlation of back extensor strength with thoracic kyphosis and lumbar lordosis in estrogen-deficient women" AM. J. PHYS. MED. REHABIL. 1996 Sep-Oct;75(5):370-4, NLM ID. 97027582,

S141 Smith B,J., Buxton J,R., Dickeson J., Heller R.F., Centre for Clinical Epidemiology and Biostatistics, University of Newcastle, NSW, Australia, "Does beclomethasone dipropionate suppress dehydroepiandrosterone sulphate in postmenopausal women? AUST N. Z. J. MED. 1994 Aug;24(4):396-401, NLM CIT. ID: 95071070,

S150 SmithKline Beecham Consumer Healthcare "Tums Tapped as Safe Calcium Supplement", (http://biz.yahoo. com/prnews/97/02/07/sbh_y0022_1.html)

S160 Snead, E.L., SAY NO! TO HERPES, AIDS AND CHRONIC FATIGUE, AUM Publicastions, 1993

S161 Snead, E.L., SOME CALL IT AIDS,...I CALL IT MURDER, AUM Publications, 1991

S170 Sogaard C.H., Wronski T.J., McOsker J.E., Mosekilde L., Department of Connective Tissue Biology, University of Aarhus, Denmark, "The positive effect of parathyroid hormone on femoral neck bone strength in ovariectomized rats is more pronounced than that of Estrogen or Bisphosphonates", ENDOCRINOLOGY 1994 Feb, 134(2):650-7, NLM CIT. ID: 94130809

S180 Sokol R.J., McKim J.M Jr., Devereaux M.W., "alpha-tocopherol ameliorates oxidant injury in isolated copper-overloaded rat hepatocytes", Department of Pediatrics, University of Colorado School of Medicine, USA, PEDIATR. RES. 1996 Feb;39(2):259-63, NLM CIT. ID: 96423196,

S190 Srivastava et al., "Tooth lead concentration as an Indicator for environmental lead pollution in Agra City, India" BULL. ENVIRON. CONTAM. Toxicol. (1992) 48(3):334-336.

S200 Standford University Medical Center,"Many Effects of aging can now be reversed, bring about dramatic rejuvenating results in older people" PSYCHO-NEURO ENDOCRINOLOGY, Vol.. 17, No. 4, 1992

S210 Stein M.S., Scherer S.C., Walton S.L., Gilbert R.E., Ebeling P.R., Flicker L., Wark J.D., Department of Medicine, University of Melbourne, Victoria, Australia,"Risk Factors for secondary hyperparathyroidism in a nursing home Population" CLIN. ENDOCRINOL. (OXF) 1996 Apr., 44(4):375-83, NLM CIT. ID: 96296991,

S211 Steinberg K.K., Freni-Titulaer L.W., DePuey E.G., Miller D.T., Sgoutas D.S., Coralli C.H., Phillips D.L., Rogers T.N., Clark R.V., Environmental Health Laboratory Sciences, Center for Environ- mental Health and Injury Control, Atlanta, Georgia, "Sex Steroids and bone density in premenopausal and perimenopausal women",J. CLIN. ENDOCRINOL. METAB. 1989 Sep;69(3): 533-9, NLM CIT. ID: 89340787,

S211 Stevenson J.C; Hillyard C.J; MacIntyre I; Cooper H; Whitehead M.I., "A physiological role for calcitonin: protection of the maternal skeleton", LANCET 1979 Oct 13;2(8146):769-70 NLM CIT. ID: 80031595

S220 Sugiyama Y; Hamamoto H; Takemoto S; Watanabe Y; Okada Y, "Systemic production of foreign peptides on the particle surface of tobacco mosaic virus" FEBS LETT 1995 Feb 13;359 (2-3):247-50

S230 Suzuki T., Nagai H., Yoshida H., Kusumoto A., Ayano H., Kumagai S., Watanabe S., Shibata H., Yasumura S., Haga H., Department of Epidemiology, Tokyo Metropolitan Institute of Gerontology, "Appropriateness and limitations of bone mineral measurements by DXA (dual energy x-ray absorptiometry) in the elderly—comparison with x-ray findings", NIPPON KOSHU EISEI ZASSHI 1995 Jun;42(6):385-97, NLM ID. 95375292,

S231 Swerdloff R.S., Wang C., Hines M., Gorski R., Harbor-UCLA Medical Center, Torrance 90502, "Effect of Androgens on the Brain and other organs during development and Aging", PSYCHONEUROENDOCRINOLOGY 1992 Aug;17(4):375-83, NLM CIT. ID: 93066856,

S240 Swierczynski J., Kochan Z., Mayer D., Department of Biochemistry, Medical University of Gdansk, Poland, "Dietary alpha-tocopherol prevents dehydroepiandrosterone-induced lipid peroxidation in rat liver microsomes and mitochondria", TOXICOL. LETT. 1997 Apr 28;91(2):129-36, NLM CIT. ID: 97318912,

T010 Taggart H.M., Do drugs affect the Risk of hip fracture in elderly women? [see comments], Department of Geriatric Medicine, Queen's University of Belfast, Northern Ireland, 1988 Nov;36(11):1006-10, J. AM. GERIATR. SOC., NLM CIT. ID: 89009396, COMMENT: J. AM. GERIATR. SOC.,1990 Jun;38(6):727-8,

T020 Taggart H.M., Do drugs affect the Risk of hip fracture in elderly women? [see comments], Department of Geriatric Medicine, Queen's University of Belfast, Northern Ireland, 1988 Nov;36(11):1006-10, J. AM. GERIATR. SOC., NLM CIT. ID: 89009396, COMMENT: J. AM. GERIATR. SOC.,1990 Jun;38(6):727-8,

T030 Tamburini, M., Divisione di Ricerche Psicologiche, Istituto Nazionale Tumori, Milano, Italy) "Qualty of Life Assessment in Medicine", (Twenty years of research on the evaluation of quality of life in medicine) http://www.glamm.com/ql/elenco.htm

T040 Tell I., Somervaille LJ., Nilsson U., Bensryd I., Schutz A., Chettle D.R., Scott M.C., Skerfving S., Department of Occupational and Environmental Medicine, University Hospital, Lund, Sweden, "Chelated Lead and bone lead", SCAND. J. WORK ENVIRON. HEALTH. 1992 Apr., 18(2):113-9, NLM CIT. ID, 92294817,

T050 Tertrin-Clary., Roy M., de la Llosa P. "Action of Mn2+ and vanadium compounds on Hormone and forskolin induced stimulation of juvenile rat ovarian adenylate cyclase", BIOCHEM. INT. 1986 Dec;13(6):1019-35, NLM CIT. ID: 87100243

T051 Tice R.R., Yager J.W., Andrews P., Crecelius E., Integrated Laboratory Systems, Research Triangle Park, NC 27709, USA, "Effect of hepatic methyl donor status on urinary excretion and DNA Damage in B6C3F1 mice treated with sodium arsenite", MUTAT. RES. 1997 Jun;386(3):315-34, NLM CIT. ID: 97363244,

T060 Tijburg L.B., Haddeman E., Kivits G.A., Weststrate J.A., Brink E.J., Unilever Research Laboratory, Vlaardingen, The Netherlands, "Dietary linoleic acid at high and reduced dietary fat level decreases the Faecal excretio of vitamin E in young rats", BR. J. NUTR. 1997 Feb;77(2):327-36, NLM CIT. ID: 97281068,

T061 Torring O., Isberg B., Sjoberg HE., Bucht E., Hulting A.L., Department of Endocrinology, Karolinska Hospital and Institute, Stockholm, Sweden, "Plasma calcitonin, IGF-I levels and vertebral bone mineral density in hyperprolactinemic women during bromocriptine treatment", ACTA ENDOCRINOL (Copenh) 1993 May;128(5):423-7, NLM CIT. ID: 93304046,

T070 Trachtenbarg D.E., "Treatment of Osteoporosis. What is the Role of Calcium? University of Illinois, College of Medicine, Peoria 61603, POSTGRAD. MED. 1990 Mar;87(4):263-6, 269-70, NLM CIT. ID: 90192546,

T071 TRICKEY, R. (1994) "Alternative therapies for menopausal problems" in BLACK, C. (ed.) Menopause: The Alternative Way. Facts and Fallacies of the Menopause Industry", Australian Women's Research Centre, Geelong, Victoria. pp. 62-80.

T072 Tsuchita H., Sekiguchi I., Kuwata T., Igarashi C., Ezawa I., Central Research Institute, Meiji Milk Products Co., Ltd., Higashimurayamashi, Japan, "The Effect of casein phosphopeptides on calcium utilization in young ovariectomized rats", Z. ERNAHRUNGSWISS. 1993 Jun;32(2):121-30, NLM CIT. ID: 93392519,

T073 Tsuchiya H., Bates C.J., MRC Dunn Nutrition Unit, Cambridge, Br. J. Nutr. 1994 Nov;72(5):745-52, NLM CIT. ID: 95127612, ABSTRACT"Ascorbic acid deficiency in guinea pigs: contrasting effects of tissue ascorbic acid depletion and of associated inanition on status indices related to Collagen and Vitamin D",

T080 Tsuchiya H., Bates C.J., "Vitamin C and copper interactions in Guinea-Pigs and a Study of collagen cross-links", MRC Dunn Nutrition Unit, Cambridge, BR. J. NUTR. 1997, Feb;77(2):315-25, NLM CIT. ID: 97281067

T081 Tsutsumi N., Central Research Laboratories, Kissei Pharmaceutical Co., Ltd., Nagano, Japan, "Effect of Coumestrol on bone metabolism in organ culture", BIOL. PHARM. BULL.1995, Jul., 18(7):1012-5, NLM CIT. ID: 96080771,

T090 Turner J.A., Denny M.C., "Do antidepressant medications relieve chronic low back pain?" Department of Psychiatry and Behavioral Sciences, University of Washington School of Medicine, Seattle 98195, J. Fam. Pract. 1993 Dec;37(6):545-53, Unique Identifier: MEDLINE 94065606

U009 U.S. Department of Health and Human Services, Public Health Service, Agency for Toxic Substances and Disease Registry (ATSDR). 1992. Toxicological profile for barium. Atlanta, GA

U010 U. S. Food and Drug Administration, Center for Food Safety and Applied Nutrition, "Lead Acetate Used in Hair Dye Products", OFFICE OF COSMETICS FACT SHEET, February 5, 1997 (www), Hypertext updated by dms 2/8/97

U020 U. S. Food and Drug Administration, Center for Food Safety and Applied Nutrition, Office of Cosmetics Fact Sheet, February 23, 1995 (www)

U030 U.S. Department of Health and Human Services, Public Health Service, Agency for Toxic Substances and Disease Registry (ATSDR). 1992. Toxicological profile for barium. Atlanta, GA:

U040 U.S. Department of Health and Human Services

U050 United States District Court; District of New Jersey. 12/4/95.
http://www.tiac.net/users/mgold/ bgh/bst- free.txt

U060 United States Department of Agriculture, Human Nutrition Information Service, "Composition of Foods: Legume and Legume Products", AGRICULTURE HANDBOOK, Number 8-16. Revised December 1986.

U070 University of California at San Francisco

U080 Unknown, "Arthritis and Your Love Life," 8, Men's Health, 1989.

U081 "Arthritis and Diet," Arthritis Foundation, 1314 Spring Street, N.W., Atlanta, GA 30309

U090 Unknown,"Association of osteoporotic vertebral compression fractures with impaired functional status"(NATURE January 20, 1994).

U091 Unknown, "Can Diet Relieve Arthritis," University of California, Berkeley, Wellness Letter, Volume 6, Issue 8

U092 Unknown,Complementary Medical Products Ltd. may be reached by e-mail at: reiddds@reiddds.com

http://www3.sympatico.ca/debmar/WHATTENS.HTM

U100 Unknown, "Constitutional Law and Vermont's dairy labeling law enjoined".NEW YORK LAW JOURNAL 8/27/96. p.21.

U101 Unknown, DATE OF PUBLICATION OF THIS PACKAGE INSERT: APRIL 1980. Code 809-5601-01/ Rosside 28063, Information presented by Malahyde Information Systems © Copyright 1996,1997, Hosted by Intekom (Pty) Ltd.
(http://home.intekom.com/pharm/index/index_G_calcium_carbonate.shtml)

U110 Unknown, "Dye Products", OFFICE OF COSMETICS FACT SHEET, February 5, 1997 (www), Hypertext updated by dms 2/8/97

U111 Unknown, "FDA approves BST for cows". FDA Consumer. Jan-Feb 1994. v28 n1 p2.

U120 Unknown, "Medicine for the Layman - Arthritis," Clinical Center Office of Clinical Reports & Inquiries,

U121 Unknown, Natural Medical Solutions, Copyright 1997, http://www.natmedsol.com/Condits/Menopaus.htm

U122 Unknown, NEW JERSEY DEPARTMENT OF HEALTH Right to Know Program, CN 368, Trenton, NJ, 08625-0368

U130 Unknown, "Obesity and post-menopausal bone loss: the influence of obesity on vertebral density

U140 Unknown, "Osteoporosis and osteoarthritis (osteoarthrosis). Anthropometric distinctions"

U141 Unknown, "Osteoporosis in Transplant Recipients: Initiate Treatment asSoon as Possible", Drugs & Therapy Perspectives [TM], DRUGS & THER. PERSPECT. 10(8): 7-10, 1997. © 1997 Adis International Limited, Produced by Medscape, Inc. All material on this server Copyright © 1994-1997 by the publishers involved.

U142 Some of this material was mailed to me, its sources are, allegedly Stephen B. Edelson, M.D., F.A.A.F.P., F.A.A.E.M. • Environmental and Preventive Health Center of Atlanta, 3833 Roswell Road, Suite 110 • Atlanta, GA 30342 • (404) 841-0088 • FAX: (404) 841-6416, The Chelation Phenomenon: A Natural Biochemical Process. Home Page (http://www.EnvPrevHealthCtrAtl. com) and ©1990 Leon Chaitow, N.D., D.O.

U150 Unknown, "State bills focus on Labeling of dairy products from BST-treated cows Food Labeling News v5n19; 2/13/97.

U151 Unknown, "Use of bovine somatotropin (BST) in the United States: its potential effects". January 1994.

U160 Unknown,"Vermont won't appeal denial of enforcement of milk hormone label law". MEALEY'S LITIGATION REPORTS: BIOTECHNOLOGY. v1n1; 11/8/96.

U170 Unknown "Lead Information." Internet. Netscape 2.0.

U180Unknown "Lead Paint Poisoning of Children." Internet. Netscape 2.0: http://www.civil-rights. com/leadpaint.html

U190 Unknown, "Quale trattamento oggi?" MINERVA PEDIATR 1994;46:437-43.

U200 Unknown "The UCD-PCC Answer Book - Lead Poisoning." Internet. Netscape 2.0: http://edison.ucdmc. ucdavis.edu/poison_control/leadpois.html

U210 Unknown "White, Wet and.?" THE ECONOMIST. V336, n7932; p35.

V010 Vaananen H.K., Harkonen P.L., Department of Anatomy and Biocenter, University of Oulu, Finland,"Estrogen and bone metabolism", MATURITAS 1996 May;23 Suppl:S65-9, NLM CIT. ID: 97018527 []

V020 Van Vort W.B., Rubenstein M., Rose R.P., Department of Psychiatry, University of California, Los Angeles School of Medicine "Osteoporosis with pathologic hip fractures in major depression", J. GERIATR. PSYCHIATRY. NEUROL. 1990 Jan-Mar;3(1):10-2, NLM CIT. ID: 90267606

V021 Vedi S., Compston J.E., Department of Medicine, University of Cambridge Clinical School, UK, "The Effects of long-term hormone replacement therapy on bone remodeling in post-menopausal women", BONE,1996 Nov;19(5):535-9, NLM CIT. ID: 97081410

V030 Veldhuis J.D., "Mechanisms subserving hormone action in the ovary: role of calcium ions as Assessed by steady state calcium exchange in cultured swine granulosa cells", ENDOCRINOLOGY 1987 Feb;120(2):445-9, NLM CIT. ID: 87105275Reddy R.L., Reddy B.V., Reddy P.R. School of Life Sciences, University of Hyderabad, India, "Effects of vanadyl sulphate on ornithine decarboxylase and progesterone levels in the Ovary of Rat", BIOCHEM. INT. 1989 Feb;18(2):467-74, NLM CIT. ID: 89351024

V031 Venezian R., Shenker B.J., Datar S., Leboy P.S., Department of Biochemistry, School of Dental Medicine, University of Pennsylvania, Philadelphia 19104-6003, USA., "Modulation of chondrocyte proliferation by ascorbic acid and BMP-2", J. Cell. Physiol. 1998 Mar;174(3):331-41, NLM CIT. ID: 98122527, ABSTRACT

V040 Vickery B.H., Avnur Z., Cheng Y., Chiou S.S., Leaffer D., Caulfield J.P., Kimmel D.B., Ho T., Krstenansky J.L, Inflammatory Disease Unit, Roche Bioscience, Palo Alvo, California, USA, J. Bone Miner. Res. 1996 Dec;11(12):1943-51, "RS-66271, a C-terminally substituted analog of human parathyroid hormone-related protein (1-34), increases trabecular And cortical bone in ovariectomized, osteopenic rats, NLM CIT. ID: 97125825

V041 Villalobos C., Nunez L., Garcia-Sancho J., Universidad de Valladolid y CSIC, Departmento de Bioquimica y Biologia Molecular y Fisiologia, Facultad de Medicina, Valladolid, Spain, "Mechanisms for stimulation of rat anterior pituitary cells by arginine and other amino acids" J. PHYSIOL. (Lond) 1997 Jul 15;502 (Pt 2):421-31, NLM CIT. ID: 97409560

V050 Vucenik I., Yang G.Y., Shamsuddin A.M., Department of Medical and Research Technology, University of Maryland School of Medicine, Baltimore 21201-1192, USA, "Inositol hexaphosphate and inositol inhibit DMBA-induced rat mammary cancer" ,CARCINOGENESIS 1995 May;16(5):1055-8, NLM CIT. ID: 95285513

W000 Walshe J.M., Department of Neurology, Middlesex Hospital, London, "Copper: "not too little, not too much, but just right" Based on the triennial Pewterers Lecture delivered at the National Hospital for Neurology, London, on 23 March 1995 [see comments]" J. R. COLL. PHYSICIANS. Lond. 1995 Jul-Aug;29(4):280-8,, NLM CIT. ID: 96003069 COMMENT: J R Coll Physicians Lond 1995 Sep-Oct;29(5):449 ,

W010 Warrell, R. P., MD. (1995), "Gallium for Treatment of Bone Diseases", (Guy Berthon, editor), HANDBOOK OF METAL-LIGAND INTERACTIONS IN BIOLOGICAL FLUIDS - BIOINORGANIC MEDICINE, Volume 2, Marcel Dekker, Inc., New York, pages 1253 - 1265.

W020 Washington, DC: American College of Obstetricians and Gynecologists; 1992. ACOG Technical

W030 Waters D.J., Caywood D.D., Trachte G.J., Turner R.T., Hodgson S.F., Department of Small Animal Clinical Sciences, College of Veterinary Medicine, University of Minnesota, St. Paul, "Immobilization increases bone prostaglandin E. Effect of acetylsalicylic acid on disuse osteoporosis studied in Dogs", ACTA ORTHOP. SCAND. 1991 Jun;62(3):238-43, NLM CIT. ID: 91253385,

W040 Watkins B.A., Xu H., Turek J.J., Department of Food Science, Lipid Chemistry, Purdue University, West Lafayette, Indiana 47907-1160, USA,"Linoleate impairs collagen synthesis in primary cultures of avian chondrocytes" PROC. SOC. EXP. BIOL. MED. 1996 Jun;212(2):153-9, NLM CIT. ID: 96236102

W050 Watson R.R., Huls A., Araghinikuam M., Chung S., Arizona Prevention Center, University of Arizona, School of Medicine, Tucson, USA, rwatson@ccit.arizona.edu, DRUGS AGING 1996 Oct, 9(4):274-91, NLM CIT. ID: 97049797

W05a Wegger I., Palludan B., Department of Anatomy and Physiology, Royal Veterinary and Agricultural University, Frederiksberg C, Denmark, "Vitamin C deficiency causes hematological and skeletal abnormalities during fetal development in Swine.", J. NUTR 1994 Feb;124(2):241-8, NLM CIT. ID: 94141553, ABSTRACT

W051 West D.P., Worobec S., Solomon L.M., "Pharmacology and Toxicology of infant skin", J. INVEST. DERMATOL., 1981 Mar;76(3):147-50, NLM CIT. ID: 81216757,

W060 White, Edward R. M.D.,RR2 Box 4500, Damariscotta, ME 04543, Phone: (207) 563-1040, FAX: (207) 563-1039, E-Mail: ewhite@lincoln.midcoast.com, "Octobers [sic] Newsletter from Dr. White in Switzerland", The Osteoporosis Initiative

W061 Whitten P.L, Lewis C, Russell E, Naftolin F., Department of Anthropology, Emory University, Atlanta, GA. 30322, "Potential adverse effects of Phytoestrogens", J. NUTR. 1995 Mar, 125(3 Suppl):771S-776S, NLM CIT. ID: 95190657,

W062 Whitten P.L; Lewis C; Russell E; Naftolin F., Department of Anthropology, Emory University, Atlanta, Georgia 30322, "Phytoestrogen Influences on the Development of Behavior and Gonadotropin Function", PROC. SOC. EXP. BIOL. MED. 1995 Jan;208(1):82-6, NLM CIT. ID: 95199381,

W063 Wild R.A., Buchanan J.R., Myers C., Demers L.M., Department of Obstetrics and Gynecology, Milton S. Hershey Medical Center, Pennsylvania State University, Hershey 17033, "Declining adrenal androgens: an association with bone loss in aging women", PROC. SOC. EXP. BIOL. MED. 1987 Dec;186(3):355-60, NLM CIT. ID: 88097505,

W068 Wilson A.K., Bhattacharyya M.H., Center for Mechanistic Biology and Biotechnology, Argonne National Laboratory, Illinois 60439-4833, USA, "Effects of Cadmium on Bone: an in vivo model for the early response", TOXICOL. APPL. PHARMACO.L 1997 Jul;145(1):68-73, NLM CIT. ID: 97364876,

W069 Wilson A.K,. Cerny E.A,. Smith B.D,. Wagh A,. Bhattacharyya M.H., Center for Mechanistic Biology and Biotechnology, Argonne National Laboratory, Illinois 60439-4833, USA, "Effects of cadmium on osteoclast formation and activity in vitro", TOXICOL. APPL. PHARMACOL. 1996 Oct;140(2):451-60, NLM CIT. ID: 97042236,

W070 Wilson C.; Anglmayer R.; Vicente O.; Heberle-Bors E., "Molecular cloning, functional expression in Escherichia Coli, and Characterization of Multiple mitogen-activated-protein kinases from Tobacco" EUR. J. BIOCHEM. 1995 Oct 1;233(1):249-57:

W080 Wolinsky-Friedland M., Associated Internists of Danbury, Connecticut, USA,"Drug-induced metabolic bone disease" ENDOCRINOL. METAB. CLIN. NORTH. AM. 1995 Jun;24(2):395-420, NLM CIT. ID: 95385698

W090 Wu B., Xu B., Huang T.Y., Dept. of Pharmacoeogy, Medical and Pharmaceutical Research Institute of 999 Enterprise Group, Guangdong, "Effect of Kanggusong in Prevention and Treatment of retinoic acid induced osteoporosis in Rats", CHUNG KUO CHUNG HSI I CHIEH HO TSA CHIH 1996 Jan;16(1):32-6, NLM CIT. ID: 96331876 []

W100 Wu J., Norris L.A., Wen Y.C., Sheppard B.L., Feely J., Bonnar J., Department of Obstetrics and Gynaecology, Trinity College, Centre for the Health Sciences, Coombe Women's Hospital, Dublin, Ireland, "The Effects of hormone replacement therapy on plasma vitamin E levels in post-menopausal women"EUR. J. OBSTET. GYNECOL. REPROD. BIOL. 1996 Jun;66(2):151-4, NLM CIT. ID: 96330728

W110 www (World Wide Web)

W120 www University of Iowa

X010 Xintaras, Charlie / chx1@cdc.gov

X020 Xu X., Wang H.J., Murphy P.A., Cook L., Hendrich S.: Department of Food Science and Human Nutrition, Iowa State University, Ames 50011, J. NUTR 1994 Jun, 124(6):825-32

Y008 Yamaguchi M., Ehara Y., Laboratory of Endocrinology and Molecular Metabolism, Graduate School of Nutritional Sciences, University of Shizuoka, 52-1 Yada, Shizuoka City 422, Japan, "Effect of essential trace metal on bone metabolism in the femoral-metaphyseal tissues of Rats with skeletal unloading: comparison with zinc-chelating dipeptide", CALCIF. TISSUE. INT. 1996 Jul;59(1):27-32, NLM CIT. ID: 96269847,

Y009 Yamashita H., Kitagawa M., Department of Pathology, Toyama Medical and Pharmaceutical University, Japan, "Histomorphometric Study of Ribs with looser zones in Itai-itai disease", CALCIF. TISSUE INT. 1996 Mar;58(3):170-6, NLM CIT. ID: 97005261,

Y010 Yang, Jwing-Ming, "Chinese Medical Perspective" WWW

Z000 Zava D.T., Duwe G., Aeron Biotechnology, Inc., San Leandro, CA 94577, USA, "Estrogenic and antiproliferative properties of Genistein and other Flavonoids in human breast cancer cells in Vitro", NUTR. CANCER. 1997;27(1):31-40, NLM CIT. ID: 97125075, ABSTRACT

Z010 Zhitnikov AIa; Mazhuga P.M., "Changes in the Metabolism of Chondrocytes after chronic intake of Phenol and Lead", ARKH. ANAT. GISTOL. EMBRIOL. 1986 Jan;90(1):72-6, NLM CIT. ID: 86158372,

Z020 Zofkova I., Kancheva R.L., Institute of Endocrinology, Prague, Czech Republic, "Effect of estrogen status on bone regulating hormones", BONE 1996 Sep;19(3):227-32, NLM CIT. ID: 97027876,

ALPHABETICAL INDEX

For Other Titles Call (800) 729-4131 or email: global@nidlink.com